Cardiorespiratory and Cardiosomatic Psychophysiology

NATO ASI Series

Advanced Science Institutes Series

A series presenting the results of activities sponsored by the NATO Science Committee, which aims at the dissemination of advanced scientific and technological knowledge, with a view to strengthening links between scientific communities.

The series is published by an international board of publishers in conjunction with the NATO Scientific Affairs Division

A	**Life Sciences**	Plenum Publishing Corporation
B	**Physics**	New York and London
C	**Mathematical and Physical Sciences**	D. Reidel Publishing Company Dordrecht, Boston, and Lancaster
D	**Behavioral and Social Sciences**	Martinus Nijhoff Publishers
E	**Engineering and Materials Sciences**	The Hague, Boston, and Lancaster
F	**Computer and Systems Sciences**	Springer-Verlag
G	**Ecological Sciences**	Berlin, Heidelberg, New York, and Tokyo

Recent Volumes in this Series

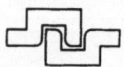

Series A: Life Sciences

Cardiorespiratory and Cardiosomatic Psychophysiology

Edited by

P. Grossman

Institute for Stress Research
and Free University
Amsterdam, The Netherlands

K. H. L. Janssen

Tilburg University
Tilburg, The Netherlands

and

D. Vaitl

University of Giessen
Giessen, Federal Republic of Germany

Plenum Press
New York and London
Published in cooperation with NATO Scientific Affairs Division

Proceedings of a NATO ASI on
Cardiovascular-Respiratory and -Somatic Integration in Psychophysiology,
held November 17–19, 1983,
in Schloss Rauischholzhäusen, University of Giessen, Giessen,
Federal Republic of Germany

Library of Congress Cataloging in Publication Data

NATO ASI on Cardiovascular-Respiratory and -Somatic Integration in Psycho-
    physiology (1983: Schloss Rauischholzhausen, Germany)
    Cardiorespiratory and cardiosomatic psychophysiology.

    (NATO ASI series. Series A, Life sciences; v. 114)
    "Proceedings of a NATO ASI on Cardiovascular-Respiratory and -Somatic
Integration in Psychophysiology, held November 17–19, 1983, in Schloss
Rauischholzhausen, University of Giessen, Giessen, Federal Republic of Ger-
many"—T.p. verso.
    "Published in cooperation with NATO Scientific Affairs Division."
    Includes bibliographies and index.
    1. Arrhythmia—Psychosomatic aspects—Congresses. 2. Nervous system,
Vasomotor—Congresses. I. Grossman, P. II. Janssen, K. H. L. III. Vaitl, D.
(Dieter) IV. North Atlantic Treaty Organization. Scientific Affairs Division. V. Ti-
tle. VI. Series. [DNLM: 1. Arrhythmia, Sinus—congresses. 2. Heart
Rate—congresses. 3. Psychosomatic Medicine—congresses. 4. Respiration—congresses. 5. Somatoform Disorders—congresses. WG 330 N279c
1983]
RC685.A65N36   1983   616.1′2808   86-21252

ISBN 978-1-4757-0362-7   ISBN 978-1-4757-0360-3 (eBook)
DOI 10.1007/978-1-4757-0360-3

© 1986 Plenum Press, New York
Softcover reprint of the hardcover 1st edition 1986

A Division of Plenum Publishing Corporation
233 Spring Street, New York, N.Y. 10013

ACKNOWLEDGMENT

Both our original meeting and this volume were made possible by a grant of the NATO Scientific Affairs Division. University of Giessen's Schloss Rauischholzhausen proved a most agreeable place for the meeting. We would, furthermore, like to thank Ineke Hermanns-Vervaert and the rest of the secretarial staff of the Department of Experimental Psychology, the Free University of Amsterdam, for their very helpful and tangible contributions. We also acknowledge the secretarial and technical assistance of Tinie Aarts-Poulussen and of Christa Kansog, Baerbel Schmitt, and Dr. Harald Lachnit at the Psychology Departments of Tilburg University and University of Giessen.

CONTENTS

BIOFEEDBACK AND SELF-REGULATION

CLINICAL APPLICATIONS

INTRODUCTION AND THEORETICAL OVERVIEW

P. Grossman, K. H. Janssen and D. Vaitl

This volume derives from the proceedings of the 'First International Symposium on Cardiovascular-Respiratory and -Somatic Integration in Psychophysiology', held in Schloss Rauischholzhausen, West Germany on November 17-19, 1983. This conference, sponsored by NATO's Scientific Affairs Division and the University of Giessen, provided for experts from diverse disciplines to come together to discuss various aspects of the psychophysiology of cardiovascular integration with respiratory and somatomotor systems.

A major premise of both the meeting and the present collection of papers is that cardiovascular processes within the well-functioning organism, are fundamentally integrated with respiratory and somatomotor functions. To neglect this fact would be to miss the essential biological functionality, acquired through evolution, that binds physiology to behavior. Changing behavioral states and transactions mirror altered adaptational demands for respiratory, cardiovascular and somatomotor control systems, all of which must be closely coordinated in order to maintain homeostatic functioning. Within this framework, the cardiovascular system can be conceived as playing an intermediary role: whereas respiratory processes provide for adequate gas exchange between the atmosphere and the internal environment, and somatomotor mechanisms serve as the effector of behavior, the cardiovascular system primarily ensures optimal regional gas exchange to body tissues. The immense variety of behavioral adjustments for coping with environmental contingencies implies, therefore, equally complex and flexible patterns of respiratory, cardiovascular and somatomotor coordination.

Cardiovascular psychophysiologists, in recent years, have paid greater heed to the biological significance of behavioral-cardiovascular interactions (e.g. the adaptive value of specific patterns of cardiac responses to particular psychological or behavioral activities). However, there seems to be somewhat less awareness of certain important developments in physiology that have occurred over the last ten years: a formidable amount of evidence has been gathered, leading many to reconsider the independent nature of cardiovascular control mechanisms in favor of an integrative model whereby cardiovascular control forms one component of a higher-order system (Koepchen, Hilton and Trzebski, 1980; Miyakawa, Koepchen and Polosa, 1984; Schlaefke, Koepchen and Seer, 1983). More specifically, there appear to be different mechanisms uncovered by which coupling of physiologically distinct processes can be realized - common central commands, common inputs from the periphery, interconnections between functionally associated neural structures, and brainstem centers that differentially influence more than one effector system. These latest advances in physiological research have, in fact, led to an altered understanding of the organization and adaptive significance of lower brain centers. Interactional phenomena between systems (e.g. respiratory sinus arrhythmia), once thought to be unimportant epiphenomena due either to spillover among distinct brainstem centers or peripheral mechanical interference, have now been shown to possess significant control functions (e.g. the modulation of cardiac vagal efferent control). Hence it appears that at every neural level, from central nervous system to periphery, autonomic response components of individual physiological systems do not occur in isolation, but rather there are coordinated patterns of alterations involving a number of organs and systems and aimed at maintenance of the total organism.

From a psychophysiological point of view, there may be particularly attractive aspects of an integrated respiratory and somatic approach to behavioral-cardiovascular interactions. Cortical contributions to both somatomotor and respiratory activity are acknowledged to exert their impact by way of direct effects or in interplay with lower brain mechanisms. Cortical influences upon the cardiovascular system seem to be more indirect and often are produced through the effects of these other more consciously controlled functions. Therefore, the cardiovascular system can be considered as an automatic regulatory energy transport system in series with, and juxtaposed between, two other energy transport processes which are greatly influenced by higher brain functions. With this conception in mind, the only adequate physiology of cardiovascular processes is one that relates cardiac and circulatory adjustments to variations in behavior. Thus primary aims of psychology and physiology merge. Inclusion of a more integrative physiological perspective may serve to better ground psychophysiological theory.

Along another line, a major topic in psychophysiology is breakdown in adaptive responses to stressful conditions, both over short- and long-term periods. The focus of interest is upon behavioral, as well as physiological, dysregulation, and a prime emphasis, within this context, is currently placed upon cardiovascular disorders as presumable consequences of breakdowns in behavioral adaptation. Explanatory mechanisms for these relations, however, often remain vague and unsubstantiated. On the other hand, breakdown in behavioral adaptation to stress may be linked to impaired coordination between respiratory, cardiovascular and somatomotor activities. This makes good sense if we consider the central control mechanisms simultaneously guiding behavior and physiological functioning. Furthermore, there is much evidence of uncoupling of cardiovascular, respiratory and somatic mechanisms occurring in various cardiovascular disease states and under acute psychologically stressful conditions. A greater research orientation in this direction could provide important clues into how psychological stress responses may contribute to cardiovascular risk.

This volume represents an initial stage in the development of a psychophysiology of cardiorespiratory and cardiosomatic integration. As such, it is embryonic: often relatively undifferentiated. Still we have gathered together a group of chapters which we believe illustrate the promise of this approach for basic theoretical, methodological, research and clinical applications. Many of the papers contain valuable information that has not yet been readily available to psychophysiologists and other professional audiences. Other more familiar lines of research reported here may benefit the reader by being cast in the light of the general theoretical framework of this volume.

In the section on physiological mechanisms, Langhorst and his group provide evidence concerning the morphological substrate of a system which regulates and controls cardiovascular, respiratory, and somatomotor processes and influences the degree of cortical activity. Summarizing their investigations, they find the reticular formation to be a multi-functional common brainstem center which is not diffusely organized: although single neurons of the reticular formation do have multifunctional properties and are concerned with control functions of various effector systems, distinct types of functional organization can be observed.

The effects of muscular exercise on circulatory parameters and neural control are discussed in the Chapter by Gelsema. He sheds new light upon both reflex mechanisms and central efferent activity (i.e. central command hypothesis) involved in the control of cardiovascular function during muscular exercise. One conclusion that may be derived from this Chapter is that both neural mechanisms may participate under normal circumstances.

In order to study the influence of parasympathetic activity upon heart rate variability, Karemaker's Chapter has been guided by the innovative book by A. T. Winfree, The Geometry of Biological Time (1980). Using Winfree's topological concepts, Karemaker stresses the importance of the timing of naturally occurring vagal efferent discharge in each heart period for its effectiveness in controlling or altering heart rate. From animal research and basic physiology, Karemaker argues that changes in amplitudes of heart rate variability (e.g. respiratory sinus arrhythmia) may not unambiguously index changes in modulation of vagal activity.

The Section on Quantification and Validation of Models is specifically oriented to aspects of the quantification of cardiac signal variability, how parameters can be used to assess neural processes and what the present and potential research and clinical applications may be. The overwhelming emphasis is upon issues related to respiratory sinus arrhythmia. Rompelman addresses basic concerns in the analysis and treatment of cardiac time series, guiding the reader along the steps from initial acquisition of the ECG signal through sampling and conversion of the signal from an event series to an equidistant or continuous signal, ready for spectral analysis. All along the way he aptly points out the potential problems that may be encountered and suggests solutions.

In the next Chapter, Kitney applies a systems theory approach to the rhythmic oscillations that occur in heart rate. He describes fundamental properties and phenomena of oscillating systems in general, such as stable entrainment, nonlinear modulation and frequency pulling. By using computer modeling and spectral analytic techniques, he then attempts to demonstrate that these same general properties obtain with the physiological oscil-lating systems reflected in cyclic fluctuations in heart rate. Finally he explains how these mechanisms may account for the neural basis of respir-atory sinus arrhythmia.

In a somewhat different approach to respiratory sinus arrhythmia (RSA), Porges mainly addresses the usefulness of the phenomenon for assessing parasympathetic chronotropic cardiac effects. The author begins by presenting the physiological grounds for consideration of RSA as an index of vagal control and then attempts to justify a specific quantifi-cation method for deriving an estimate of vagal tonus. Finally, on the basis of certain clinical evidence, an argument is made for the possibility that RSA magnitude may also reflect general aspects of the status of the central nervous system.

The following Chapter by Grossman and Wientjes examines certain funda-mental issues related to RSA quantification, applications and inferences which can be made concerning RSA as mirror of neural processes: different RSA quantification methods are compared with respect to their established sensitivities to cardiac vagal variations; evidence is cited indicating that RSA may not always reflect status of central processes; and the respiratory contribution to RSA levels and variations in parasympathetic control is empirically evaluated.

In the last Chapter of this Section, Turpin examines cardiac-respiratory interactions with regard to their implications for analysis and interpretation of attentional cardiac phasic responses. The manner by which RSA fluctuations and stimulus-elicited respiratory changes may interfere with estimation of independent phasic cardiac responses is critically analyzed, with the help of a careful review of the available literature, and a plea is made for further study of cardiorespiratory interactions in regard to stimulus-elicited phasic responses.

Psychophysiological approaches have focussed upon different environmental events, psychological processes, and behavioral activities, such as eliciting, maintaining or fractionating factors for the different modes of cardiovascular, respiratory and somatomotor interactions. Engel presents in his Chapter a synopsis of his laboratory's extensive work on operant conditioning of cardiovascular and somatic functions in primates. He discusses evidence showing that, under certain circumstances, it is possible to modify cardiovascular and somatomotor-cardiovascular inter-actions by altering contingencies of primate behavior. Using physical exercise and operant conditioning of heart rate slowing, this research indicates that cardiosomatic interactions are less invariant than previously assumed and are clearly dependent upon environmental conditions.

There are various factors which may influence the covariation of heart rate and somatomotor-mediated oxygen consumption. In a series of animal experiments, Brener lends support to the notion that cardiac activities that covary with metabolic rate are primarily produced by feedback from striate muscular activity. In contrast, changes in cardiac activity that occur independently of metabolic processes are mainly produced by higher nervous system processes acting directly upon the medullary systems involved in cardiac control.

Langer et al. address the issue of integration of cardiac and metabolic responses to both exercise and behavioral stress. Reviewing the available literature and summarizing their own research, these authors present evidence suggesting a dissociation of cardiac and metabolic func-tions to occur under certain forms of psychological stress. This cardio-vascular-metabolic uncoupling, probably due to beta-adrenergic responses, may create systemic overperfusion and consequently elicit autoregulatory reflexes which could contribute to cardiovascular risk.

The integration of cardiovascular and respiratory systems appears to be realized by a hierarchy of coupling mechanisms which depends upon the functional state of the organism. Raschke distinguishes in his Chapter two modes of cardiac-respiratory coupling, modulation and phase coordination (phase coupling): both modes of coupling vary in response to degrees of physical and psychological activation.

Svebak's Chapter uniquely illustrates how integrated physiological responses can be related to theoretical psychological constructs. Drawing from both Apter's recent reversal theory of motivation and classical psychophysiological experimental approaches, Svebak addresses the manner by which intrinsic task-related and extrinsic motivational factors influence cardiovascular, respiratory, and somatic activity. Psychophysiological responses seem to differ in a systematic manner with respect to both dispositional and situational characteristics. Furthermore, the results indicate promise for the use of reversal theory constructs in cardio-respiratory and -somatic psychophysiology.

The study of cardiovascular-respiratory and -somatic interactions also suggests new clinical approaches and techniques. One possible development here is the clinical application of biofeedback from cardiovascular and pulmonary parameters. The Chapter by Stoney and colleagues sets out with evidence that the effects on heart rate obtained in biofeedback paradigms are related largely to respiratory and somatomotor activity. Furthermore, a cardiopulmonary stress response is discussed which apparently occurs together with an increase in ventilation, and it is later shown that with cardiac feedback, it is possible effectively to modify this ventilatory increase. Additional data are used to suggest that one prominent source of intersubject variation in cardiopulmonary response to stress, may be attributed to the Type A dimension.

Johnston et al. discuss whether cardiovascular biofeedback leads to very specific physiological effects, or to an overall pattern of neural and metabolic adjustments. To that end, they present findings on the use of a combined parameter composed of both heart rate and pulse transit time. Evidence is then reported suggesting that in contrast to dynamic exercise, the cardiovascular response to static exercise cannot be reduced by cardio-vascular feedback. The clinical implications of this research are discussed in terms of the possible application of self-control procedures to the treatment of exercise-related cardiovascular disorders such as angina pectoris.

Sinus tachycardia is another area where cardiovascular biofeedback may find useful clinical applications. Janssen and Beckering describe how the question of respiratory and somatomotor mediation has influenced the development of clinical heart rate feedback and discuss this issue in relation to sinus tachycardia. They also examine neurophysiological mechanisms that may underlie biofeedback effects in this disorder: evidence is presented that vagal control is often deficient with sinus tachycardia and that heart rate feedback may result in shifts in cardiac vagal tone.

The perspective of a well-tuned interaction of cardiovascular, respiratory and somatic functions as necessary for the functioning of the healthy organism, may lead to new insights into the pathophysiology of several disorders. As we shall see in the last Section, this may not only apply to stress-related disorders, but also to some conditions that are traditionally conceived of as purely organic disorders.

Mortensen et al. describe the use of hyperventilation as a diagnostic test for patients with Prinzmetal's variant angina (PVA), as well as those with other types of chest pain. It is shown that voluntary hyper-ventilation among PVA patients elicits a similar pattern of coronary vasospasm, ECG abnormalities and chest pain as typically seen during a spontaneous PVA episode. Inferences are drawn from this data concerning how stress-induced hyperventilation may compromise the health of PVA patients.

The relationship between ischemic heart disease and hyperventilation is further dealt with in the contribution by Freeman. She discusses the role of hyperventilation in the development and exacerbation of various organic cardiovascular disorders. Furthermore, psychophysiological mechanisms responsible for interactions between cardiovascular processes and hyperventilation are explored, and a possible behavioral treatment is described for alleviating hyperventilation.

5

Vasovagal syncope is another cardiovascular disorder in which respiratory processes may play a significant role. Sledge and Janssen's Chapter provides support for this hypothesis by summarizing recent pathophysiological findings: vasovagal fainting does not appear to be simply a vasomotor failure, but instead is strongly associated with emotional excitation of the parasympathetic nerves to the heart and with vasodilatory effects in the muscles. Based on evidence of an apparent specificity in the presymptom cognitions and affect in many of these patients, a model is presented concerning how these several physiological, affective, cognitive and psycho-environmental aspects may interact in the genesis of vasovagal syncope.

Kitney, in his second Chapter, directs his control theory model to cyclic heart rate variability in neonates and individuals with autonomic neuropathy. Once again utilizing spectral analytic techniques, various physiological deductions are made concerning how these groups differ from normal adults. Kitney, furthermore, suggests the usefulness of his approach for assessing autonomic neuropathy among different populations.

REFERENCES

Koepchen, H. P., Hilton, S. M., and Trzebski, A., 1980, Central Interactions between Respiratory and Cardiovascular Control Systems, Springer, New York.
Miyakawa, K., Koepchen, H. P., and Polosa, C., 1984, Mechanisms of Blood Pressure Waves, Springer, New York.
Schlaefke, M. E., Koepchen, H. P., and See, W. R., 1983, Central Neurone Environment and the Control Systems of Breathing and Circulation, Springer, New York.
Winfree, A. T., 1980, The Geometry of Biological Time, Springer, New York.

PHYSIOLOGICAL MECHANISMS

INTEGRATIVE CONTROL MECHANISMS FOR CARDIORESPIRATORY
AND SOMATOMOTOR FUNCTIONS IN THE RETICULAR FORMATION
OF THE LOWER BRAIN STEM

P. Langhorst, G. Schulz and M. Lambertz

Institute of Physiology
The Free University of Berlin
Arnimallee 22, D-1000 Berlin 33, FRG

INTRODUCTION

From the functional point of view it is well accepted that only close
interactions between cardiorespiratory and somatomotor control systems
guarantee the integrity of organisms in all conditions of everyday life
[30,31,83]. Characteristic modes of coordinations of somatomotor and
autonomic innervation patterns determine the actual behavior. Both
components of behavior – somatomotor and autonomic – are not merely running
parallel, but depend on each other. Adequate autonomic innervation enables
the organism to realize somatomotor activity. On the other hand, the
somatomotor nervous system assists the autonomic nervous system in
homeostatic regulation. The functional synergy of the autonomic and the
somatomotor nervous system was distinctly elaborated by W. R. Hess and by
W. B. Cannon [15,30,31]. W. R. Hess discerned two functional states: an
ergotropic one in which the autonomic nervous system supports the somatomotor system during intensive physical work and a trophotropic one in which
the somatomotor system supports the autonomic nervous system in regulating
assimilation and restitution of cell energy. This requires nervous structures responsible for integration of somatomotor and autonomic nervous
activity. The nature of the investigations of the nervous structures
integrating the body functions during regulation was determined by two
controversial concepts: the idea of narrow localizations of different
functions in the brain and the concept of the brain as a single dynamic
entity.

The idea of cerebral localization of mental faculties was first
suggested by L. C. A. Meyer (1779) [63]. Gall formulated the concept of
brain centers in 1825, and the first description of isolated areas lesions
of which led to disturbances of isolated functions was presented by Broca
in 1861 [11,25]. The idea that the brain is an "aggregate of separate
organs" (see Luria [59]) included no suggestions for the mechanisms integrating the isolated functions under physiological conditions. Therefore
this concept was rejected by Haller in 1769 [28]. He postulated that the
brain is a single organ composed of parts of equal importance. Flourens
supported this concept in 1824 with the results of his physiological experiments [23]. Jackson in 1869 observed that lesions of circumscribed areas
of the brain were never followed by a complete loss of function [38]. He
concluded that every control function of the brain is not performed by just
one localized group of nerve cells. He elaborated the concept of a

vertical organization of neurons in the brain responsible for control functions. He postulated that the first representation of neurons involved in the control mechanisms is located at a spinal and brainstem level. The control functions exerted by brainstem neurons are re-represented in higher brain structures. Although the concept of the brain as a single dynamic entity was propagated by physiologists on the basis of experiments (see Luria [59]), the neurophysiological investigations in the last century were mainly determined by the hypothesis of brain centers [10].

LOCALIZATION

Although numerous investigations have emphasized the importance of higher brain structures and the spinal cord, the central role of the lower brainstem for cardiovascular, respiratory and somatomotor regulation is beyond question [2,34,44,48,72,73,77,88,92]. The first investigations were done with the aid of classical transection, ablation and lesion experiments of central nervous tissue. These experiments have revealed that neurons for cardiorespiratory and somatomotor regulation are localized in the reticular formation of the lower brainstem in a rostralcaudal extension between upper pons and a few millimeters caudal of the obex [16,26,57,58, 69,74,86,89]. Relying upon their hypotheses [3,5,7,18,19], investigators tried to narrow down a precise localization of the "centers" in question.

However, neither with anatomical nor with lesion experiments was it possible to distinguish the location of respiratory and vasomotor cells from that of neurons responsible for other reticular effects (see [46,49, 75]).

Another methodological approach to identify cardiovascular, respiratory and somatomotor centers consisted in circumscribed electrical stimulations within the central nervous system. An accumulation of effective stimulation sites was found in the same area of the lower brainstem in which lesions resulted in loss of autonomic rhythms and of sympathetic tone, in an exaggeration of extensor muscle tone and in synchronization of EEG waves [4,12,66]. Rossi and Zanchetti stated in 1957 that "stimulation experiments give little more than an inventory of the influences exerted by the reticular formation on other parts of the nervous system" [75]. Thus neither lesion nor stimulation techniques resulted in distinct local discriminations between cardiovascular, respiratory and other centers.

Since it cannot be denied that the neurones responsible for the various basic control functions are located in the reticular formation of the lower brainstem, the question arises whether these neurones are not organized in closely circumscribed centers with specific control functions. Many reported experimental results can be explained by the assumption that the neurones of the 'centers' are intermingled or that these 'centers' overlap. There are results reported in the literature emphasizing the existence of one system that regulates several functions, so to say a multi-functional center. Hering concluded in 1869 form his investigations of blood pressure waves that there is a close relationship between cardiovascular and respiratory centers [29]. Boothby described in 1915 the possibility of a common center for the regulation of circulation and respiration [9]. Hess concluded from stimulation experiments that there exists a common brainstem mass for the regulation of respiration and circulation [32].

The observation that extensor muscle tone increases during the inspiratory phase, that the patellar tendon reflex and the Achilles reflex oscillate with the "respiratory rhythm" and that a respiratory rhythm exists in the activity of alpha motor neurons supports the holistic concept

10

that one and the same neuronal network influences respiratory and somato-motor neurons [39,64,80]. Mollica et al. (1953) observed synchronous oscillations in reticular neuronal activity, extensor muscle tone and the degree of synchronization of the EEG. These characteristic rhythms in different systems convinced them that there are functional relations between such systems [65]. The findings supported the functional concept of Moruzzi and Magoun that a reticular neuronal system controls the states of sleep and wakefulness [67]. Stimulation of the Ascending Reticular Activiating System (ARAS) induces a desynchronization of the EEG. This pattern of the EEG is representative of an arousal reaction or an alerting response. Magoun completed this concept by describing ascending influences on cortical structures and corresponding descending actions on the spinal cord from the same brainstem regions [62].

MORPHOLOGY

The term "reticular formation" was used by the old anatomists and physiologists to describe the morphological properties of the neuronal network in the core of the brainstem seen by the light microscope. The structure is characterized by aggregations of nerve cells of different size enclosed by bundles of fibers travelling in many directions of the trans-verse section and thereby forming a reticular structure [13,41]. Detailed descriptions of the cyto-architecture of the reticular formation were given by the Scheibels, Valverde and Taber [79,90,91]. In the medial two-thirds, they described large cells with long axons often dichotomizing shortly after the origin in an ascending and a descending branch. This finding was confirmed with electrophysiological methods by Magni and Willis. With the aid of intracellular recordings they were able to show that one and the same neuron could be invaded antidromically from rostral as well as from spinal cord levels [61].

Moreover, short collaterals of these neurons contact other neurons of the same type in the neighborhood. The neurons are the morphological substrate which simultaneously influence rostral brain structures and the spinal cord neurons [12]. The dendritic trees of these neurons are highly developed and oriented chiefly in a plane perpendicular to the longitudinal axis of the brainstem [79]. Such dendrites extend over large areas of the cross-section of the brainstem, partly invading specific nuclei and con-tacting specific and unspecific sensory pathways. The dendritic fields of neighboring neurons overlap to a large degree. According to the morpho-logical properties and to their first electrophysiological investigations, Scheibel et al. [78] considered the reticular neuronal network to be a functionally unspecific system.

ELECTROPHYSIOLOGICAL INVESTIGATIONS OF SINGLE RETICULAR NEURONS

The advent of microrecording techniques encouraged several investi-gators to try to record the activity of neurons of cardiovascular and respiratory centers. Others tried to study the functional organization of the neuronal network constituting the ARAS. The neurons were classified according to the afferents influencing their discharge patterns. Cardio-vascular neurons should be influenced by blood pressure variations [42,72,77]. Reticular neurons were labelled as somatosensory neurons if they could be influenced by somatosensory afferents [70]. Respiratory neurons should be influenced by activities from receptors measuring changes of blood gas composition and lung volume. The spontaneous activity of neurons of the respiratory oscillator is characterized by a fixed temporal relation to the respiratory cycle [5,7,26]. Neurons which changed their activity in relation to an arousal reaction were labelled as neurons of the ARAS [60,65].

11

The first extracellular recordings of such reticular neuronal activities revealed that somatosensory afferents from different receptor types and different sites of the body [4] converge at single neurons [3,84]. The influence from cortical and cerebellar neurons on the same reticular neurons is described in the literature [6]. Scheibel et al. [78] reported that the afferent spectra were different from neuron to neuron. These results induced the concept of the unspecific brainstem system.

A comparison of the numerical occurrence of the different types of neurons reported reveals that a separation of different types is purely arbitrary. Siegel made a compilation of the results of such investigations and found that the percentages of different cell types add up to far more than 100%, i.e. one group described 77% of their neurons to be somatosensory in function, another described 91% of neurons to belong to supraspinal motor control, and a third group believed 36% of the neurons to be respiratory ones [87]. We could show that 88% of such reticular neurons were influenced by baroreceptor afferents. According to the criteria mentioned above, these neurons have the properties of "cardiovascular neurons" [55].

All the neurons described by different investigators were distributed in the medial two-thirds of the reticular formation of the lower brainstem. A concentration of neurons with so defined functions in circumscribed reticular areas could not be proved. It must be assumed that the various investigators recorded the activity of the same neurons under a narrow point of view, neglecting other possible viewpoints. Therefore, one can phypothesize that individual reticular neurons have multifunctional properties. This hypothesis is supported by the morphological properties described above.

SINGLE RETICULAR NEURONS WITH INPUTS FROM ENTEROCEPTORS
AND SOMATOSENSORY RECEPTORS

We have investigated the physiological properties of reticular neurons to test the hypothesis of a multifunctional brainstem system. Extracellular recordings of single neurons of the reticular formation of the lower brainstem were made in dogs anesthetized with chloralose urethane. The methods applied were described in detail in previous publications [55]. All data were recorded simultaneously on magnetic tape and on a Schwarzer polygraph. Auto- and cross-covariance histograms, power spectra and cross-power spectra and interval historgrams were calculated from the tape recordings. In most cases the neurons could be recorded continuously for several hours. By means of a delay circuit, the entire courses of the action potentials were displayed on a storage oscilloscope to control the constancy of wave form and amplitude of the recorded unit. This ensured that over the entire period, one and the same neuron was recorded. All neurons investigated by us during this program over the last two decades were located in the medial two-thirds of the reticular formation in an area reaching from several millimeters rostral of the obex to 4 mm caudal of the obex.

The spontaneous activity of typical neurons of the reticular formation could be changed by experimental changes of hemodynamic parameters. Inflating a balloon in the thoracic aorta increased the activity of baroreceptors. Neuron no. 60/8, the activity of which is shown in Figures 1 and 5, reacted each time with a decrease of its discharge frequency to the rhythmically repeated increases of arterial pressure. The result of this intervention shown in part A of Figure 1 also demonstrates a decrease of respiratory frequency and depth, and an increase of the degree of synchronization of the EEG with each blood pressure increase. Part B of Figure 1

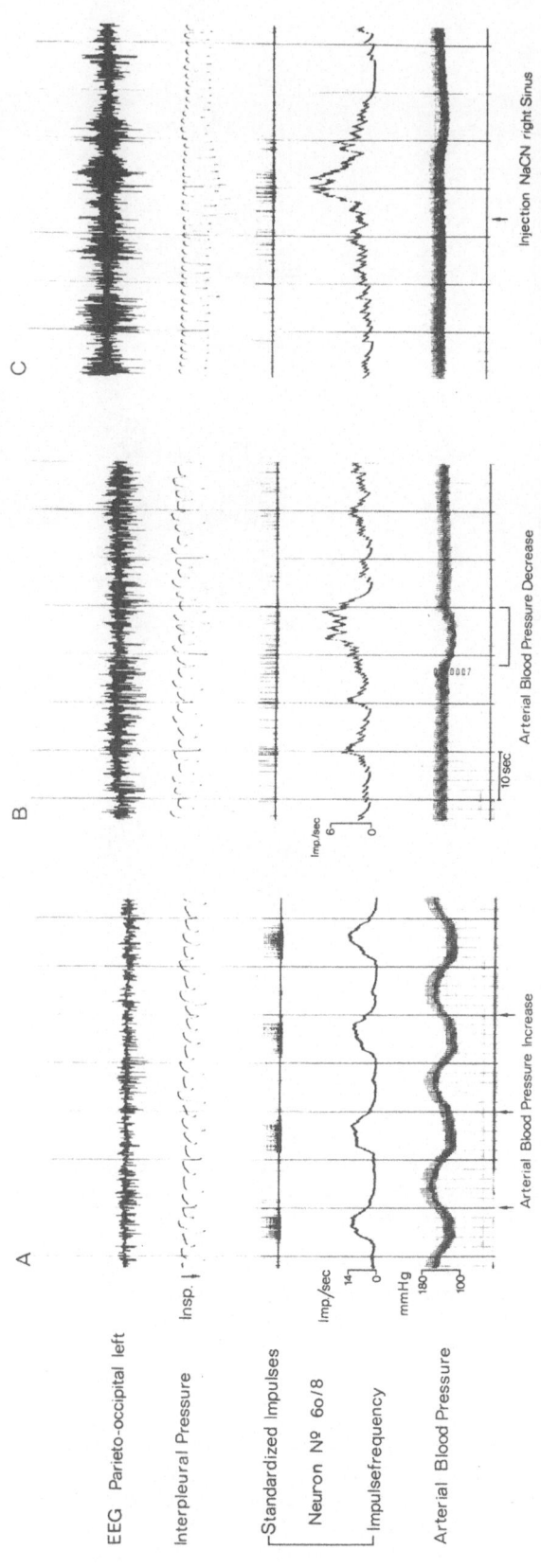

Fig. 1. Response of a reticular neuron (60/8) to stimulation of arterial presso- and chemoreceptors. On the poly-graphic registration the neuronal activity is represented by standardized impulses and a leaky integrated frequency curve together with arterial blood pressure; respiration, measured as interpleural pressure and the ipsilaterally recorded EEG waves. A: Inflating a balloon in the abdominal aorta rhythmically induces artific-ial blood pressure increases thereby increasing pressoreceptor afferent activity. During the rising phases of the pressure waves the neuron reduces its discharge frequency, which increases again during the falling phases. This experiment demonstrates that pressoreceptors have an activity-decreasing effect on reticular neurons. B: Inflating a balloon in the caval vein reduced venous return to the heart and thereby arterial pressure. This procedure leads to an increase of the discharge frequency of the neuron. Note that respiratory modulation of the discharge frequency becomes more prominent at this time. C: Injection of a low dose of NaCN into the right carotid sinus (blind sac preparation) stimulates arterial chemoreceptors mildly. This leads to an increase of respiratory depth and frequency. At the same time neuronal activity increases markedly, together with arterial blood pressure. The discharge pattern of the neuron does not become distinctly respiratory modulated, indicat-ing that the chemoreceptor effect onto this neuron is not mediated by respiratory neurons. This example demonstrates that pressoreceptor and chemoreceptor afferents converge onto single neurons in the reticular formation.

13

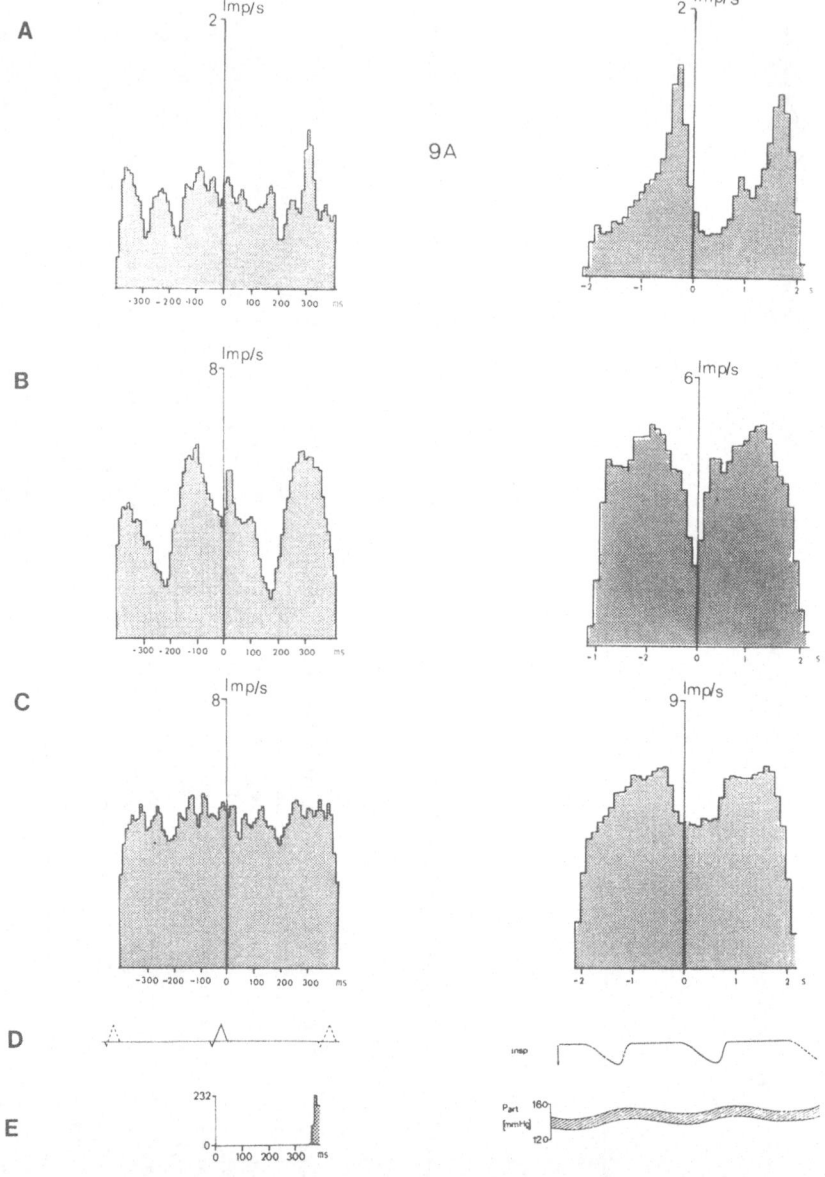

Fig. 2.   Investigation of respiratory and pulse-rhythmic modulations of the
discharge patterns of three neighboring reticular neurons recorded
simultaneously with one electrode by ECG- and inspiration-
triggered post-event-time histograms.   Left side: A-C: Histograms
triggered by the R-deflection of the ECG.   D: Schematic course of
the ECG.   E: Distribution of trigger signals.   Mean R-R interval
is 386 msec; histograms are computed for 776 heart cycles.   The
histograms show the temporal relation of the discharges of the
three different neurons before (left to the ordinate) and after
the respective R-wave of the ECG (right to the ordinate).   The
basic activity in all three histograms indicates that the neurons
discharge at any moment of the cardiac cycle.   The three histograms have a trough approximately 170 to 200 msec after the
beginning of the cardiac cycle, which demonstrates that the
activity of the neurons is rhythm modulated by the heart.   All
three neurons reduced their discharge frequencies when blood

pressure was artificially elevated. The results show that pressoreceptor afferents modulate the activity of reticular neurons.
Right side: A-C: Histograms triggered by the beginning of inspiration. D: Schematic course of interpleural pressure related to
the histogram. E: Schematic course of blood pressure waves
related to the histogram. Histograms are computed for 132
respiratory cycles, mean duration of respiratory cycle, 2248 msec.
The histograms give the temporal relation of the discharge of the
three neurons before and after the beginning of respiratory cycle.
A-C: All three histograms have a trough of different duration
during the inspiratory phase of the respiratory cycle.
This example demonstrates that the activity of neighboring
reticular neurons can be modulated by pressoreceptor afferents and
respiratory activity at the same time.

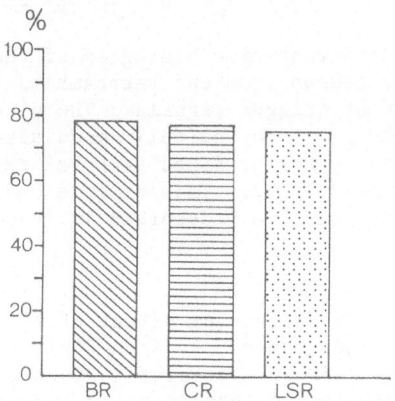

Fig. 3. Positive reactions of reticular neurons to adequate stimulations
of baroreceptors (BR), chemoreceptors (CR) and lung stretch
receptors (LSR) in percent of tested units. The diagram indicates
that nearly 80% of tested neurons respond to stimulation of
afferents in vegetative systems.

shows the result of experimental blood pressure decrease induced by
inflating a balloon in the orifice of the right atrium. During experimental blood pressure decrease, the discharge frequency of the neuron
rises, at the same time respiratory frequency and depth increase, and the
EEG shows a desynchronization. Oscillations with respiratory frequency can
be observed in the integrated frequency curve during high discharge rates.
These findings demonstrate that this neuron received pressoreceptor
afferents. In addition, such influences could be detected in many cases
with the aid of ECG-triggered post-event-time histograms of neuronal
activity. A pulse-related rhythm is indicated by a higher or lower number
of counts in several successive bins deviating from the mean value of the
histogram in temporal relation to the R-deflection of the ECG. The left
half of Figure 2 gives three examples of such histograms computed from the
activity of three reticular neurons. These three neurons were recorded
simultaneously with one electrode. The influence of afferents from baroreceptors on the discharge rates could be detected in 93% of tested
neurons. Stimulation of chemoreceptors activated 77% of the same neurons,
and 75% of these neurons decreased their activity during experimental lung
inflations. These results are summarized in Figure 3. These findings
demonstrate that a labelling of reticular neurons as cardiovascular or
respiratory neurons according to the afferents from cardiovascular and
respiratory systems is not suitable. These receptors exert a generalized
influence on reticular neurons.

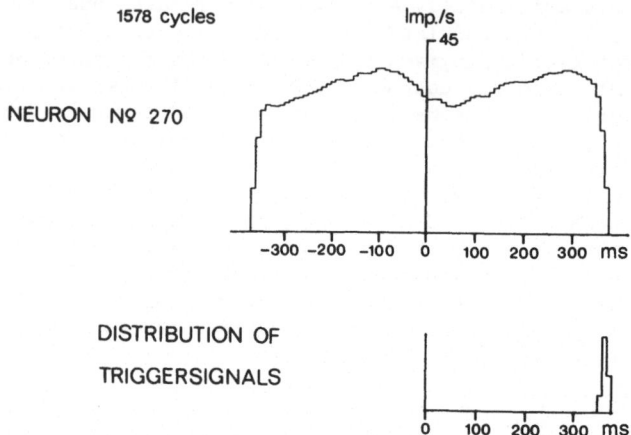

Fig. 4. ECG-triggered post-event-time histogram of the neuronal activity of an expiratory neuron from the retroambigual respiratory area and distribution of trigger signals. The discharge pattern of the neuron is clearly heart-rhythmically modulated. At this time of the recording, there was no fixed temporal relation between respiration and heart rate. This example shows that pressoreceptor afferents exert a widespread influence on many neurons.

The generalized activity-decreasing effect of afferents from pressoreceptors is a well-known phenomenon. E. Koch [40] induced sleeping behavior by inflating a balloon in the carotid sinus of unanesthetized dogs. Physiological excitation of baroreceptors has reduced respiratory parameters [33], the excitability of cortical neurons [8] and spinal motor neurons [81]. This generalized activity-decreasing effect is conveyed by the reticular system and can be proved also in typical expiratory neurons (Figure 4).

The same neurons can be influenced by afferents from somatorsensory receptors. An example is given in Figure 5. This is the same neuron, the activity of which is shown in Figure 1 reacting to inputs from enteroceptors. The neurons reacted to stimulation of afferents from different receptor types and different sites of the body. Each neuron can be influenced by a limited number of such afferents. The combinations of effective afferents from somatosensory receptors converging on single neurons change from neuron to neuron is already described by Scheibel et al. [78]. Our results concerning somatosensory afferents correspond with the data reported in the literature [70], but there are no reports from other groups describing the additional influence from cardiovascular and pulmonary receptors on the same neurons [55,82].

EVIDENCE FOR EFFERENT INFLUENCES OF THE RETICULAR SYSTEM

The question of the efferent relations of reticular neurons cannot be investigated by the aid of stimulation experiments as discussed above. The relations between reticular neurons and their effector systems can be analyzed by detecting reticular rhythms in the activity of these effectors. The spontaneous activity of the reticular neurons is marked by characteristic rhythms. These rhythms are partly the result of rhythmical afferents to the reticular neurons. Such a rhythm is, for example, the cardiac rhythm. The cardiac rhythmic afferent activity of the baroreceptors affects the various body systems via the reticular neurons, as discussed

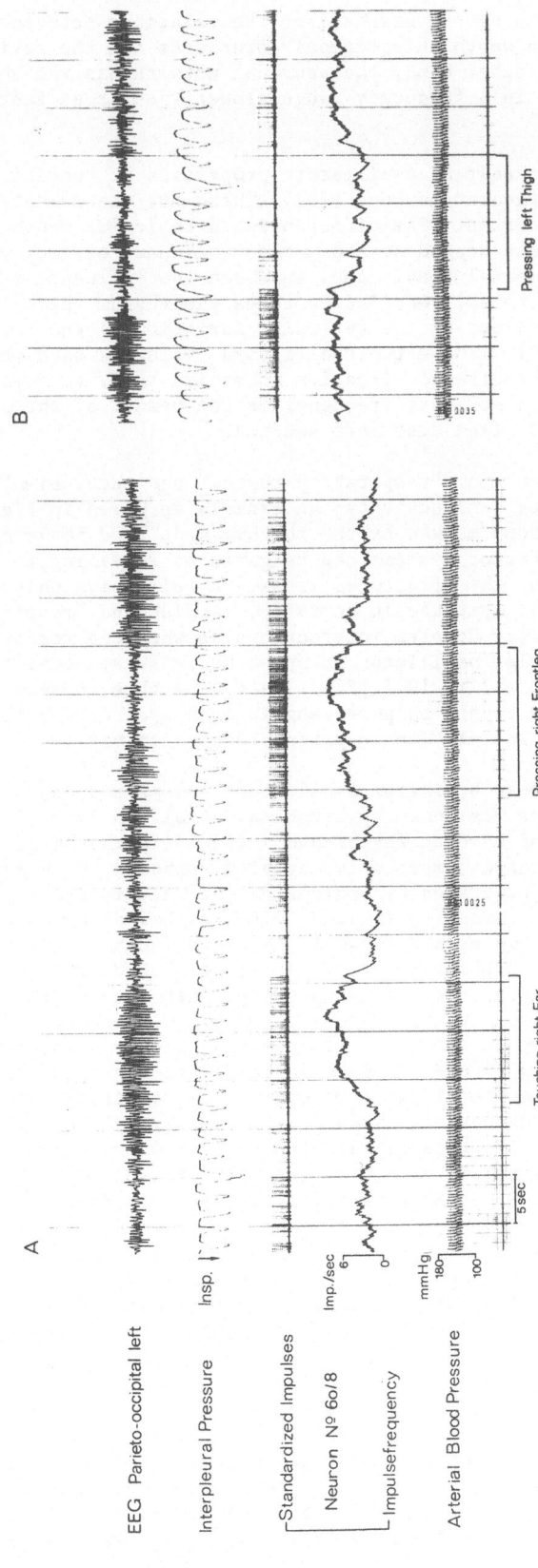

Fig. 5. Response of the reticular neuron shown in Figure 1 to stimulation of afferents from skin and muscles (same presentation of signals as in Figure 1). A: Touching the right ear and the right foreleg increases the discharge frequency of the neuron. B: Pressing the left thigh has an activity-decreasing effect onto the neuron. At the same time the EEG becomes desynchronized. The results show that single reticular neurons can be influenced by afferents from somatosensory systems in different ways and from different parts of the body.

17

above. Similar conditions can be assumed for the relations between the delta-theta oscillator in septal hippocampal structures and the reticular neuronal system. On the other hand, the neuronal network has the ability to generate oscillations in a frequency range slower than or as fast as respiration.

Ventilation is the result of oscillatory properties of specialized and functionally separate reticular neurons [76]. These are the so-called respiratory oscillator neurons. The differentiated reticular neurons of the respiratory oscillators depend on the marked influence of lung volume receptors. Under experimental conditions, in which the influence of lung volume receptors is eliminated, ventilation takes the rhythm which is generated by the other neurons of the reticular formation of the lower brainstem [20,21,22,51,56]. These two oscillators influence each other following the rules of relative coordination according to E. v. Holst [36,37]. Sinus arrhythmia of heart frequency is the result of the inter-action of both oscillators (see also last section).

The cardiac rhythm and the "respiratory rhythm" can occur simul-taneously in reticular neuronal activity; an example is given in Figure 2. A demonstration that neurons marked by the rhythms mentioned above exert influences on various effector systems can be given by revealing the same rhythms in the activity of the effector systems. A well-known phenomenon is that in post-ganglionic sympathetic activity, cardiac and "respiratory" rhythms are visible [1,17]. Complex interactions between the respiratory oscillator and the reticular oscillator in sympathetic nerve activity were demonstrated by Gebber et al. in 1977 [27]. They were able to show that the so-called respiratory rhythm in post-ganglionic sympathetic activity occurs with phase-shifts in relation to phrenic nerve activity.

The interaction between brainstem oscillator neurons and neurons of the respiratory oscillator was shown by Langhorst et al. in 1977 [51,56]. Simultaneous occurrence of cardiac rhythm and delta-theta rhythm in reticular and post-ganglionic sympathetic activity supports the hypothesis that sympathetic tone is generated by neurons of the multifunctional system in the brainstem. [14]. Neuronal activities with rhythmical components temporally related to EEG waves are shown in Figure 6. Both simultaneously recorded neurons exhibit an EEG-rhythmical pattern of 2.8 Hz. In the given example the delta-theta rhythm is partly congruent with the cardiac rhythm. Very often both rhythms could be observed with slight differences in fre-quency [50]. The same two rhythms exist in post-ganglionic sympathetic nerve activity as shown in Figure 7. Experimental interventions which temporarily remove baroreceptor input completely lead to disapperance of the cardiac rhythmical component in sympathetic activity. Then only the delta-theta rhythm can be observed but its frequency now changes. These observations are another example of the interaction of two oscillators according to the rules of E. v. Holst's relative coordination. In this example one of the oscillators is not a nervous structure but the heart. The heart is not only the oscillator acting on nervous structures but also the effector of nervous influences originating in the same structures. The physiological properties of these functional relations can be analyzed only in the intact system. That is why the reductionistic approach of open loop analyses can yield misleading results.

The temporal relations between the two oscillators change depending upon their input. This means that the oscillatory properties of the reticular network are determined also by the incoming afferents. The discharge behavior of the single neurons thus depends on at least three factors: (1) on the influence of afferents from enteroceptors and from somatosensory receptors; (2) on the influence from other nerve cells of the reticular formation; and (3) on inflows from higher brain structures.

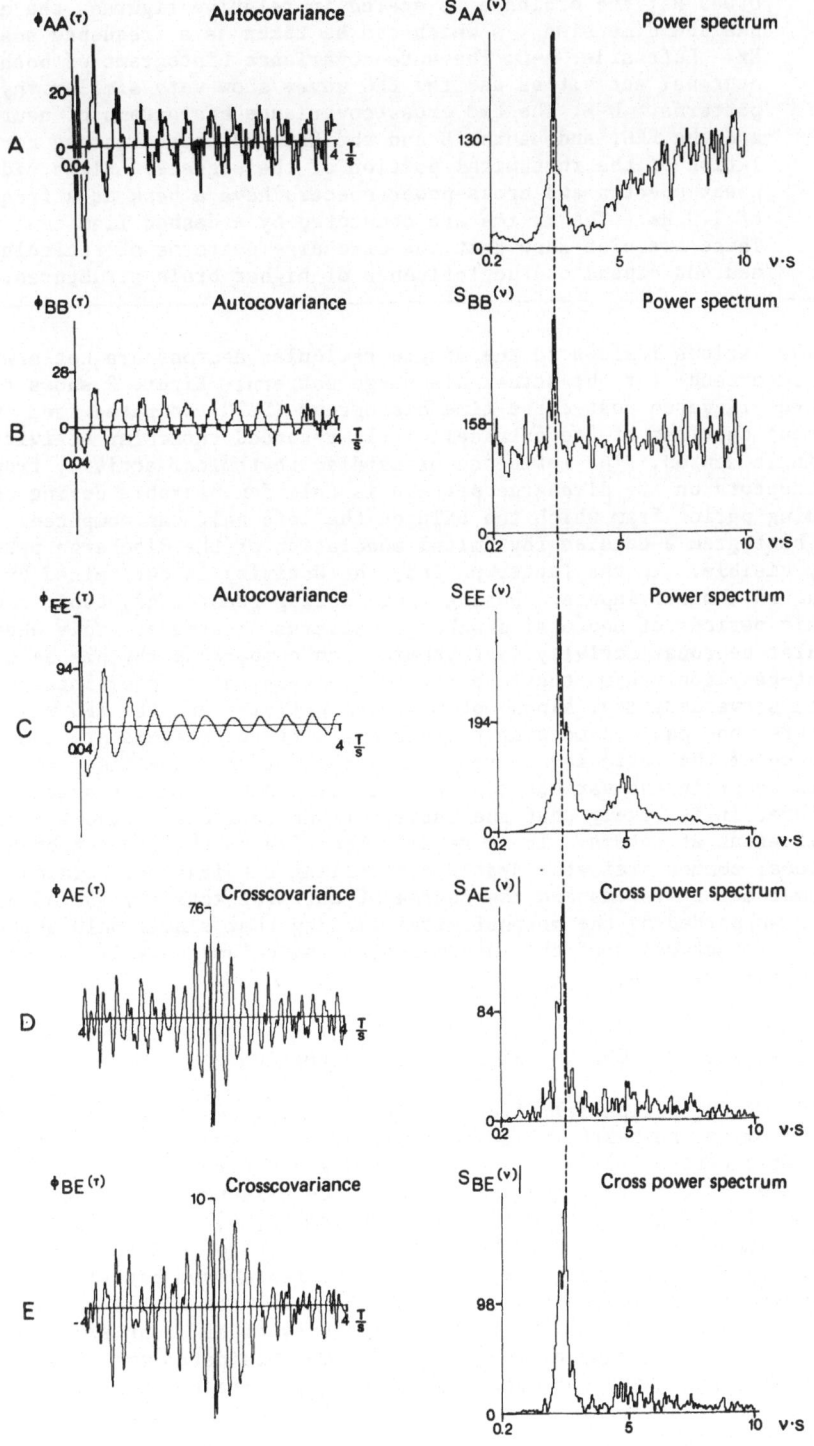

Fig. 6. Investigations of the temporal relations between the discharges of
two neighboring reticular neurons and the ipsilaterally recorded
cortical EEG waves by means of auto- and cross-covariance histograms and power spectra. τ_{max} : 10.24 sec; bin width of auto- and
cross-covariance histograms: 20 msec, the abscissa is equivalent
to the mean value of the histogram; bin width of power spectra:
(continued)

0.049 Hz; the ordinate is scaled in relative figures, the abscissa has the dimension ν·s which can be taken as a frequency scale in Hz. Left side: A-C: The auto-covariance histograms of both neuronal activities and the EEG waves show very similar rhythmical patterns. D-E: The two cross-covariance histograms of neuron A and the EEG, and neuron B and the EEG indicate a strong correlation of the rhythmical portion of the signals. Right side: All power spectra and cross-power spectra have a peak at a frequency of 2.8 Hz. The maxima are connected by a dashed line. These examples show that the discharge patterns of reticular neurons depend on the influence of higher brain structures.

The various inflows to the single reticular neurons are not always of equal importance for the actual discharge pattern. Figure 8 shows two ECG-wave-triggered post-event-time histograms (PETH) computed from two different sections of the extracellularly recorded reticular activity of one single neuron. The influence of cardiac rhythmical activity from baroreceptors on the discharge pattern is only demonstrable during the recording period from which the PETH on the left half was computed. In the right histogram a cardiac rhythmical modulation of the discharge pattern is hardly visible. In the latter period, the activity is determined by non-cardiac rhythmical inputs. During long-lasting recordings, tonic and rhythmic periods of neuronal discharge patterns alternate. Only when the reticular neuronal activity is rhythmic, can comparable rhythms be observed in post-ganglionic sympathetic activity, in respiratory oscillator neurons, phrenic nerve activity, alpha-motor neuron activity and the EEG waves. Therefore, one can assume that the various effector systems are under the influence of the reticular neuronal network. At the same time, comparable rhythms occur in the various central and peripheral effector systems. Therefore, it is likely that the entity of the reticular network acts on the different effectors. These results have led to the concept of a multifunctional common brainstem system controlling respiration, cardiovascular and somatomotor systems and the degree of cortical activity [52,53,55,82]. This is supported by the morphological finding that single bulbospinal neurons contact cells of the intermediolateral column as well as neurons of the ventral horn [35].

PARASYMPATHETIC NEURONS IN THE RETICULAR FORMATION

One of the peripheral effectors of the multifunctional common brainstem system is the heart, which is innervated by sympathetic and parasympathetic nerves [47,71]. Both components exert reciprocal effects on heart rate. During rest the influence of the parasympathetic nerve is dominant, inducing respiratory sinus arrhythmia [24]. The main difference between sympathetic and parasympathetic components of heart innervation consists in their reciprocal reaction to afferents from baroreceptors. Parasympathetic tone of cardiac branches is mainly generated by baroreceptor afferents which inhibit tonic activity of efferent sympathetic nerves. Multifunctional neurons of the common brainstem system which can act as parasympathetic tone-generating neurons increase their discharge frequency under afferents from baroreceptors. That means that in conditions in which the activity of the common brainstem system is predominantly determined by baroreceptor inputs, sympathetic tone and parasympathetic tone-generating neurons can be discerned. An example of two neighboring reticular neurons which can be candidates for the parasympathetic tone-generating neurons is shown in Figure 9. Both neurons increase their discharge frequencies during experimental blood pressure elevations. Neuron A mirrors the experimental blood pressure waves better than neuron B. Parallel to the experimental blood pressure increases,

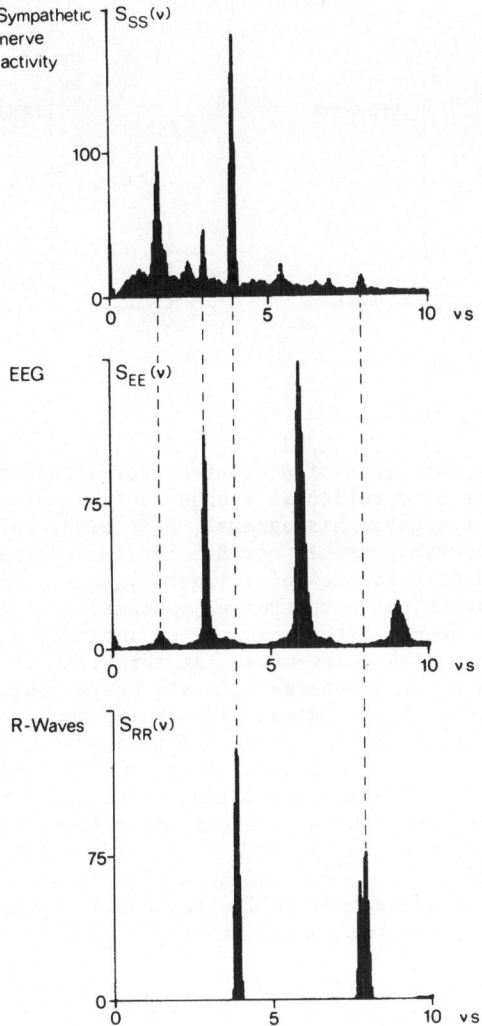

Fig. 7. Demonstration of the simultaneous occurrence of cardiac and EEG
rhythm in post-ganglionic renal sympathetic activity by means of
frequency analysis (ordinate of power spectra scaled in relative
figures, the abscissa has the dimension $\nu \cdot s$ which can be taken as
a frequency scale in Hz). The power spectrum of sympathetic nerve
activity contains several maxima, two of which coincide with
maxima of the power spectrum of EEG waves, and two others are
related to maxima of the power spectrum of the ECG.
This example demonstrates that at the same time, two rhythms of
different frequencies and origin can exist in sympathetic
activity.

respiratory depth and frequency are reduced. Stimulations of arterial
chemoreceptors produce not only an increase of efferent phrenic nerve
activity, but also an increase of the discharge rates of both neurons
(Figure 10). The ECG-triggered post-event-time histograms of the activity
of the same neurons shown in Figures 9 and 10 reveal a strong influence of
baroreceptor activity on the discharging of the neurons in that phase from
which the PETH were computed (Figure 11). Respiratory-triggered PETH of
the same neuronal activity shows a marked respiratory modulation of discharge frequency (Figure 12). Both neurons could be influenced by

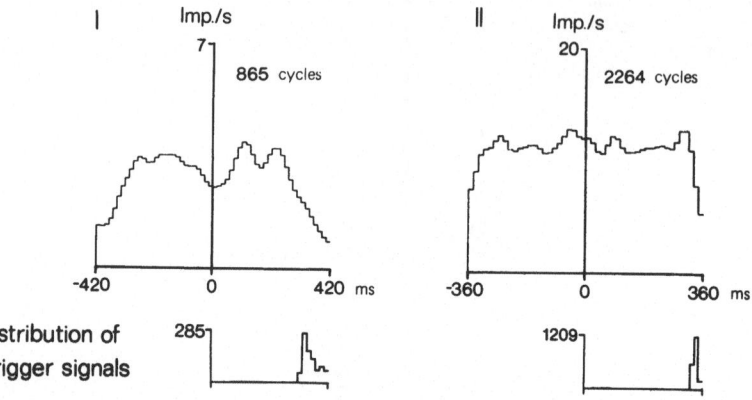

Neuron № 8

Fig. 8. Changes of the influence of pressoreceptor afferents on the discharge behavior of a reticular neuron in the course of time shown
by pulse-wave-triggered histograms. Left side: Pulse-wave-
triggered histogram computed for 865 cardiac cycles, mean duration
(395 msec) and distribution of trigger signals. The histogram
indicates a marked pulse-rhythmical modulation of the discharge
pattern of the neuron with a minimum of activity during the late
systolic phase of the pulse-wave. At this time of the recording
the neuron had a low discharge rate and heart frequency showed a
marked sinus arrhythmia. Right side: Pulse-wave-triggered histogram computed of another portion of the recording with 2264
cardiac cycles, mean duration 348 msec. In this histogram a
cardiac-rhythmical modulation of the discharge pattern is hardly
visible. Now the neuron has a higher discharge frequency; heart
rate has increased and sinus arrhythmia is reduced.
This example shows that the influence of pressoreceptor afferents
on the discharge pattern of reticular neurons is not a constant
one but changes over the course of time.

afferents from somatosensory receptors. These two neurons, like all others
of this type, have properties of the multifunctional reticular neurons.
The only difference is their reaction to baroreceptor activity. A labelling as parasympathetic tone-generating neurons is only possible under the
conditions in which their discharge pattern is mainly determined by baroreceptor inputs [54]. This means that according to the criteria discussed
above, it is possible to label a small amount of reticular neurons in a
dynamic way as parasympathetic tone-generating neurons.

SIMILARITIES OF THE PROPERTIES OF NEIGHBORING NEURONS

The proposed concept of a multifunctional common brainstem system
explains many of the seemingly controversial results. This multifunctional
system has to guarantee the optimal adjustment of the somatomotor and
autonomic systems of the body to cover the whole range of activity from
sleep to high levels of attention. This requires a highly flexible coordination of the activities of the nervous cells on the brainstem level.
The principles of such a functional organization can be investigated only
when several neurons are recorded simultaneously and thereby under
identical conditions [55]. This experimental approach seems to be the only
possibility for the investigation of the interactions between single

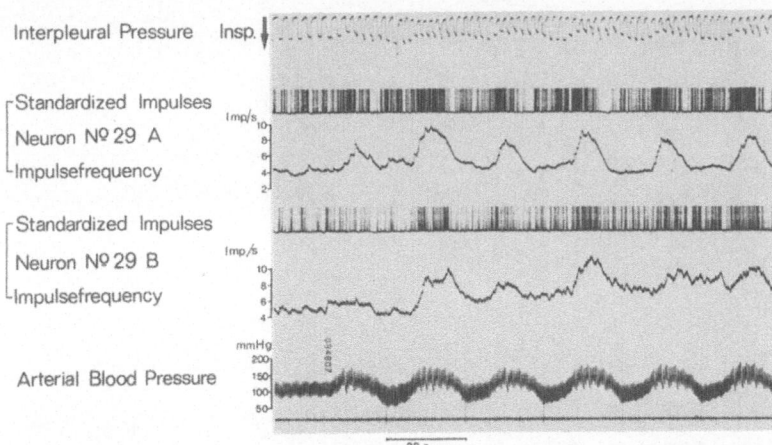

Fig. 9. Influence of increased pressoreceptor activity on the discharge
frequency pattern of two neighboring neurons with properties of
parasympathetic tone-generating neurons. Arterial blood pressure
is varied rhythmically by inflating a balloon in the abdominal
aorta. During phases of elevated blood pressure the discharge
frequencies of both neurons increase. Note the reduction of
respiratory depth and frequency parallel to blood pressure
increase.

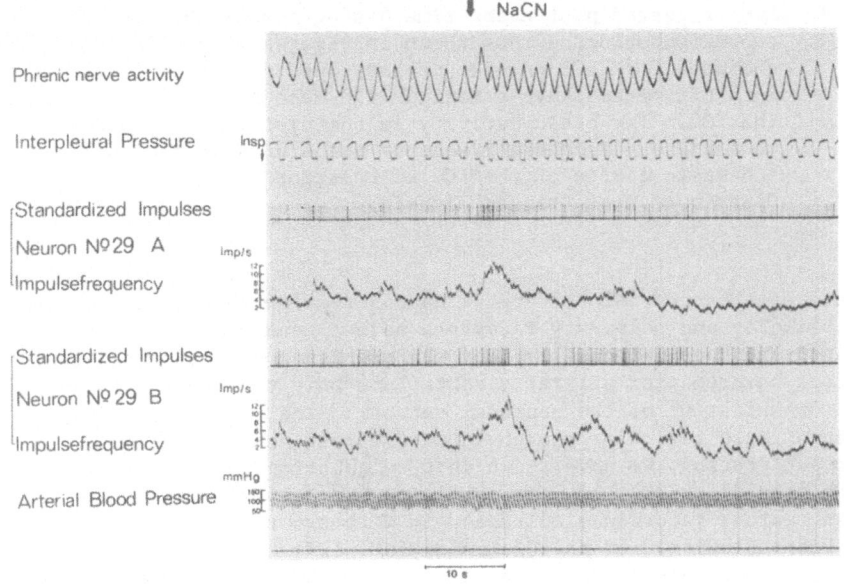

Fig. 10. Reaction of the two neurons shown in Figure 9 to stimulation of
arterial chemoreceptors. After injection of NaCN into the right
carotid sinus, phrenic nerve activity and thereby respiration
increases. At the same time both neurons increase their discharge rates.

23

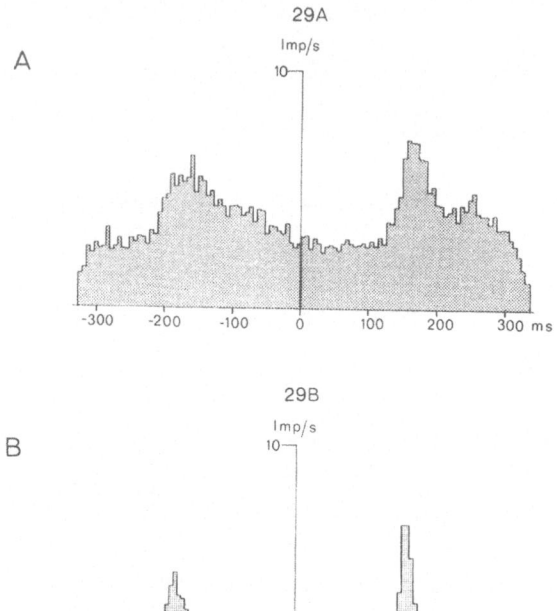

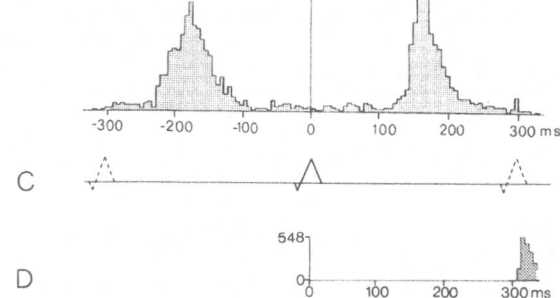

Fig. 11.   ECG-triggered post-event-time histograms of the activities of the
two neighboring neurons shown in Figures 9 and 10.   Histograms
computed for 2528 cardiac cycles, mean duration 320 msec.   A-B:
Both histograms have a maximum 150 msec after the R-deflection of
the ECG.   The basic activity in the histogram of neuron A is due
to a higher discharge frequency compared with neuron B.   C:
Schematic course of the ECG in relation to the histogram.   D:
Distribution of trigger signals.

elements of the neuronal network.   The observation that afferents from
cardiovascular and pulmonary receptors have a generalized effect on 90% of
the single neurons was confirmed by the simultaneous recordings [55].
Therefore baroreceptor afferents contribute only to a more uniform functional organization of the neuronal network.   The concept that the afferent
spectra of each reticular neuron is unique must be reconsidered.   In a
recent publication, we have shown that neighboring neurons receive 41% to
100% (mainly 91 - 100%) of afferents from the same somatosensory receptors,
whereas neurons recorded simultaneously with two electrodes from different
sites reacted only in 0% to 40% (mainly 0 - 10%) of the cases to the same
somatosensory afferent input.   An example of the reaction patterns of
simultaneously recorded neighboring neurons is given in Figure 13.   Whenever the discharge behavior is mainly determined by common somatosensory
afferents, neighboring neurons are coupled to form functional units [82].
The number of neurons which are organized in such a subpopulation depends
on the number and type of incoming afferents and on the level of pre-
existing activity in the neuronal network.

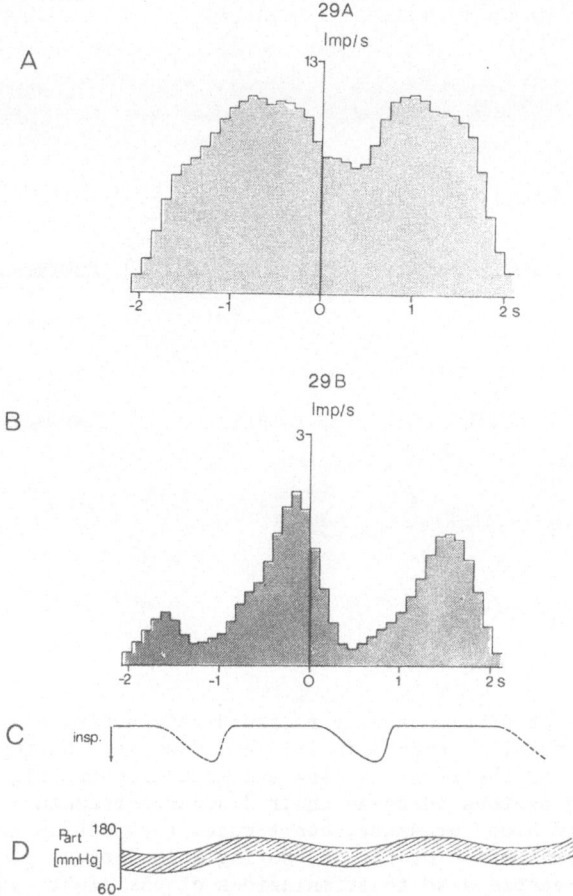

Fig. 12.   Inspiration-triggered histograms showing the temporal relation
between the discharges of the neurons and the respiratory cycle.
Histograms were computed for 403 respiratory cycles with a mean
duration of 2012 msec. A-B: During inspiration both histograms
show a minimum of discharges. C: Schematic course of interpleural pressure in temporal relation to the histogram. D:
Schematic course of blood pressure waves related to the interpleural pressure.

     The same stimulus was not effective at each time presented. This type
of changing susceptibility [52] is described as dynamic specificity. These
findings are completed by analyzing mean discharge frequencies, interval
distributions and the coordinations of discharge times of the neurons
functionally organized into subpopulations. Three different discharge
frequency ranges of reticular neurons can be discerned. Each of these
three frequency ranges is characterized by typical forms of interval
histograms (Figure 14). In the low level of activity, neurons discharge
with up to 7 impulses/sec. Then the interval histograms are of a bi- or
trimodal shape (part A of Figure 14). This is a functional state in which
neuronal activity is frequently modulated parallel to EEG waves. In the
second frequency range of 8 - 16 impulses/sec, the interval histograms have
an exponential course (part B). In this state a functional organization of
reticular neurons by afferents from somatosensory receptors to subpopulations can be observed. Symmetrical shapes of the interval histograms
are observed when the neurons discharge with more than 16 impulses/sec

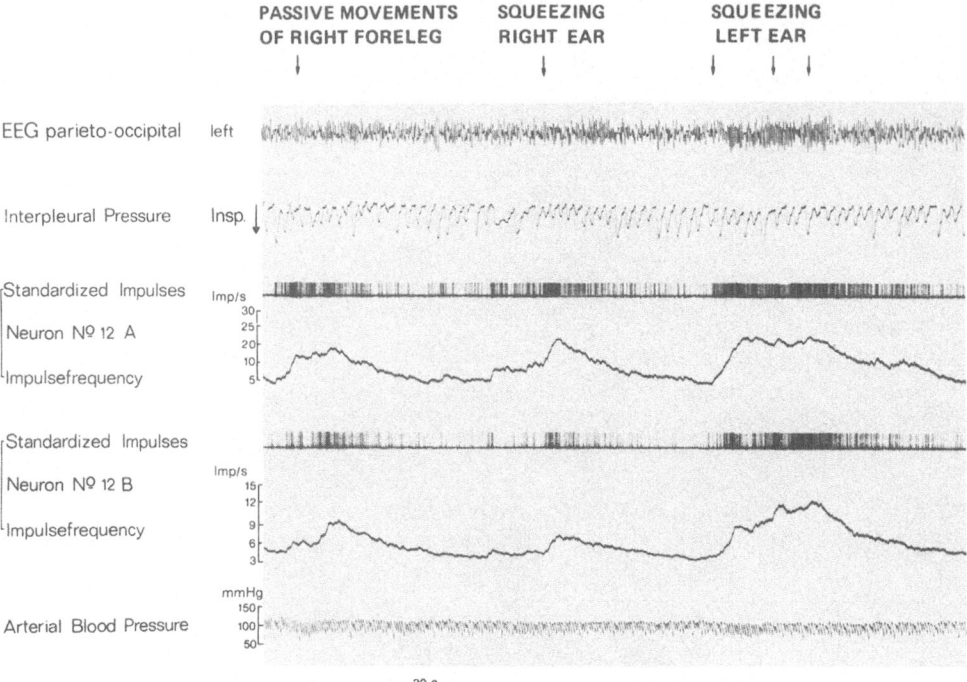

PASSIVE MOVEMENTS OF RIGHT FORELEG   SQUEEZING RIGHT EAR   SQUEEZING LEFT EAR

EEG parieto-occipital   left

Interpleural Pressure   Insp.

Standardized Impulses
Neuron № 12 A
Impulsefrequency

Arterial Blood Pressure

20 s

Fig. 13.   Reactions of simultaneously recorded neighboring neurons to
stimulation of receptors in skin and muscles. During passive
movements of the right foreleg and squeezing the right and left
ear, both neurons increase their discharge frequencies. Note
changes of blood pressure, heart rate, respiration and the degree
of synchronization of the EEG during stimulation. The same
neurons reacted also to stimulations of the right and left back
and to passive movements of the other three extremities.

(part C). Neurons recorded simultaneously with one electrode or recorded
at different sites with two electrodes at the same time displayed similar
interval histograms. In the course of long-lasting recordings, the neurons
changed spontaneously or were experimentally induced to change their discharge frequency, and thereby the distribution of intervals changed, too.

The coordination of the discharge times and patterns of neighboring
neurons were investigated by the computation of cross-covariance histograms
to get information about the intrinsic organization of the common brainstem
system. Similar to the three different types of interval distributions and
discharge frequency ranges, three different major forms of coordinated
discharging were observed.

In the low frequency range between 0.5 - 7 impulses/sec, the cross-
covariance histograms show a rhythmic pattern with a broad maximum strad-
dling the ordinate. The neurons then discharge rhythmically coupled
(Figure 17). This type of correlated discharge behavior could be observed
not only between neighboring but also between neurons recorded simultaneously from different sites in the medulla. This again indicates that
the rhythmic discharge behavior is a wide-spread phenomenon; so organized,
the brainstem acts as a single system composed of equally important parts.
Moruzzi supposes that in this state the brainstem system acts mainly as an
energizer for higher brain structures and the spinal cord, maintaining the

26

Neuron № 14   Neuron № 7   Neuron № 26

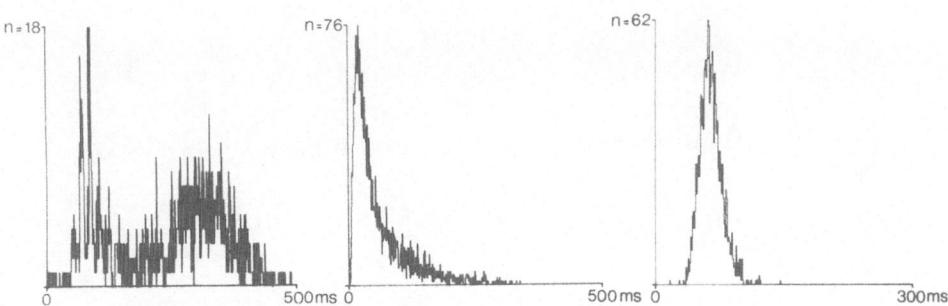

Fig. 14. Distribution of discharge intervals of three different neurons
          firing with different mean frequencies. Analysis done by first
          order interval histograms; bin width 1 msec, ordinate counts/bin,
          abscissa scales in milliseconds.

Spike train statistics:

	neuron 14	neuron 7	neuron 26
mean frequency [impulses/sec]	4	14	18
mean interval [msec]	246	68	54
interval minimum [msec]	2	2	16
interval maximum [msec]	2445	336	145

A: The first-order interval histogram has a bimodal shape which
is typical for neurons discharging rhythmically with mean
frequencies below 8 Hz. B: The histogram has an exponential
course which was always found when the neurons discharged with
irregular intervals in a range of 8-16 Hz. C: The histogram is
of symmetrical shape. This was observed only when the neurons
discharged with more than 16 impulses/sec.

basic level of activity necessary for adequate execution of different tasks
in the advent of new situations [68].

In the intermediate frequency range, very often the discharges of
neighboring neurons are strongly coupled; then the cross-covariance
histograms have sharp maxima with durations of 2 - 5 msec right or left of
the ordinate (Figure 16). This is interpreted to be the result of the
influence of somatosensory afferents acting on these neurons [82a].
Moruzzi suggested that in the intermediate frequency range, the reticular
formation is organized into functional units. This suggestion is confirmed
by the experimental data described above. In this intermediate level of
activity, the output of the network is highly differentiated, and the
common brainstem system exerts different influences on different effector
systems and has thus the largest regulatory potency [68].

In the range of high-frequency discharging, neurons discharge independently of each other, which is indicated by flat cross-covariance histograms. The differentiated type of organization of the common system is
lost (Figure 15). In this state the system acts, e.g. as in an emergency
reaction [15].

CONCLUDING REMARKS

The reticular formation is the morphological substrate for a system
which regulates and controls cardiovascular, respiratory and somatomotor

Autocovariances

Crosscovariances

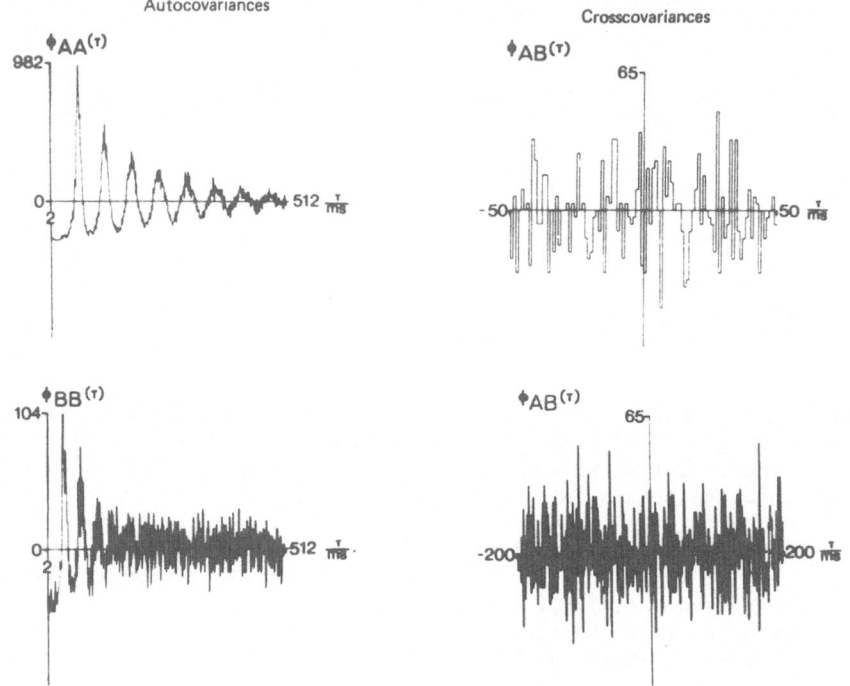

Fig. 15.   Analyses of the temporal coordination of the discharges of two
           neighboring neurons recorded simultaneously with one electrode by
           the aid of auto- and cross-covariance histograms. All covari-
           ances in this and the subsequent two figures are computed for
           latencies of τ_{max} = 512 msec. Histograms have a bin width of
           1 msec. Abscissa scales in msec, ordinate in counts/bin related
           to bin width and time of evaluation. Left side: Autocovariance
           (ACH) histograms of the two neurons. Both histograms have
           similar forms with a rapid decline of the maxima. This indicates
           that the neurons discharge regularly with fluctuating intervals.
           Right side: Cross-covariance histograms plotted for τ = ±50 msec
           (top) and for τ = ±200 msec (bottom). The bin counts fluctate
           around the abscissa without reaching an outstanding maximum
           indicating that the neurons discharge independently of each
           other.

systems, together with the degree of cortical activity. Single neurons of
the reticular formation have multifunctional properties. Each can be
concerned with control functions of various effector systems. This multifunctional common brainstem system is not diffusely organized. According
to mean discharge frequencies, interval distributions, discharge behavior
and coordination of the discharge times of the neurons, three types of
functional organization can be discerned in the given matrix of the
reticular formation.

    In the discharge frequency range of 8 - 16 impulses/sec, the spon-
taneous activity is characterized by irregular tonic discharging. The
shapes of the interval histograms are of an exponential type and the cross-
covariance histograms reveal a strong coupling of neighboring neurons on a
time scale of a few milliseconds. In this type of functional organization,
the reticular formation is organized in subpopulations and has a high
regulatory potency. The functional organization to subunits is maintained
by somatosensory afferents to those neurons. In the highest discharge

28

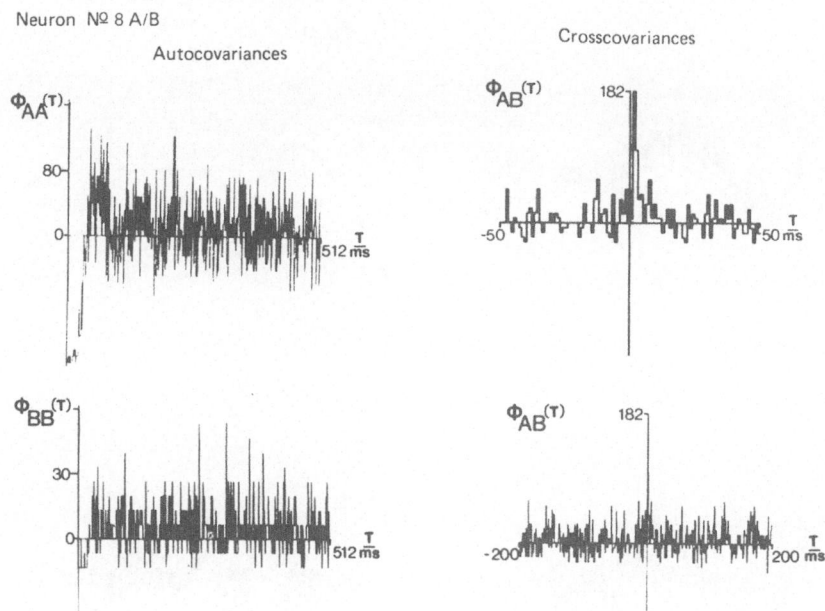

Neuron № 8 A/B

Autocovariances

Crosscovariances

Fig. 16.   Auto- and cross-covariance histograms of the activities of two
neighboring neurons with strongly coupled discharges. Right top:
The CCH has a sharp peak right to zero lag. Right bottom: The
peak in the second bin is not repeated in longer lags. Both
ACH's have no pronounced pattern indicating quite irregular
discharges in a frequency range between 8-16 impulses/sec.

frequency range of above 16 impulses/sec, the common brainstem system is no
longer able to maintain differentiated activities and regulatory influences.   Interval histograms are of symmetrical shape indicating quite
regular discharge intervals.   The cross-covariance histograms reveal an
independency of the occurrence of action potentials in neighboring neurons.
This type of functional organization shows all properties of the nervous
control substrates responsible for extreme levels of activity well-known to
be characteristic during emergency reaction [15].

In the lowest frequency range of up to 7 impulses/sec, spontaneous
activity is characterized by rhythmic discharge patterns.   Those rhythms
can be observed in the activity of various peripheral and central systems
controlled by the common brainstem system.   In heart frequency, the respiratory sinus arrhythmia is an expression of rhythmic discharge behavior of
the common brainstem system.   Further details will be discussed in the
following Section.   The interval histograms are of bi- or trimodal shapes.
Action potentials are rhythmically coupled in frequency ranges of heart/
delta-theta rhythm of the EEG and of respiratory/reticular rhythm.   This
form of coupling can be observed not only in the activity of neighboring
neurons, but also of neurons from other sites of the reticular formation of
the lower brainstem.   In this type of functional organization, the common
brainstem system acts as an entity, and the discharge patterns of the
neurons are predominantly determined by the other neurons of the network.

The dynamic organization of reticular neurons in subpopulations and
the coordination of the activity of these populations are thought to be the

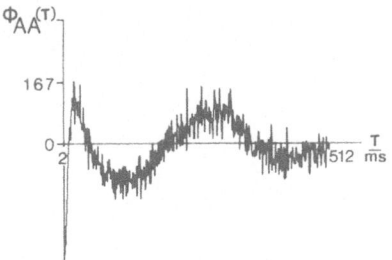
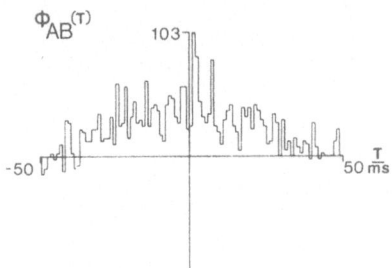

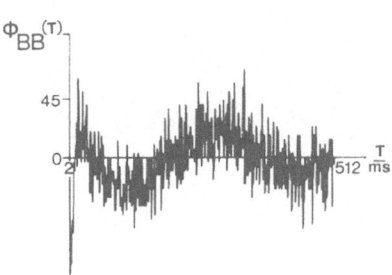
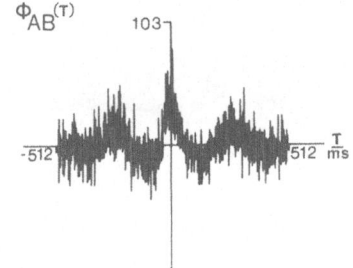

Fig. 17. ACH and CCH of the activity of a pair of neurons discharging rhythmically coupled. Both ACH's have a distinct rhythm with a period duration of around 300 msec. Right bottom: The CCH has also a rhythmic course for positive and negative lags. The frequency of this rhythm is identical with that of the ACH's. Right top: The broad maximum, symmetrical to both sides of the ordinate, indicates that there are no phase shifts between the rhythmic signals of the two activities.

mechanism which permits coordinated regulation of respiratory, cardiovascular and somatomotor systems in the adaptation of the organism to different functions.

BLOOD PRESSURE WAVES AS THE RESULT OF INTERACTIONS BETWEEN THE RESPIRATORY OSCILLATOR AND THE OSCILLATING COMMON BRAINSTEM SYSTEM

The neurons of the multifunctional common brainstem system tend to discharge with rhythms similar to the respiratory rhythm. Such rhythmical discharge patterns occur when the neurons of the network are functionally coupled to an entity and discharge in low-frequency ranges as described above. During long-lasting recordings of reticular neuronal activities, it could be observed that the activity changed several times from rhythmic to tonic discharge patterns.

Figure 18 gives a typical example of three phases of neuronal discharge frequency modulation with period durations around 6 sec. In general, the frequencies of this reticular rhythm range from about 0.25 Hz to 0.1 Hz. The periods of rhythmic discharges in Figure 18 are interrupted by two short phases of tonic activity. During the phases of tonic discharges, respiratory frequency is higher than during the phases of rhythmic discharges. Blood pressure waves become more prominent during reticular rhythmical discharge patterns. The period durations of these oscillations of neuronal activity are clearly different from the period durations of respiratory cycles. The rhythmic oscillations of discharges have period durations of 6.7 sec. The respiratory cycles in Figure 18 have period durations of 3 sec. Such relations between the discharge frequencies of reticular neurons and the frequency of the respiratory oscillator were seen regularly. The relations between rhythmical events in neuronal activity, respiration and blood pressure were analyzed with the aid of covariance histograms and power spectra. Figures 19 and 20 show results from such analyses. The autocovariances and power spectra computed from a part of recorded activity in which the neurons discharge more tonically are shown in Figure 19. The blood pressure waves mirror the respiratory rhythm at 0.41 Hz together with a more pronounced rhythm of 0.088 Hz. This rhythm is related to the oscillatory properties of smooth muscles of the blood vessels. These findings suggest that under conditions in which the neuronal activity of the common brainstem system is not rhythmically modulated, the blood pressure waves are the result of interactions between the respiratory oscillator and the oscillating smooth muscles of the vessels.

The reticular and the respiratory oscillator have a permanent interrelation obeying the rules of relative corodination according to E. v. Holst [36,37]. Between periods in which no relations can be detected and periods in which both oscillators are completely coupled, a broad spectrum of interrelations can be observed. In the periods with no observable relation the eigen-frequencies of the oscillators are quite stable and clearly different, whereby the frequency of the reticular oscillator is slower than that of the respiratory one. In the periods of observable interrelations the frequencies of the oscillators are less stable, and the variability of both period durations increases. In such cases, the frequency of the reticular oscillator increases and that of the respiratory oscillator decreases. In these fluctuating interrelations, the oscillators prefer definite phase couplings in which they tend to persist for longer periods. All cases of extreme deviations of the actual oscillator frequencies are followed by abrupt phase shifts to establish stable relations. E. v. Holst named this the "magnetic effect". Observations of such effects in the arterial blood pressure waves were described thoroughly by Koepchen in 1962 [43].

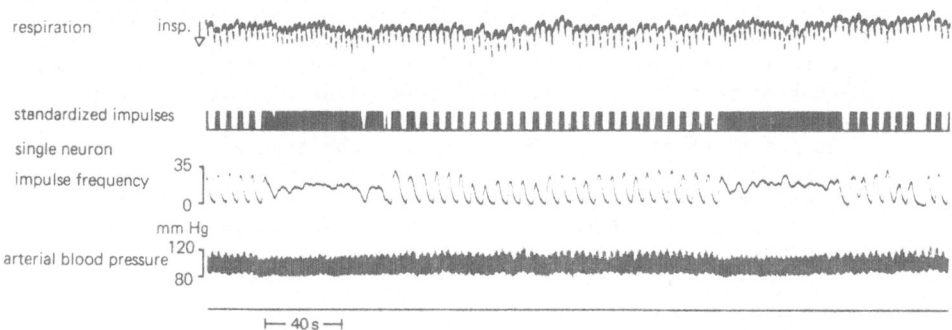

Fig. 18. Polygraph registration of spontaneous oscillations of the discharge frequency of a reticular neuron, together with respiration and arterial blood pressure. Phases of rhythmic discharge with period durations of 6.7 sec are interrupted by short phases of tonic activity. During the phases of tonic discharges, respiratory frequency is higher than during the phases of rhythmic discharges. Blood pressure waves become more prominent during rhythmic discharges. The relation between respiratory frequency and neuronal oscillations is approximately 2:1.

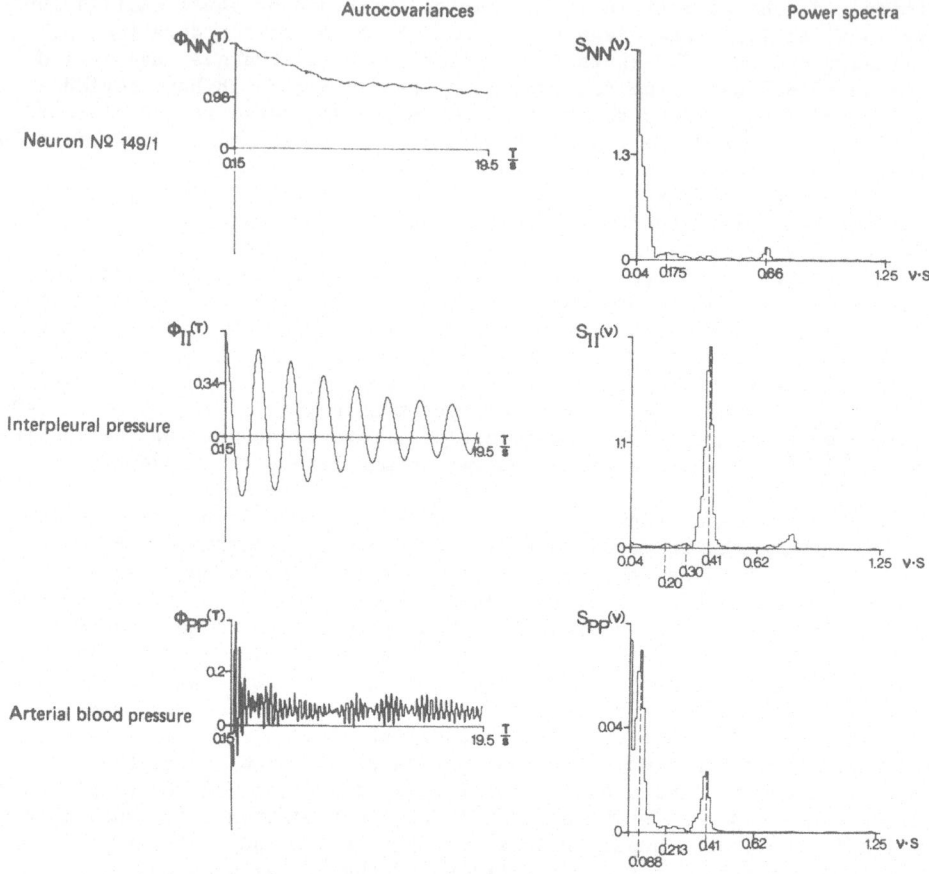

Fig. 19. Autocovariance histograms (ACH) (left side) and power spectra
(PS) (right side) of the activity of a single reticular neuron,
of interpleural pressure and of arterial blood pressure. The
ordinate is scaled in relative figures and the abscissa is scaled
dimensionless by multiplying the frequency with its inversed
dimension (sec). The numbers give the actual values of the
frequencies. The ACH of neuron 149 shows a rhythm with a period
duration of 1.52 sec. In the PS this rhythm appears with a small
peak at 0.66 Hz. In the PS of interpleural pressure the main
peak is at 0.41 Hz equivalent to a period duration of 2.44 sec.
In the PS of arterial blood pressure the frequency of respiration
appears at 0.41 Hz. The dominant frequency of blood pressure is
found at 0.088 Hz (period duration 11.36 sec). The PS is cut off
at 1.25 Hz, therefore the frequency of pulse waves is not
visible.

The power spectra of the neuronal activities of the oscillators or
their effector systems, blood pressure and respiration, show in these cases
a broadening of the peaks or the appearance of new peaks. The effects of
respiratory and reticular oscillators on the arterial blood pressure are
the stronger, the more these frequency ranges overlap. Figure 20 gives an
examples of a period in which overlapping is visible. Compared with the
results in Figure 19, the respiratory rhythm has become slower and its
frequency is nearly identical with that of the reticular oscillator. The
effect on the arterial blood pressure is now dominant. The blood pressure
fluctuations induced by the oscillations of the smooth muscles of the blood

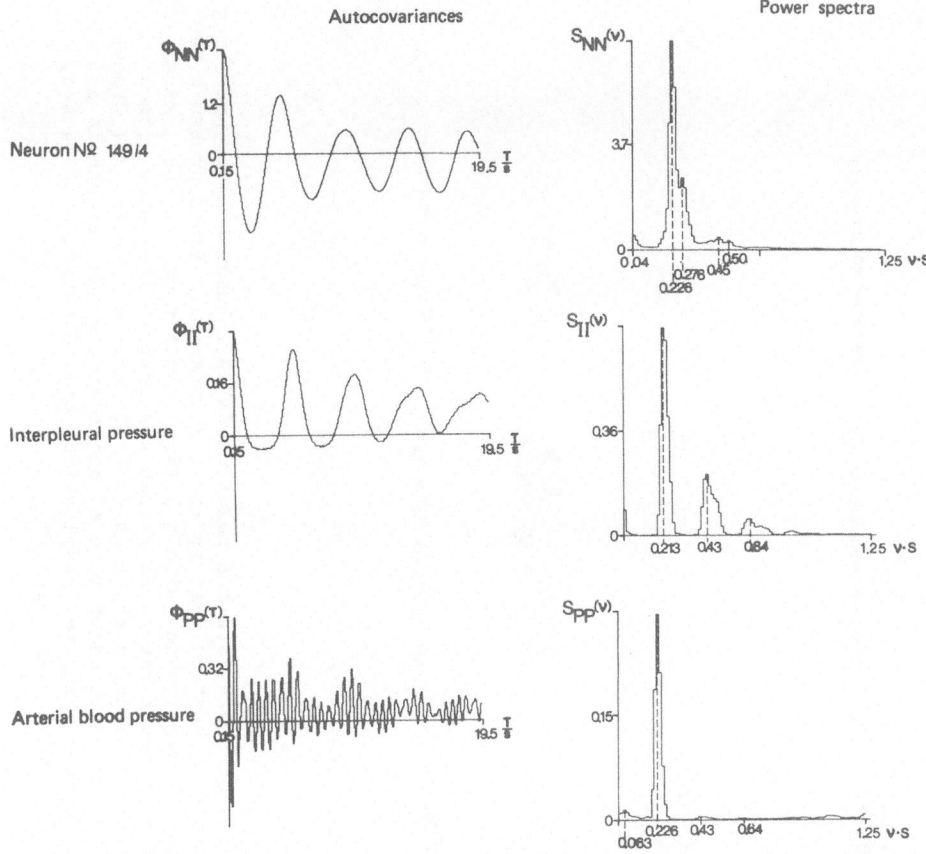

Fig. 20. ACH and PS of another part of the registration of neuron 149.
The ACH of the neuronal activity shows oscillations of the discharge frequency with a period duration of 4.7 sec. This is
equivalent to the peak at 0.226 Hz in the PS. The ACH of interpleural pressure shows oscillations with a period duration of
about 4.7 sec, equivalent to the peak at 0.213 Hz in its PS. The
ACH of blood pressure shows pulse waves with a frequency of 1.7
Hz. The PS is cut off at 1.25 Hz, therefore the frequency of
pulse waves is not visible.

vessels are highly reduced. The peak of the power spectrum of arterial
blood pressure at 0.088 Hz in Figure 19 has become very small and shifted
to 0.063 Hz.

   Similar results as obtained by experiments in anesthetized dogs can be
raised by investigations of alert humans. In man, these properties of the
oscillators have been investigated indirectly by measuring arterial blood
pressure, resiration and heart frequency. The frequency ranges of optimal
overlapping of the respiratory and reticular oscillator can be determined
by voluntary variations of respiratory frequency. Sinus arrhythmia and
blood pressure waves show their largest fluctuation when the voluntary
breathing is in a state of resonance with the reticular oscillator.

   An example is given in Figure 21. The preset period durations of
respiration were 3, 10, and 15 sec. The resonance frequency of the
reticular oscillator determined by this approach is at 0.1 Hz. At this
frequency, blood pressure waves and sinus arrhythmia have the largest

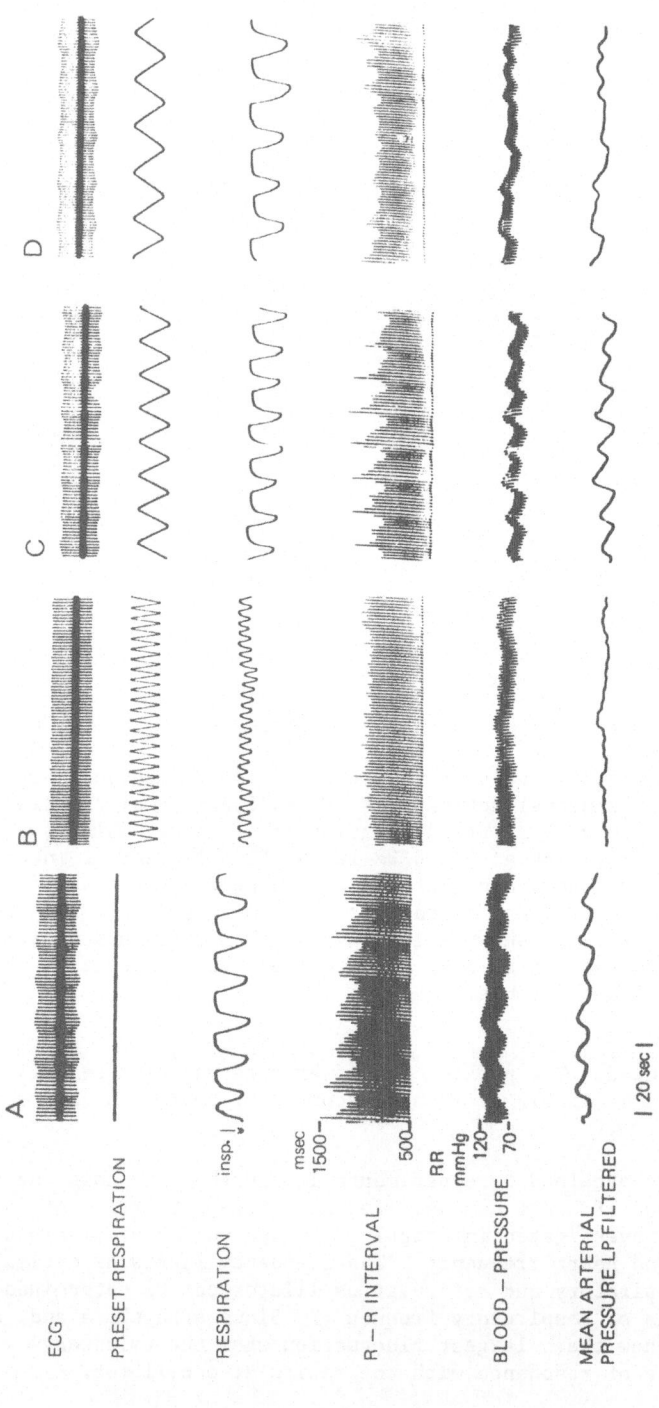

| 20 sec |

Fig. 21. Recording of ECG, ventilatory movements, variations of heart rate and pulse waves in a human subject breathing at different frequencies. Heart rate was measured from beat to beat by the R-R interval. Blood pressure was low-pass-filtered to show slow waves. A: Spontaneous respiration with a period duration of 11.4 sec, mean heart rate 63 beats/min, sinus arrhythmia 30% of mean heart rate. B: Preset respiratory frequency with a period duration of 3 sec, mean heart rate 66 beats/min, sinus arrhythmia 7.6% of mean heart rate. C: Preset respiratory frequency with a period duration of 10 sec, mean heart rate 66 beats/min, sinus arrhythmia 33% of mean heart rate. D: Preset respiratory frequency with a triggered respiration, period duration of 14 sec, mean heart rate 72 beats/min, sinus arrhythmia 15% of mean heart rate.

amplitudes (part C of Figure 21). In part A of Figure 21, the relations between blood pressure waves and sinus arrhythmia during spontaneous breathing are shown. The results are similar to that shown in C. This shows that in quiet relaxation, the subject breathes involuntarily with a frequency of 0.1 Hz, which is close to the optimal frequency range of the overlapping oscillators.

It is widely accepted that the respiratory sinus arrhythmia is mainly determined by parasympathetic nervous activity [47,71]. The arterial blood pressure waves depend, among other factors, on rhythmic patterns of efferent sympathetic activity [45,85]. Therefore one has to assume that both nervous activities depend on the oscillator of the common brainstem system.

REFERENCES

1. E. B. Adrian, D. W. Bronk, and G. Phillips, Discharges in mammalian sympathetic nerves, J. Physiol. (London), 74:115-133 (1932).
2. R. S. Alexander, Tonic and reflex functions of medullary sympathetic cardiovascular centers, J. Neurophysiol., 9:205-217 (1946).
3. V. E. Amassian, and R. V. De Vito, Unit activity in reticular formation and nearby structures, J. Neurophysiol., 17:575-603 (1954).
4. L. M. N. Bach, Relationship between bulbar respiratory, vasomotor and somatic facilitatory and inhibitory areas, Am. J. Physiol., 171:417-435 (1952).
5. H. L. Batsel, Localization of bulbar-respiratory center by micro-electrode sounding, Exp. Neurol., 9:410 (1964).
6. R. v. Baumgarten, A. Mollica and G. Moruzzi, Modulierung der Entladungs-frequenz einzelner Zellen der Substantia reticularis durch corticofugale und cerebelläre Impulse, Pflügers Arch. ges. Physiol., 259:56-78 (1954).
7. R. v. Baumgarten, A. v. Baumgarten and K. P. Schaefer, Beitrag zur Lokalisationsfrage bulboreticulärer respiratorischer Neurone der Katze, Pflügers Arch. ges. Physiol., 264:217 (1957).
8. M. Bonvallet, P. Dell and D. Hiebel, Tonus sympathique et activité électrique corticale, EEG clin. Neurophysiol., 6:119-144 (1954).
9. W. M. M. Boothby, The determination of the circulation rate in men at rest and work, Am. J. Physiol., 37:383-415 (1915).
10. M. A. Brazier, The historical development of neurophysiology, in: "Handbook of Physiology, Section I, Neurophysiology, vol. 1", J. Field, H. W. Magoun and V. E. Hall, eds., American Physiological Society, Washington (1959).
11. P. Broca, Remarques sur le siège de la faculté du langage articulé, Bull. Soc. Anthrop., 6 (1861).
12. A. Brodal, The reticular formation of the brain stem. Anatomical aspects and functional correlations, in: "The Henderson Trust Lecture", Oliver & Boyd, Edinburgh (1957).
13. S. Ramón y Cajal, Contribución al estudio de los ganglios de la substancia reticular del bulbo, citation in: Trab. Laborat. Invest. Biol. Univ., 7 (1909).
14. H. Camerer, M. Stroh-Werz, B. Krienke and P. Langhorst, Post-ganglionic sympathetic activity with correlation to heart rhythm and central cortical rhythms, Pflügers Arch. ges. Physiol., 370:221-225 (1977).
15. W. B. Cannon, Bodily changes in pain, hunger, fear and rage. An account of recent researches into the function of emotional excitement, Appleton, New York, London (1929).
16. M. I. Cohen, Neurogenesis of respiratory rhythm in the mammal, Physiol. Rev., 59:1105-1173 (1979).

17. W. Delius, K. E. Hagbarth, A. Hongell and B. G. Wallin, General characteristics of sympathetic activity in human muscle nerves, Acta Physiol. Scand., 84:65–81 (1972).

18. P. Dell, M. Bonvallet and A. Hugelin, Tonus sympathique, adrénaline et contrôle de la motricité spinale, EEG clin. Neurophysiol., 6:599–618 (1954).

19. C. Dittmar, Über die Lage des sogenannten Gefäßzentrums in der Medulla oblongata, Ber. Verh. sächs. Ges. Wiss. Leipzig, Math. Phys Cl., 25:449–469 (1873).

20. K. Dittmar, Aktivitätsmuster reticulärer Hirnstammneurone mit Beziehungen zu Änderungen des arteriellen Blutdrucks, des Interpleuraldrucks und des Synchronisationsgrades des EEGs, Thesis, Berlin (1977).

21. K. Dittmar, M. Werz, H. Camerer, and P. Langhorst, Relations between discharge patterns of rhythmically active neurons in the reticular formation and simultaneously occurring rhythmic events in EEG, blood pressure and respiration, Pflügers Arch. ges. Physiol., 339:R78 (1973).

22. K. Dittmar, P. Langhorst, and M. Werz, Relations between the degree of rhythmicity of single reticular brain stem neurons and arterial blood pressure, respiration and EEG, Pflügers Arch. ges. Physiol., 347:R19 (1974).

23. M. J. P. Flourens, Recherches expérimentales sur les propriétés et les fonctions du système nerveux dans les animaux vertébrés, Crebot, Paris (1824).

24. F. M. Fouad, R. C. Tarazi, C. M. Ferrario, S. Fighaly, and C. Alicandri, Assessment of parasympathetic control of heart rate by a noninvasive method, Am. J. Physiol., 246:H838–H842 (1984).

25. F. J. Gall, Sur les fonctions du cerveau et sur celles de chacune de ses parties, 6 vols., Baillière, Paris (1825).

26. R. Gesell, J. Bricker, and C. Magee, Structural and functional organization of the central mechanism controlling breathing, Am. J. Physiol., 117:423–452 (1936).

27. G. L. Gebber, and S. M. Barman, Brainstem vasomotor circuits involved in the genesis and entrainment of sympathetic nervous rhythms, Prog. Brain Res., 47:61–75 (1977).

28. A. Haller, Elementa physiologiae corporis humani, Lausanne (1769).

29. E. Hering, Über Atembewegungen des Gefäßsystems, S. Ber. Akad. Wiss. Wien, Math.–Naturwiss. Cl., 2, Abt. 60:829–836 (1869).

30. W. R. Hess, Über die Wechselbeziehungen zwischen psychischen und vegetativen Funktionen, Schweiz. Arch. Neurol. Neurochir. Psychiatr., 15:260–277 (1924).

31. W. R. Hess, Über die Wechselbeziehungen zwischen psychischen und vegetativen Funktionen, Arch. Neurol., 16:36–55 (1925).

32. W. R. Hess, Das physiologische Zusammenspiel von Kreislauf und Atmung, Verh. Dt. Ges. Kreislaufforsch., 8, Tagung (1935).

33. C. Heymans, and J. J. Bouckaert, Sinus caroticus and respiratory reflexes, J. Physiol. (London), 69:254–266 (1930).

34. S. M. Hilton, and K. M. Spyer, Participation of the anterior hypothalmus in the baroreceptor reflex, J. Physiol. (London)., 218:271 (1971).

35. G. Holstege, H. G. J. M. Kuypers, and R. C. de Boer, Anatomical evidence for direct brainstem projections to the somatic moto-neuronal cell groups and autonomic pre-ganglionic cell groups in cat spinal cord, Brain Res., 171:329–333 (1969).

36. E. v. Holst, Über olen Prozeß der zentralnervösen Koordination, Pflügers Arch. ges. Physiol., 236:149–158 (1935).

37. E. v. Holst, Die relative Koordination als Phänomen und als Methode zentralnervöser Funktionsanalysen, Erg. Physiol., 42:228–306 (1939).

38. J. H. Jackson, Evolution and dissolution of the nervous system, in: "Selected Writings of John Hughlings Jackson", (Croonian Lectures, 1884), J. Taylor, ed., Basic Books, New York (1958).

39. L. E. King, E. M. Blair, and W. E. Garrey, The inspiratory augmentation of proprioceptive reflexes. A study of the knee jerk and the Achilles reflex, Am. J. Physiol., 97:329-342 (1931).

40. E. Koch, Die Irradiation der pressoreceptorischen Kreislaufreflexe, Klin. Wschr., 2:225-227 (1932).

41. A. Koelliker, "Handbuch der Gewebelehre des Menschen, Bd. 2: Nervensystem des Menschen und der Tiere", Engelmann, Leipzig (1896).

42. H. P. Koepchen, P. Langhorst, and P. H. Wagner, Methodik und erste Ergebnisse extracellulärer Mikroableitungen aus dem Rhombencephalon des Hundes, Pflügers Arch. ges. Physiol., 272:76 (1960).

43. H. P. Koepchen, "Die Blutdruckrhythmik", Steinkopff-Verlag, Darmstadt (1962).

44. H. P. Koepchen, P. Langhorst, H. Seller, J. Polster, and P. H. Wagner, Neuronale Aktivität im unteren Hirnstamm mit Beziehungen zum Kreislauf, Pflügers Arch. ges. Physiol., 294:40-64 (1967).

45. H. P. Koepchen, H. Seller, J. Polster, and P. Langhorst, Uber die Fein-Vasomotorik der Muskelstrombahn und ihre Beziehung zur Ateminnervation, Pflügers Arch. ges. Physiol., 264:285 (1968).

46. H. P. Koepchen, P. Langhorst, and H. Seller, The problem of identification of autonomic neurones in the lower brain stem, Brain Res., 87:375-393 (1975).

47. H. P. Koepchen, Zentralnervöse und reflektorische Steuerung der Herzfrequenz, in: "Autonome Innervation des Herzens", B. Brisse, and F. Bender, eds., Steinkopff-Verlag, Darmstadt (1982).

48. P. I. Korner, Integrative neural cardiovascular control, Physiol. Rev., 51:311-367 (1971).

49. P. Langhorst, and M. Werz, Concept of functional organization of the brainstem "cardiovascular center", in: "Central Rhythmic and Regulation", W. Umbach, and H. P. Koepchen, eds., Hippokrates-Verlag, Stuttgart (1974).

50. P. Langhorst, M. Stroh-Werz, K. Dittmar, and H. Camerer, Facultative coupling of reticular neuronal activity with peripheral cardiovascular and central cortical rhythms, Brain Res., 87:407-418 (1975).

51. P. Langhorst, M. Lambertz, K. Dittmar, G. Schulz, and B. Schulz, Oscillations of discharge frequency of blood pressure dependent neurones in the lower brainstem of the dog similar to respiratory rhythm, Proc. Int. Union Physiol. Sci., vol. XIII:1263 (1977).

52. P. Langhorst, B. Schulz, M. Lambertz, G. Schulz, H. Camerer, and M. Stroh-Werz, Dynamic characteristics of the "unspecific brainstem system", in: "Central Interactions between Respiratory and Cardiovascular Control Systems", H. P. Koepchen, S. M. Hilton, and A. Trzebski, eds., Springer-Verlag, Berlin, Heidelberg, New York (1980).

53. P. Langhorst, G. Schulz, M. Lambertz, and B. Krienke, Funktionelle Organisation eines gemeinsamen Hirnstammsystems für Kreislauf-, Atmungs- und allgemeine Aktivitätssteuerung, in: "Zentralvegetative Regulationen und Syndrome", R. Schiffter, ed., Springer-Verlag, Berlin, Heidelberg, New York (1980).

54. P. Langhorst, M. Lambertz, and G. Schulz, Central control and interactions affecting sympathetic and parasympathetic activity, J. Auton. Nerv. Syst,. 4:149-163 (1981).

55. P. Langhorst, B. Schulz, G. Schulz, and M. Lambertz, Reticular formation of the lower brainstem. A common system for cardiorespiratory and somatomotor functions: discharge patterns of neighboring neurons influenced by cardiovascular and respiratory afferents, J. Auton. Nerv. Syst., 9:411-432 (1983).

56. P. Langhorst, G. Schulz, and M. Lambertz, Oscillating neuronal network of the "common brainstem system", in: "Mechanisms of Blood Pressure Waves", K. Miyakawa, H. P. Koepchen, and C. Polosa, eds., Springer-Verlag, Berlin, Heidelberg, New York, pp. 257-275 (1984).

57. P. Lindgren, Localization and function of the medullary vasomotor center in infracollicularly decerebrated cats, Circulat. Res., 9:250 (1961).

58. T. Lumsden, Observations on the respiratory centers in the cat, J. Physiol. (London), 57:153-160 (1922/23).

59. A. R. Luria, "Higher cortical functions in man", Basic Books Inc. Publishers, New York (1980).

60. X. Machne, I. Calma, and H. W. Magoun, Unit activity of central cephalic brainstem in EEG arousal, J. Neurophysiol., 18:547-558 (1953).

61. F. Magni, and W. B. Willis, Identification of reticular formation neurons by intracellular recording, Arch. ital. Biol., 101:681-702 (1963).

62. H. W. Magoun, Caudal and cephalic influences of the brainstem reticular formation, Physiol. Rev., 30:459-474 (1950).

63. L. C. A. Meyer, "Anatomisch-physiologische Abhandlungen vom Gehirn", Berlin, Leipzig (1779), citation in: A. R. Luria, "Higher cortical functions in man", Basic Books Inc., New York (1980).

64. J. Meyer-Lohmann, Respiratory influence upon the lumbar extensor motor system of decerebrated cats, in: "Central Rhythmic and Regulation", W. Umbach, and H. P. Koepchen, eds., Hippokrates-Verlag, Stuttgart (1974).

65. A. Mollica, G. Moruzzi, and R. Naquet, Décharges réticulaires induites par la polarisation du cervelet. Leur rapports avec le tonus postural et la réaction d'eveil, Erg. clin. Neurophysiol., 5:571-584 (1953).

66. M. Monnier, Les centres végétatives bulbaires, Arch. int. Physiol., 49:455-463 (1939).

67. G. Moruzzi, and H. W. Magoun, Brainstem reticular formation and activation of the EEG, EEG clin. Neurophysiol., 1:455-474 (1949).

68. G. Moruzzi, The functional significance of the ascending reticular system, Arch. ital. Biol., 96:17-28 (1958).

69. P. H. Owsjannikow, Die tonischen und reflektorischen Zentren der Gefäßnerven, Ber. Verh. Sächs. Ges. Wiss. Leipzig, Math. Phys. Cl., 23:135-148 (1871).

70. O. Pompeiano, Reticular formation, in: "Handbook of Sensory Physiology, vol. 2: Somato-Sensory System", A. Iggo, ed., Springer-Verlag, Berlin, Heidelberg, New York (1973).

71. S. W. Porges, P. M. McCabe, and B. G. Yongue, Respiratory heart rate interactions: psychophysiological implications for pathophysiology and behavior, in: "Perspectives in Cardiovascular Psycho-physiology", J. T. Cacioppo, and R. E. Petty, eds., Guilford Press, New York (1982).

72. N. N. Preobrazhenskii, Microelectrode recording of activity from neurones in vasomotor centre, Fed. Proc., 25:T18-22 (1966).

73. A. C. Przybyla, and S. C. Wang, Neurophysiological characteristics of cardiovascular neurones in the medulla oblongata of the cat, J. Neurophysiol., 30:645-660 (1967).

74. P. Rhines, and H. W. Magoun, Brainstem facilitation of cortical motor response, J. Neurophysiol., 9:219-229 (1946).

75. G. F. Rossi, and A. Zanchetti, The brainstem reticular formation. Anatomy and physiology, Arch. ital. Biol., 95:203-435 (1957).

76. G. C. Salmoiraghi, and B. D. Burns, Notes on mechanism of rhythmic respiration, J. Neurophysiol., 23:14-26 (1960).

77. G. C. Salmoiraghi, "Cardiovascular" neurons in the brainstem of the cat, J. Neurophysiol., 25:182-197 (1962).

78. M. E. Scheibel, A. B. Scheibel, K. Mollica, and G. Moruzzi, Convergence and interaction of afferent impulses on single units of reticular formation, J. Neurophysiol., 18:309-331 (1955).

79. M. E. Scheibel, and A. B. Scheibel, Structural substrates for integrative patterns in the brainstem core, in: "Reticular Formation of the Brain", Henry Ford Hospital Symposium, H. H. Jasper, and L. D. Proctor, eds., Little, Brown & Co., Boston (1958).

80. W. Schmidt-Vanderheyden, L. Heinich, and H. P. Koepchen, Investigations into the fluctuations of proprioceptive reflexes in man, I: Fluctuations of the patellar tendon reflex and their relation to the vegetative rhythms during spontaneous respiration, Pflügers Arch. ges. Physiol., 317:72-83 (1970).

81. F. J. Schulte, H.-D. Henatsch, and W. Busch, Uber den Einfluß der Carotis-sinus-Sensibilität auf die spinalmotorischen Systeme, Pflügers Arch. ges. Physiol., 259:248-263 (1959).

82. B. Schulz, M. Lambertz, G. Schulz, and P. Langhorst, Reticular formation of the lower brainstem. A common system for cardio-respiratory and somatomotor functions: discharge patterns of neighboring neurons influenced by somatosensory afferents, J. Auton. Nerv. Syst., 9:433-449 (1983).

82a. G. Schulz, M. Lambertz, B. Schulz, and P. Langhorst, Reticular formation of the lower brainstem. A common system for cardio-respiratory and somatomotor functions: cross-correlation analysis of discharge patterns of neighboring neurons, J. Auton. Nerv. Syst., 12:35-62 (1985).

83. S. Schweitzer, "Die Irradiation autonomer Reflexe", Verlag von S. Karger, Basel (1937).

84. J. P. Segundo, T. Takenaka, and H. Encabo, Somatic sensory properties of bulbar reticular neurons, J. Neurophysiol., 30:1221-1238 (1967).

85. H. Seller, P. Langhorst, D. Richter, and H. P. Koepchen, Uber die Abhängigkeit der pressoreceptorischen Hemmung des Sympathicus von der Atemphase und ihre Auswirkung in der Vasomotorik, Pflügers Arch. ges. Physiol., 302:300 (1968).

86. C. S. Sherrington, Decerebrate rigidity and reflex coordination of movement, J. Physiol. (London), 22:319 (1898).

87. J. M. Siegel, Behavioral functions of the reticular formation, Brain Res. Rev., 1:69-105 (1979).

88. O. A. Smith, Reflex and central mechanisms involved in the control of the heart and circulation, Ann. Rev. Physiol., 36:93 (1974).

89. J. M. Sprague, and W. W. Chambers, Control of posture by reticular formation and cerebellum in the intact anesthetized and unanesthetized decerebrated cat, Am. J. Physiol., 176:52-64 (1954).

90. E. Taber, The cytoarchitecture of the brainstem of the cat, I: brainstem nuclei of cat, J. comp. Neurol., 116:27-70 (1961).

91. F. Valverde, Reticular formation of the pons and medulla oblongata. A Golgi study, J. comp. Neurol., 116:71-99 (1961).

92. H. Weidinger, L. Fedina, H. Kehrel, and H. Schaefer, Uber die Lokalisation des "bulbären sympathischen Zentrums" und seine Beeinflussung durch Atmung und Blutdruck, Z. Kreisl.-Forsch.., 50:229 (1961).

A PHYSIOLOGICAL REVIEW OF MECHANISMS INVOLVED IN THE

CARDIOVASCULAR CORRELATES OF MUSCULAR ACTIVITY

A. J. Gelsema*

Interfaculty of Physical Education, Free University
and Department of Physiology, University of Amsterdam
Amsterdam, The Netherlands

INTRODUCTION

In psychophysiological research concerning the mechanisms underlying
behavioral reactions to stimuli of widely different origins, it is not
uncommon to use heart rate (HR) or its inverse, cardiac cycle length, as a
measure of the mental events involved in the processing of those stimuli.
On the other hand, it has been recognized that the rhythm of our heart beat
is continuously controlled by neural, humoral and mechanical factors in
order to adjust its function to the variable needs of the organism's
tissues. Among these, one of the most variable types of demand arises from
skeletal muscles. It is our daily experience that our heart beats the more
frequently, the more intense the physical exertion. This phenomenon is
only the most conspicious of a series of events that occur in order to
adapt the circulation to the muscles' need of blood. The physiology of the
control mechanism underlying this adaptation will be the subject of the
present paper.

Traditionally, muscular exercise is classified in two categories:
dynamic, also called rhythmic or isotonic, exercise, when the muscular
force is used to cause a considerable shortening of muscle length
accompanied by movements of joints, such as in bicycling, rowing and running; and static, or isometric, exercise, when the muscular force is not
used for the movements of joints or limbs, but merely as force or tension
without overt muscle shortening, hence isometric. Activities that require
this latter kind of force development occur in lifting, pushing, and grasp-
ing, for example. The cardiovascular adjustment to these two kinds of use
of our striate musculature is different, especially when the changes of
blood pressure during lasting exercise is concerned. However, if we
restrict ourselves to the description of the phasic changes in HR at the
onset of either form of exercise, the subdivision into dynamic and static
contractions is redundant, as quantitatively similar reactions of the HR
occur in both instances.

A major part of the physiological literature concerning the phasic
reaction of heart rate describes results from experiments where static

---

*Present address: Dept. of Physiology, Health Science Center, University of
Western Ontario, London (Ont), Canada N6A 5C1.

contractions were performed. The present paper reviews the published results of such human and animal experimentation. Both types of investigation have their drawbacks: Experiments using human volunteers cannot be as incisive as the experimenter would like to have it, while experiments on animals frequently need the use of anesthetics that may suppress central nervous activity, especially in the brainstem, and thus the cardiovascular responses to neural inputs may be distorted. Nonetheless we will deal with the available literature and, where necessary, clarify results that seem contradictory.

In the course of history, the phenomenon of the increased heart rate during exercise was initially described merely; at the turn of the century, investigations were begun to elucidate the underlying mechanism. We shall follow this course in the next pages, starting with a description of the cardiovascular response to exercise and subsequently dealing with the proposed mechanisms that seem fundamental to it. For a more comprehensive treatise of the subject the reader is referred to the proceedings of a recent symposium (Mitchell et al., 1981) and to the Handbook of Physiology (Mitchell and Schmidt, 1983; Lind, 1983).

CIRCULATORY CHANGES TO ISOMETRIC CONTRACTIONS

At the onset of isometric exercise, heart rate (HR) and arterial blood pressure (BP) both increase immediately. The rise in HR in humans has frequently been reported to occur within a cardiac cycle (Freyschuss, 1970; Petro et al., 1970; Hollander and Bouman, 1975). In our laboratory, human volunteers were connected by their wrist to a dynamometer and had their lower arm flexed 90° with respect to the horizontally fixed upper half. When they were invited to contract their upper arm flexors maximally for less than 1 sec in response to an acoustic signal, the cardiac cycle following the one in which the contraction started was shortened in 95% of all cases. Moreover, the very cycle during which the contraction started was shortened in those cases when the onset of the contraction occurred during the first half of that cycle. Further investigation showed that, in man, a latency of about 550 msec exists between the onset of the contraction and the first detectable significant shortening in cardiac cycle length (Hollander and Bouman, 1975). During these experiments, visual or acoustic signals were used as a command to the volunteers to perform a contraction. It was excluded in subsequent experiments that anticipation or perception of the signal per se might be responsible for the instantaneous rise in HR (Borst et al., 1972). Also the influence on HR of a sudden change in respiration preceding or during the contraction was excluded.

Following short-lasting (<1 sec) maximal isometric contractions, a peak cycle length shortening was found at approximately 2 sec after the onset of contraction (Figure 1). The amount of cycle length shortening varied between individuals from 5 to 20% (Petro et al., 1970; Borst et al., 1972; Hollander and Bouman, 1975). With longer lasting isometric contractions, the increase in HR and BP depends on the intensity and duration of the effort. There is as yet no unanimity regarding the relation between the magnitude of the circulatory responses and the force of muscular contraction. Some authors believe that a relation exists between the HR and BP responses and the relative force of contraction, expressed as a percentage of the maximal voluntary contraction (MVC) of a particular muscle or muscle group. Lind and McNicol (1967) showed for example that handgrip contractions, thigh muscle contractions or adduction of a single finger, all performed at 20% of their maximal effort, resulted in identical increases in BP, although the absolute tension that developed differed obviously widely. This finding also shows the independency of the responses to the amount of muscle mass involved. Another rather surprising

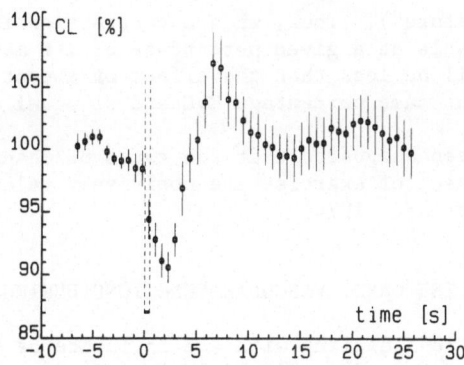

Fig. 1. Proportional cardiac cycle length (CL) response in a standing
         human volunteer to a maximal handgrip contraction of 0.5 sec
         duration. The contraction was performed 25 times. The duration
         of 10 cardiac cycles preceding and 37 cycles following the <u>onset</u>
         of each contraction (occurring at t=0) was measured. The duration
         of all cycles preceding the contraction (25 x 10) was averaged,
         yielding a basic cycle length (BCL) of 703 msec. This value was
         used as a reference level (100%). Subsequently the mean duration
         (± SE) of each consecutive cycle was plotted proportionally.
         Note that the cycle in which the contraction started is already
         shortened; at 2.5 sec after the onset of contraction, a maximum
         shortening of 10% is reached, after which the CL returns to the
         resting level.

result of their investigations was that the effects of simultaneously
contracting muscle groups were not additive. When for example persisting
bilateral handgrip contractions were performed, the cardiovascular effect
was identical to that observed with a contraction of a single hand. Similar results were obtained from experiments with short-lasting (i.e. <1 sec)
unilateral and bilateral ankle flexions of maximal force (Borst et al.,
1972).

     As contrasted with the preceding opinion, recent reports claim that
the increases in HR and BP depend on the absolute force developed (Mitchell
et al., 1980; Schibye et al., 1981). Isometric finger movements, handgrip
contractions, knee extensions, and combined handgrip plus knee extensions,
all performed at 40% MVC, resulted in increasing hemodynamic changes. A
clear linear relation between the responses and the force developed, however, could not be shown. Moreover, the authors did not take into account
the different endurances among the muscles used in their investigation (see
below). Clearly, more work in this field is necessary before unanimity
will be reached.

     Although the main subject of this review is the HR response to short-
lasting isometric contractions, it is important to note that also the
<u>duration</u> of the effort determines the extent of the circulatory changes.
With non-fatiguing contractions (i.e. less than 10-15% MVC) the HR will
climb rapidly, reach a plateau within the first minute and remain on this
level throughout the duration of the contraction. With stronger contractions of long duration, however, HR (and BP) will continue to rise during
the contraction, reaching their peak values at the moment that fatigue
occurs or, when the contraction ends earlier, at the moment of release.
This implies that the sizes of the cardiovascular responses also depend on
the type of muscles used, i.e. fatiguable ("white musculature") or fatigue-

resistant ("red musculature"). Thus, when a contraction is performed using a fatigue-resistant muscle at a given percentage of its maximal effort, the effect on HR and BP will be less than the effect of a contraction using a fatiguable muscle at the same percentage MVC and of equal duration.

Finally, it has been suggested that the rates of change of the circulatory events at the onset of exercise are positively related to the force developed (Funderbirk et al., 1974).

MECHANISMS CONTROLLING THE CARDIOVASCULAR FUNCTIONS DURING STATIC EXERCISE

In his article of 1895 dealing with the influence of induced muscular activity on the respiratory and cardiac functions in dogs and rabbits, Johansson listed the mechanisms that were possibly involved. In summary, HR could be influenced by exercise through the following mechanisms:

1. Co-activation of the "cardiac centers" in the brainstem by impulses radiating from "higher motor centers" when activating the required musculature. Later this mechanism was called central (or cortical) irradiation, or plainly, central command.

2. Activation of those "cardiac centers" by neural impulses arising in the joints, tendons, skin or in the activated muscles themselves due to the contraction. At present this mechanism is known as somatomotor feedback (Obrist, 1981), reflex activation, or, as far as the cardiac acceleration to muscle afference is concerned, the muscle-heart reflex.

3. Activation of those "cardiac centers" or of the heart itself by metabolic products released by the contracting musculature and transported via the circulation.

4. Mechanical influences of the muscle contractions via the bloodstream (such as by a sudden increase in venous return) or the influence of increased respiratory activity on the heart.

On the strength of his results, Johansson excluded the latter 3 mechanisms from an involvement during induced muscular exercise. This view was confused by a report of Athanasiu and Carvallo (1898) who observed the absence of HR acceleration in human paraplegic subjects that were instructed to perform contractions with the disabled limbs. In the same paper, the authors described consistent HR accelerations in anesthetized animals upon electrically induced muscle contractions. Although the use of data resulting from experimentation on unhealthy human subjects is dangerous (did the patients really cooperate, being aware of the infeasibility of the instruction? What was the extent of the lesions?), the results from their experimentations on anesthetized animals seemed to exclude the participation of central command.

In 1917, Krogh and Lindhard tried to decide between the theories of central command and the reflex mechanism. Voluntary and electrically induced muscular contractions in human volunteers were followed by identical responses in HR. The onset of cardiac acceleration was faster during voluntary than during electrically induced contractions. This led the authors to the ambivalent conclusion that the response is normally of central origin, but is reflexive with induced muscular work.

The first clear evidence for the existence of a reflex from the active muscles was provided by Alam and Smirk (1937 and 1938). In their studies human volunteers performed rhythmic exercise during circulatory occlusion of the exercising limb by inflation of a sphygmomanometer cuff. Blood pressure and heart rate rose during exercise and remained elevated upon cessation until the cuff was deflated. In preliminary observations it was shown that the circulatory occlusion per se had no influence on blood pressure or heart rate. It is now generally believed that the authors concluded correctly that some metabolites emanating from the contracting muscles elicited the cardiovascular changes reflexively by activation of receptors located in the muscle. Since then, the technique of vascular occlusion during exercise has been adopted by many investigators. Similar results have been obtained with respect to the behavior of BP; however, HR is most frequently reported to return to resting values after exercise, with the circulation still occluded through the exercising muscles (McCloskey and Streatfield, 1975; Mitchell et al., 1980; Lind, 1983).

Asmussen et al. (1943) showed increases in BP, HR, and cardiac output in humans irrespective as to whether the exercise was produced voluntarily or by electrical stimulation. They concluded that central command played no role in the control of the circulation during steady state exercise. Concerning the time course of the hemodynamic responses, Humphreys and Lind (1963) and later Lind et al. (1964) showed abrupt and marked increases in BP and HR at the start of contractions and their rapid return to resting levels upon release. Even small muscle groups were able to produce such changes. Similar results were obtained in our laboratory by Borst et al. (1972) and Hollander and Bouman (1975).

The appearance within a cardiac cycle of circulatory changes to contractions of small muscles make it highly unlikely that metabolic products discharged by the contracting muscles into the circulation would influence the cardiovascular centers in the brainstem (or, alternatively, the heart directly), as the time taken by humoral transport would be too long. This, and a mechanical influence of the contraction merely on the circulation, can also be excluded in view of the observed hemodynamic changes to exercise during circulatory arrest (Alam and Smirk, 1938; McCloskey and Streatfield, 1975; Mitchell et al., 1980).

In several studies in man, the possible influence on HR of a sudden inspiration at the onset of exercise has been recognized. Freyschuss (1970) instructed her subjects to count aloud during the contractions they performed, thus eliminating the possibility that the increase in HR found in her experiments was secondary to inspiratory activity. Borst et al. (1972) could also exclude respiratory influences by a re-examination of their experimental results that showed that the cardiac responses to short-lasting isometric contractions fell randomly throughout the respiratory cycle. These results show that the rise in HR at the onset or during isometric contractions is not caused by respiratory events.

Thus only the two alternative neural mechanisms as proposed by Johansson (see above) remain: central command and reflex activation (Figure 2). We shall concentrate now on evidence in favor of one or both of these mechanisms.

A Reflex Mechanism Mediating Contraction-induced Cardiovascular Responses

Coote et al. (1971) provided unequivocal evidence for the existence of a reflex mechanism in anesthetized and decerebrate cats. Ventral root stimulation elicited tetanic contractions of hind-limb muscles, that were accompanied by increases in BP and HR. The amount of increase in BP depended on the force developed. Sectioning of all articular and cutaneous nerves in the region of the contracting muscles did not affect the response, showing its muscular origin. The responses were, however, abolished by the administration of a neuromuscular blocking agent or by sectioning the corresponding dorsal roots. This indicates that impulses

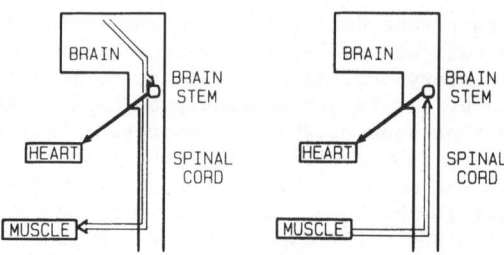

Fig. 2. Schematic drawing of 2 proposed neural mechanisms involved in the
         cardiac adaptation to exercise. Left: <u>Central command</u> (also
         central irradiation or cortical irradiation). Motor impulses
         (light open arrow), originating in higher brain centers on their
         way through the brainstem to their target, the muscle, give off
         collaterals to cardiovascular control centers. Here neural
         impulses (black arrow) arise that control the cardiac function.
         Right: <u>Reflex activation</u> (or somatomotor feedback). Afferent
         impulses, elicited by muscle contraction, ascend through the
         spinal cord (open arrow) and influence the cardiovascular brain-
         stem centers. From there, the same neural connection to the heart
         as in the left part of the figure is used.

arising in the contracting muscles and travelling via the dorsal roots to
the central nervous system mediate the circulatory responses reflexively.
McCloskey and Mitchell (1972) confirmed these results and extended them by
demonstrating that blockade of large myelinated fibers in the dorsal roots
did not affect the responses, in contrast to blockade of the small
myelinated and unmyelinated afferents, which abolished the responses completely. In another paper, it was also shown by the same group that stimulation of primary afferents of muscle spindles in the triceps surae muscle
of anesthetized or decerebrate cats had no influence on BP, HR or respiration (McCloskey et al., 1972). This is in accordance with experiments in
humans, using the same vibration technique for the specific stimulation of
Ia afferents (Gelsema and Karemaker, unpublished observations).

    The existence of a reflex mechanism in animals has been reported
consistently since the initial papers (McCloskey and Streatfeild, 1975;
Tibes, 1977; Mitchell et al., 1977; Diepstra et al., 1980; Tallarida et
al., 1981). Those reports pertain to the responses to contractions sustained for several tens of seconds. In our laboratory the initial, phasic
change in HR at the onset of brief isometric contractions was investigated.
The cardiac effect of voluntary and electrically induced, 0.5 sec lasting
handgrip contractions at 70% MVC were compared. The contractions were
accompanied by HR accelerating responses that were in both circumstances
strikingly similar in time course and magnitude (Hollander and Bouman,
1975). Hultman and Sjoholm (1982) repeated these experiments but extended
the duration (of quadriceps contractions at 20% MVC) to 5 min. These
authors also found identical responses in HR and BP to electrically and
voluntarily induced muscle contractions. It was concluded from both
studies that central command was not necessary for the occurrence of these
circulatory changes; however, the participation of such a mechanism could
not be excluded. Thus the existence of a reflex mechanism for the cardiovascular control at the onset and during exercise seems firmly established.

    Considering the details of the mechanism, the next questions to answer
is, which impulse initiates the reflex and which nervous structures compose
the reflex arc?

Possible Stimuli Initiating the Reflex

The precise character of the stimulus for the reflex mechanism is still open to debate. The experiments of Alam and Smirk, described above, suggested that the accumulation of some metabolite emanating from the contracting muscle might be involved. Lind et al. (1964) measured the changes in O_2, pH and lactate in the venous blood from contracting muscles. During the contraction there were only small changes, but larger changes were found 1 min after release, when the reflexively induced rise in BP had already subsided. The efflux of potassium ions, however, increased during the contraction and returned promptly to its resting level upon cessation of the contraction, paralleling the changes in BP.

Wildenthal et al. (1969) and McCloskey and Mitchell (1972) found that the cardiovascular responses in their experiments could be mimicked by the infusion of small amounts of K^+ in the muscle circulation. It was demonstrated that close intra-arterial injections of isotonic potassium solutions stimulate activity in small myelinated (group III) and unmyelinated (group IV) muscle afferents, which is accompanied by an increase in HR, BP and in the contractility of the left ventricle (Wildenthal et al., 1969; Hnik et al., 1969). This result was confirmed by Saltin et al. (1981) who deduced from their data that the concentration of potassium ions in the interstitial space of a contracting muscle may be responsible for the observed cardiovascular changes.

Although potassium seems to be a likely candidate for the mediation of the reflex responses to exercise, this does not preclude the existence of other stimuli. Intramuscular pressure, for example, has been shown to vary linearly with the force developed (Hill, 1948; Saltin et al., 1981; Sejersted et al., 1984), while light innocuous pressure applied locally to the exposed belly of a muscle activated preferentially about 40% of all thinly myelinated muscle afferents (Kniffki et al., 1978; Kniffki et al., 1981; Kaufman et al., 1982; Mitchell and Schmidt, 1983). Also muscle stretch activated about half of all group III afferents (Kniffki et al., 1978; Mitchell and Schmidt, 1983) and only about 10% of group IV fibers. The latter afferents, however, showed irregularity in their response. Finally, about 40% of group III muscle afferents are activated in a graded fashion by tetanic muscle contractions in the range of 20-100% MVC, while about 30% of group IV fibers fired non-proportionally upon contraction.

Thus it seems very well possible that more than one of the stimuli mentioned here will be shown to be responsible for the reflex activation of the cardiovascular changes upon muscular exercise, the more so as the time course differs with respect to the changes in HR and BP following the release of a contraction during circulatory occlusion. The rapid return of HR to precontraction levels and the persistent elevated BP which subsides only after the termination of the occlusion make the existence of at least two different stimuli likely.

Muscle Afferents Involved in the Reflex Mechanism

Table 1 summarizes the nomenclature and some of the properties of muscle afferent fibers. The data are derived from measurements in the cat. It must be stressed that boundaries between fiber groups are, in fact, non-existent, and that variations in diameters and in proportion of the fibers exist among different muscle nerves and among different species. With some adaptations, however, the data may be applied to other mammals (such as man), despite these variations.

There is abundant evidence showing that large myelinated fibers from muscle (i.e. groups I and II) are not involved in the reflex cardiovascular

Table 1. Nomenclature and Some Properties of Afferent Fibers in an
Idealized Muscle Nerve.

Fiber type	My[2]	Diameter[3] (µm)	c.v.[4] (m/s)	%[5]	Receptor structure	Function
Ia	+	9-17 max 22	50-105 max 125	10	muscle spindle, primary afferent	signals changes in muscle length
Ib	+	9-17	50-100 max 130	5	tendon organ	signals muscle tension
II	+	4-12	20-70	10	muscle spindle secondary afferent	signals actual muscle length
II	+	4-8	20	0.7	lamellated pressure sensors	signals deformation of the sensor, i.e. pressure, tension in muscle
III	+	1-7 max 11	5-30 max 40	5	free nerve endings	signals pressure, pain
III	+	1-4.5	5-20	2.5	free nerve endings in blood vessel wall	signals ischemia
IV[1]	-	≤ 1.25	< 2.5	66.6	free nerve endings	chemical state of intercellular space (?)

1) also called C-fibers   2) Myelinated fiber: + ; unmyelinated: −   3) including myelin sheath, if present   4) Conduction velocity   5) Proportion of fibers present as a percentage of all afferents in a muscle nerve
Data from Boyd and Davey, 1968, and Barker, 1974.

changes. Already mentioned are the results of McCloskey and Mitchell (1972), who found that blockade of small afferent fibers, in contrast to blockade of large myelinated afferents, abolished the cardiovascular responses to isometric muscle contractions in cats. Similar results were obtained by Tibes in the dog (1977). Also Hollander and Bouman (1975) and Gelsema et al. (1983 and 1985) presented inferential evidence that in human volunteers and in cats, the fast, vagally mediated cardiac acceleration at the onset of short-lasting muscle contractions could only be mediated by group III muscle afferents. These results, combined with the evidence presented above in favor of the activation of small muscle afferents by chemical and mechanical stimuli, point unequivocally to the involvement of group III and possibly also of group IV afferents in the reflex mechanism.

Central Pathways and Connections

There are only a few publications dealing with the ascending pathways in the spinal cord that might mediate somato-cardiovascular reflexes. In a recent study Kozelka et al. (1982) showed that the increase in HR and BP following the stimulation of a mixed nerve (the sciatic) in the hindlimb of anesthetized dogs could be completely eliminated by bilateral sectioning of the dorsolateral sulcus area in the lumbar spinal cord. On the other hand, only a reduction of the cardiovascular changes to treadmill exercise in unanesthetized dogs could be obtained by ventrally directed extensions of these lesions. The authors emphasizes that their results were not due to some damage of descending tracts from the cardiovascular centers since normal cardiovascular responses to baroreceptor activation could be obtained in animals with extensive bilateral lesions.

In an elegant study, Kalia et al. (1981) reproduced earlier findings that groups III and IV muscle afferents were most prominently responsible for the cardiovascular effects in muscular exercise. The authors demon- strated, by using standard histological techniques, that some of those afferent fibers relayed directly to the nucleus tractus solitarius (NTS) in the brainstem. Fibers originating in this area are shown to have direct access to the nucleus ambiguus in the lower brainstem, where cardiac vagal inhibitory fibers take their origin (Thomas and Calaresu, 1974). Furthermore, other fibers in the muscle nerve activated by muscular contraction were shown to terminate on ascending spino-thalamic tract neurons. Collaterals of these neurons may terminate in cardiovascular control regions of the brainstem.

In view of the recent demonstration of identical fast cardiovascular responses to muscle nerve and cutaneous nerve stimulation (Gelsema et al., 1985a, b), it is interesting to mention here that also cutaneous afferents terminate on these spinothalamic tract neurons. This finding makes the specificity of the cardiovascular response to exercise doubtful.

Additionally, inputs from group II and III somatic afferents, travelling in the spinocerebellar tracts, have been shown to elicit reflex responses in the inferior cardiac nerve (Coote and Downman, 1966). These afferents are known to project to the lateral reticular nucleus in the brainstem (Rosen and Scheid, 1973). Electrical stimulation of this nucleus elicits arterial hypertension, tachycardia and increased activity in the inferior cardiac nerve, probably by way of preganglionic sympathetic neurons emanating from this nucleus (Ciriello and Calaresu, 1977; Thomas et al., 1977).

Efferent Pathway of the Reflex

Since HR is controlled by the restraining effect of parasympathetic (vagal) activity and the stimulating effect of sympathetic activity, one might question whether HR increases in exercise are due to the withdrawal of vagal activity, to enhancement of sympathetic activity, or to a combination of both. The answer to this question is important in that it may predict the time course of the cardiac acceleration upon the onset of muscular activity or, alternatively, following a change in the intensity of a sustained effort.

The information available seems contradictory. On the one hand, authors claim that the HR response to exercise in man or in animals is vagally mediated. Hollander and Bouman (1975) showed the complete abolition of the immediate cardiac acceleration to short-lasting (<1 sec) voluntary contractions in man after the injection of atropine; Gelsema et al. (1983) repeated these observations in decerebrate cats, and showed that large infusions of an adrenergic beta-blocker (propranolol) did not diminish the HR response to induced muscular contractions. Diepstra et al. (1980) reported similar results from a study in conscious cats that were operantly conditioned to perform isometric contractions with a forelimb. On the other hand, Mitchell et al. (1977) and Crayton et al. (1979) could abolish the HR responses in animals to induced muscular exercise by the administration of propranolol. The latter authors also mentioned the minimal effect of atropine on resting HR in their preparations. Finally, some authors demonstrated cardiac accelerations in animals that could only be mediated by sympathetic activation, since the vagal nerves were sectioned for experimental reasons (Coote et al., 1971; Tallarida et al., 1981).

The differences in results in animals with intact cardiac innervation are most probably due to the use of anesthetics, which may affect parasympathetic control of the heart (Vatner et al., 1971; Kirchheim, 1976), and to extensive surgical manipulation of the animals, which causes significant somatosensory convergence upon the brainstem reticular formation (Sato and Schmidt, 1973; Schulz et al., 1983).

In conclusion, it seems very well conceivable that in normal, intact individuals, three mechanisms will appear to control HR during exercise. Immediately, i.e. within 0.5 sec after the onset of exercise, HR increases as a result of the withdrawal of vagal restraint. Then, after a delay of at least 2-5 sec (Kirchheim, 1976; Hill-Smith and Purves, 1978) following the onset of exercise, the effect of an increase of cardiac sympathetic activity may become apparent, also accelerating cardiac activity. Eventually, HR might be further controlled - predominantly during long-lasting exercise - by an increase in circulating catecholamines excreted by activation of the adrenal medulla.

The Existence of Central Command (Cortical Irradiation)

The efferent pathways discussed in the previous section could not only be activated by a peripheral reflex mechanism, but also by descending activity originating in higher motor structures in the brain and travelling through the brainstem to its target, the spinal motorneurones. In passing by the circulatory brainstem centers, it would give off collateral impulses that activate those centers (Figure 2).

There are several lines of evidence to support this concept, although detailed morphological information is lacking. Alam and Smirk (1938b) investigated the cardiovascular changes to exercise in a patient with unilateral loss of sensibility in a leg due to syringomyelia. During light exercise with either leg, the BP rose. However, after exercise and with the circulation occluded, BP remained high when the normal leg had exercised (as was reported previously in healthy individuals and in animals), but returned immediately to baseline levels when the affected leg had exercised. The authors concluded that central command was involved in the pressor response during exercise and that reflex control originating in the exercising limbs was responsible for the sustained high BP during occlusion after exercise with the normal limb.

Freyschuss (1970) compared the HR and BP responses to light handgrip contractions with the responses to intended contractions of the same muscles and the same intended force after local paralysis of the muscles involved. During paralysis she noted a HR increase that amounted on the average to 64% of the value observed during performed contractions. The corresponding mean value of the rise in BP was 52% of the control data. It was concluded that the cardiovascular changes during paralysis were elicited by central command.

Goodwin et al. (1972) investigated the cardiovascular response to isometric contractions in man. During these experiments, attempts were made to vary the central command necessary to achieve a given force of contraction by means of tendon vibration. It is known that this vibration technique predominantly activates the primary afferents of muscle spindles. Activity in these afferents excites the spinal motoneurons of the homonymous and agonist muscles, and inhibits activity in motoneurons of antagonist muscles. Consequently, when during isometric exercise the tendon of the contracting muscle is vibrated, less central command is necessary to achieve a certain level of tension, because the vibration-stimulated primary afferents "help" to achieve this level by exciting homonymous motoneurons. On the other hand, when spindle afferents are activated in the antagonist of a contracting muscle, a greater central command is required to achieve a given level of force development. It was shown in these experiments that when the effect of vibration helped to build a given force in a contracting muscle, the HR and BP responses were less than without vibration, and conversely, when the effect of vibration counter acted the achievement of a given level of tension of an antagonist, the cardiovascular responses were more than in contractions at the same level of force but without vibration. These observations suggest strongly that the cardiovascular responses are related to the required amount of central command.

In a more recent study, Freund et al. (1979) investigated the cardiovascular responses in man to a maximal effort of the quadriceps muscles during complete motor loss and lack of sensory information of the leg muscles during peridural anesthesia. No pressor responses were observed in the nadir of the anesthesia. However, during the return of strength after anesthesia, increasing pressor responses accompanied contractions of increasing force; the relation being linear. During that time no pressor responses could be obtained during rhythmic exercise with the circulation occluded, indicating the absence of reflex control. Thus the pressor responses were the result of central command.

There are other experimental results indicating the existence of central command. The notion of central command is, however, based on indirect evidence. The major problem encountered in this area is, that there exist no clear description of the term. (The description given above should be regarded as sketchy.) Consequently, it is difficult to design experiments aiming at direct proof in favor of this mechanism. On the other hand, some experimental results discussed above cannot be explained without its existence.

In conclusion, direct evidence is discussed in the present paper showing the existence of a reflex mechanism that controls the cardiovascular function from the onset of and throughout muscular exercise. The explanation of some results necessitate a second neural mechanism to be operative, and inferential evidence in favor of central command is mentioned. It is conceivable that both neural mechanisms cooperate in normal circumstances. When, for some reason, one of the mechanisms is turned off, the other will take over. Neurally spoken, this necessitates merely the (occlusive) convergence of neurones on cardiovascular brainstem centers. We must await further neurophysiologic, anatomical and pharmacological exploration before experimental results can answer the question as to the relative contributions of central and reflex mechanisms in the circulatory response to muscular exercise.

REFERENCES

Alam, M., and Smirk, F. M., 1937, Observations in man upon a blood pressure raising reflex arising from the voluntary muscles, J. Physiol. (London), 89:372-383.
Alam, M., and Smirk, F. M., 1938a, Observations in man on a pulse accelerating reflex from the voluntary muscles of the legs, J. Physiol. (London), 92:167-177.
Alam, M., and Smirk, F. M., 1938b, Unilateral loss of a blood pressure raising, pulse accelerating, reflex from voluntary muscle due to a lesion of the spinal cord, Clin. Sci., 3:247-258.
Athanasiu, J., and Carvallo, J., 1898, Le travail musculaire et le rhytme du coeur, Arch. Physiol., 2:552-567.
Asmussen, E., Nielsen, M., and Wieth-Pedersen, G., 1943, On the regulation of circulation during muscular work, Acta Physiol. Scand., 6:353-358.
Barker, D., 1974, The morphology of muscle receptors, in: "Handbook of Sensory Physiology, Vol III: Muscle Receptors"., C. C. Hunt, ed., Springer, New York.

Borst, C., Hollander, A.P., and Bouman, L. N., 1972, Cardiac acceleration elicited by voluntary muscle contractions of minimal duration, J. Appl. Physiol., 32(1):70–77.

Boyd, I. A., and Davey, M. R., 1968, Composition of Peripheral Nerves, Livingstone, London.

Ciriello, J., and Calaresu, F. R., 1977, Lateral reticular nucleus: a site of somatic and cardiovascular integration in the cat, Am. J. Physiol., 233(3):R100–R109.

Coote, J. H., and Downman, C. B. B., 1966, Central pathways of some autonomic reflex discharges, J. Physiol. (London), 183:714–729.

Coote, J. H., Hilton, S. M., and Perez-Gonzalez, 1971, The reflex nature of the pressor response to muscular exercise, J. Physiol. (London), 215:789–804.

Crayton, S. C., Aung-Din, R., Fixter, D. E., and Mitchell, J. H., 1979, Distribution of the cardiac output during induced isometric exercise in dogs, Am. J. Physiol., 236:218–223.

Diepstra, G., Gonyea, W., and Mitchell, J. H., 1980, Cardiovascular response to static exercise during selective autonomic blockade in the conscious cat, Circ. Res., 47:530–535.

Freund, P. R., Rowell, L. B., Murphy, T. M., Hobbs, S. F., and Butler, S. H., 1979, Blockade of the pressor response to muscle ischemia by sensory nerve block in man, Am. J. Physiol., 237:H433–H439.

Freyschuss, U., 1970, Cardiovascular adjustment to somatomotor activation, Acta Physiol. Scand., 342:Suppl:1–63.

Funderbirk, C. F., Hipskind, S. G., Welton, R. C., and Lind, A. R., 1974, Development of and recovery from fatigue induced by static effort at various tensions, J. Appl. Physiol., 37:392–396.

Gelsema, A. J., de Groot, G., and Bouman, L. N., 1983, Instantaneous cardiac acceleration in the cat elicited by peripheral nerve stimulation, J. Appl. Physiol., 55(3):703–710.

Gelsema, A. J., Hollander, A. P., Karemaker, J. M., and Bouman, L. N., 1985a, Mechanisms of fast rise in heart rate following short muscle contractions, in: "The Psychophysiology of Cardiovascular Control", J. F. Orlebeke, G. Mulder, and L. J. P. van Doornen, eds., Plenum Press, New York.

Gelsema, A. J., Bouman, L. N., and Karemaker, J. M., 1985b, Short-latency tachycardia evoked by stimulation of muscle and cutaneous afferents, Am. J. Physiol., 248:R426–R433.

Goodwin, G. M., McCloskey, D. I., and Mitchell, J. H., 1972, Cardiovascular and respiratory responses to changes in central command during isometric exercise at constant muscle tension, Journal of Physiology, 226:173–190.

Hill, A. V., 1948, The pressure developed in muscle during contraction, J. Physiol. (London), 107:518–526.

Hill-Smith, I., and Purves, R. D., 1978, Synaptic delay in the heart: an ionophoretic study, J. Physiol. (London), 279:31–54.

Hnik, P., Holas, M., Krekule, I., Kriz, N., Mejsner, J., Smiesko, V., Ujec, E., and Vyskocyl, F., 1976, Work induced potassium changes in skeletal muscle and effluent venous blood assessed by liquid ion-exchanger microelectrodes, Pflugers Arch., 362:85–94.

Hnik, P., Hudlicka, O., Kucera, J., and Payne, R., 1969, Activation of muscle afferents by non-proprioceptive stimuli, Am. J. Physiol., 217:1451–1458.

Hollander, A. P., and Bouman, L. N., 1975, Cardiac acceleration in man elicited by a muscle-heart reflex, J. Appl. Physiol., 38(2):272–278.

Hultman, E., and Sjoholm, H., 1982, Blood pressure and heart rate response to voluntary and non-voluntary static exercise in man, Acta Physiol. Scand., 115:499–501.

Humphreys, P. W., and Lind, A. R., 1963, Blood flow through active and inactive muscles of the forearm during sustained handgrip contractions, J. Physiol. (London), 166:120–135.

Johansson, J. E., 1894, Über die Einwirkung der Muskel thätigkeit auf die Athmung und die Herzthätigkeit, Scand. Arch. Physiol., 5:20-66.

Kalia, M., Mei, S. S., and Kao, F. F., 1981, Central projections from ergoreceptors (C fibers) in muscle involved in cardiopulmonary responses to static exercise, Circ. Res., 48:Suppl. I, 48-62.

Kaufman, M. P., Iwamoto, G. A., Longhurst, J. C., and Mitchell, J. H., 1982, Effects of capsaicin and bradykinin on afferent fibers with endings in skeletal muscle, Circ. Res., 50:133-139.

Kirchheim, H. R., 1976, Systemic arterial baroreceptor reflexes, Physiol. Rev., 56:100-176.

Kniffki, K.-D., Mense, S., and Schmidt, R. F., 1978, Responses of group IV afferent units from skeletal muscle to stretch, contraction and chemical stimulation, Exp. Brain Res., 31:511-522.

Kniffki, K.-D., Mense, S., and Schmidt, R. F., 1981, Muscle receptors with fine afferent fibers which may evoke circulatory reflexes, Circ. Res., 48:Suppl. I, 25-31.

Kozelka, J. W., Christy, G. W., and Wurster, R. D., 1982, Somato-autonomic reflexes in anesthetized and unanesthetized dogs, J. Auton. Nerv. Syst., 5:63-70.

Krogh, A., and Lindhard, J., 1917, A comparison between voluntary and electrically induced muscular work in man, J. Physiol. (London), 51:182-201.

Lind, A. R., 1983, Cardiovascular adjustments to isometric contractions: static effort, in: "Handbook of Physiology, Section 2: The Cardiovascular System Vol III: Peripheral Circulation and Organ Blood Flow, part 2", J. T. Shepherd and F. M. Abboud, eds., Am. Physiol. Soc., Bethesda, MD.

Lind, A. R., and McNicol, G. W., 1976, Influence of combined sustained and rhythmic contractions of different muscle groups on the circulatory responses to sustained handgrip contractions, J. Physiol. (London), 192:595-607.

Lind, A. R., Taylor, S. R., Humphreys, P. W., Kenelly, B. M., and Donald, K. W., 1964, The circulatory effects of sustained voluntary muscle contractions, Clin. Sci., 27:229-244.

McCloskey, D. I., Matthews, P. B. C., and Mitchell, J. H., 1972, Absence of appreciable cardiovascular and respiratory responses to muscle vibration, J. Appl. Physiol., 33(5):623-626.

McCloskey, D. I., and Mitchell, J. H., 1972, Reflex cardiovascular and respiratory respones originating in exercising muscle, J. Physiol. (London)., 224:173-186.

McCloskey, D. I., Streatfeild, K. A., 1975, Muscular reflex stimuli to the cardiovascular system during isometric contractions of muscle groups of different mass, J. Physiol. (London), 250:431-441.

Mitchell, J. H., Blomquist, C. G., Lind, A. R., Saltin, B., and Shepherd, J. T., 1981, Static (isometric) exercise: cardiovascular responses and neural control mechanisms, Circ. Res., 48, Suppl. I.

Mitchell, J. H., Payne, F. C., Saltin, B., and Schibye, B., 1980, The role of muscle mass in the cardiovascular response to static contractions, J. Physiol. (London), 309:45-54.

Mitchell, J. H., Reardon, W. C., and McCloskey, D. I., 1977, Reflex effects on circulation and respiration from contracting skeletal muscle, Am. J. Physiol., 233(3):H374-H378.

Mitchell, J. H., and Schmidt, R. F., 1983, Cardiovascular reflex control by afferent fibers from skeletal muscle receptors, in: "Handbook of Physiology, Section 2: The Cardiovascular System Vol III: Peripheral Circulation and Organ Blood Flow, part 2", J. T. Shepherd and F. M. Abboud, eds., Am. Physiol. Soc., Bethesda, MD.

Obrist, P. A., 1981, Cardiovascular Psychophysiology; a Perspective, Plenum Press, New York.

Petro, J. K., Hollander, A. P., and Bouman, L. N., 1970, Instantaneous cardiac acceleration in man induced by a voluntary muscle contraction, J. Appl. Physiol., 29(6):794-798.

Rosen, I., and Scheid, P., 1973, Patterns of afferent input to the lateral reticular nucleus of the cat, Exp. Brain Res., 18:242-255.

Saltin, B., Sjogaard, G., Gaffney, F. A., and Rowell, L. B., 1981, Potassium, lactate, and water fluxes in human quadriceps muscle during static contractions, Circ. Res., 48:Suppl. I:18-24.

Sato, A., and Schmidt, R. F., 1973, Somatosympathetic reflexes: afferent fibers, central pathways, discharge characteristics, Physiol. Rev., 53:916-947.

Schibye, B., Mitchell, J. H., Payne, F. C., and Saltin, B., 1981, Blood pressure and heart rate response to static exercise in relation to electromyographic activity and force development, Acta Physiol. Scand., 113:61-66.

Schulz, B., Lambertz, M., Schulz, G., and Langhorst, P., 1983, Reticular formation of the lower brainstem. A common system for cardiorespiratory and somatomotor functions: discharge patterns of neighboring neurons influenced by somatosensory afferents, J. Auton. Nerv. Syst., 9:433-449.

Sejersted, O. M., Hargens, A. R., Kardel, K. R., Blom, P., Jensen, O., and Hermansen, L., 1984, Intramuscular fluid pressure during isometric contraction of human skeletal muscle, J. Appl. Physiol., 56(2):287-295.

Tallarida, G., Baldoni, F., Peruzzi, G., Raimondi, G., Massaro, M., and Sangiorgi, M., 1981, Cardiovascular and respiratory reflexes from muscles during dynamic and static exercise, J. Appl. Physiol., 50(4):784-791.

Thomas, M. R., and Calaresu, F. R., 1974, Localization and function of medulary sites mediating vagal bradycardia in the cat, Am. J. Physiol., 226:1344-1349.

Thomas, M. R., Ulrichsen, R. F., and Calaresu, F. R., 1977, Function of lateral reticular nucleus in central cardiovascular regulation in the cat, Am. J. Physiol., 232(2):H157-H166.

Tibes, U., 1977, Reflex inputs to the cardiovascular and respiratory centers from dynamically working canine muscles: some evidence for involvement of group III and IV nerve fibers, Circ. Res., 41:332-341.

Vatner, S. F., Franklin, D., and Braunwald, E., 1971, Effects of anesthesia and sleep on circulatory responses to carotid sinus nerve stimulation, Am. J. Physiol., 220:1249-1255.

Wildenthal, K., Mierzwiak, D. S., Mitchell, J. H., 1969, Acute effects of increased serum osmolality on left ventricular performance, Am. J. Physiol., 216:898-904.

RELATIONS BETWEEN CHANGES IN CARDIAC PARASYMPATHETIC

ACTIVITY AND HEART RATE VARIABILITY

John M. Karemaker

Department of Physiology, University of Amsterdam
Academic Medical Center, Meibergdreef 15
1105 AZ Amsterdam, The Netherlands

INTRODUCTION

Heart rate is looked upon in psychophysiology as one of the easily obtainable tale-bearers of the autonomic system's condition. For most autonomic efference the final common pathway originates in the medulla oblongata; this region of the CNS is held responsible for the tonic activities of the sympathetic and parasympathetic system and their interplay (Koizumi and Brooks, 1980). However, the medulla is not "the" autonomic center by itself; it takes part in the complex interaction between different regions in the CNS where somatic and autonomic functions are tuned in response to environmental stimuli. Not only do we find in the medulla the motor neurons of the vagus nerve, controlling such functions as heart rate and activity of the upper intestinal tract, it also contains the centers for the automatic control of respiration.

Therefore, one should not be surprised if changes in one "system" (e.g., cardiovascular) accompany activity changes in another (e.g., respiratory). The well-known respiratory sinus arrhythmia (RSA) is an example of such a combined action of the medulla oblongata: it appears that inspiratory activity, per se, can depress efferent vagus nerve activity to the sino-atrial node, thereby increasing heart rate (Koepchen, Wagner and Lux, 1961).

It is obvious that RSA is observed only if there is some ongoing vagus nerve activity that can be modulated. If the vagus nerve to the heart is silent, due to what ever reason, it cannot be silenced further during inspiration. Therefore, the amount of RSA present is taken to represent a reliable measure of parasympathetic tone (Eckberg, 1983). This line of reasoning will hold true whether the respiration-coupled vagal modulation is of central or peripheral origin.

The objects of the present study are:

1. To show that the effect of a burst of vagus nerve impulses on heart rate depends on the moment of occurrence of the burst in the cardiac cycle.

2. To present an analysis that will explain this phenomenon in terms of the general oscillator theory developed by A. T. Winfree (1980), and the specific properties of the sino-atrial node.

3. From this it will be inferred that, depending on the circumstances, the same changes in vagus nerve activity may seem amplified or
reduced if judged from changes in heart rate.

METHODS

Animals

Experiments were performed in rabbits (New Zealand Whites) of about 3
kgs. under Nembutal anesthesia. The animals were artificially ventilated
through a tracheal canula. Activation of the atrium was detected by a
bipolar catheter electrode that was introduced via the right external
jugular vein. Both vagus nerves were dissected in the neck and cut. The
right vagus to the heart was stimulated via a miniature flexible electrode,
fitting to the size of the nerve. Electrode and nerve were embedded in
mineral oil in order to ensure stable stimulus responses.

Stimulation

Stimuli (duration 0.2 - 2.0 ms, amplitude 5 - 15 V) in bursts of
programmable duration and within-burst repetition rate were presented to
the vagus nerve. The stimulus burst was coupled to the P-wave after a
programmable delay. The bursts would be delivered either once every 15
seconds or after each P-wave.

OSCILLATOR THEORY

In order to appreciate the outcome of the experiments, we should first
look into the theoretical possibilities. The effect of a perturbation on
an oscillator, be it the menstrual cycle, circadian rhythm or pacemaker of
the heart, has found a basis in topology in the work of A. T. Winfree
(1980). The present description is just a simple presentation, limited to
the goals of this contribution.

Suppose we have an ongoing stable oscillator that triggers a flash of
light at the start of every new cycle. By applying a stimulus to this
oscillator we are able to delay the start of the next cycle, thereby delaying the next light flash. Now we may imagine two extreme situations,
depending on the characteristics of the oscillator and the applied stimulus
(see Figure 1). If the stimulus is applied once at different instants in
the cycle (ordinate in Figure 1), two basic patterns may be observed:

1. (Figure 1A) - the stimulus delays the next flash for the same
amount of time, independent of its timing in the cycle. The dashed lines
in Figure 1A indicate the moments where the lights would have flashed, had
we presented no stimulus.

2. (Figure 1B) - the stimulus resets the oscillator to a new state
and the next flash will occur at a fixed time after the stimulus, independent in which phase the oscillator was when it was hit by the stimulus.
After this perturbed cycle the oscillator returns to its original state.

Winfree has designated the type of rescheduling described under 1 as
weak rescheduling (1983) or type 1 reset (1980); the rescheduling under 2
goes by the name of strong rescheduling or type 0 reset. An essential
difference between weak and strong rescheduling is that after weak rescheduling all possible states of the oscillator may exist. In the case of
strong rescheduling only a limited set of phases exist after the stimulus,
although the whole cycle is scanned.

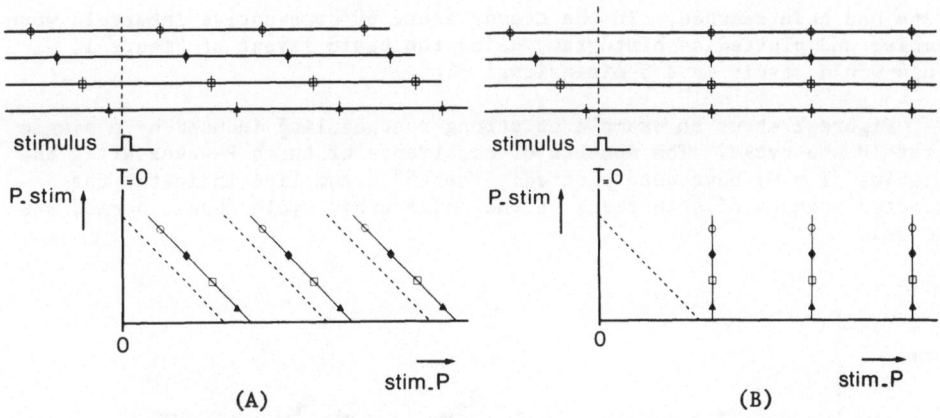

Fig. 1.   Theoretical examples of weak (A) and strong (B) rescheduling.
Top: different time tracings of the oscillator firings are
symbolized. The stimulus is applied in one cycle in each run,
progressively earlier in the cycle. Bottom: comprehensive plots
of the oscillator firings after the stimulus. Ordinate (P-stim)
denotes elapsed time since the last firing until the stimulus,
abscissa (stim-P) denotes moment of firing after the stimulus.
Dashed lines indicate expected moments of firing without stimulus.
Symbols refer to top tracings.

The most important practical consequence in the case of strong rescheduling is found if we consider Figure 1B more carefully. Suppose the
stimulus is applied gradually later in the cycle. The time between
stimulus and next flash is constant; however, the apparent prolongation of
the ongoing cycle is getting longer and longer (horizontal stretch between
dashed line and first vertical drawn line). If the stimulus is progressively advanced in the cycle, the apparent prolongation decreases. The
extremes of both situations mark the end of a cycle or the beginning of the
next cycle. It can be expected that a stimulus applied at that very moment
may have unpredictable results.

Depending on the properties of the oscillator under study and the
strength of the applied stimulus, moments in the normal cycle may exist
where the effect of the stimulus is unpredictable, where it may even
silence the oscillator for a number of periods (or forever, if one thinks
of the heart that is set to fibrillate by an electrical stimulus in the
vulnerable period).

EXPERIMENTAL RESULTS

As has been explained under methods, two types of experiments were
performed:

1. Where the vagus nerve to the heart was stimulated once every 15
seconds. This period was sufficient to have the sino-atrial node back in
steady state when the next stimulus occurred. The stimulus was shifted
progressively through the cycle and the results were plotted in the format
of Figure 1.

2. Where the vagus was stimulated once every heart period. The
stimulus was shifted to some position in the cycle (determined by the
programmable delay between previous P-wave and start of the stimulus).
After each change the stimulus timing was left unchanged until a steady

state had been reached. In the steady state 60 consecutive intervals were sampled and plotted as histogram, using the basic layout of Figure 1. (This would result in a 3-dimensional plot.)

Figure 2 shows an example of strong rescheduling induced by a single burst in one cycle. The moments of occurrence of three P-waves after the stimulus (T = 0) have been plotted. The 45° drawn line indicates the expected moments of occurrence of the undisturbed cycle (basic period was 220 ms).

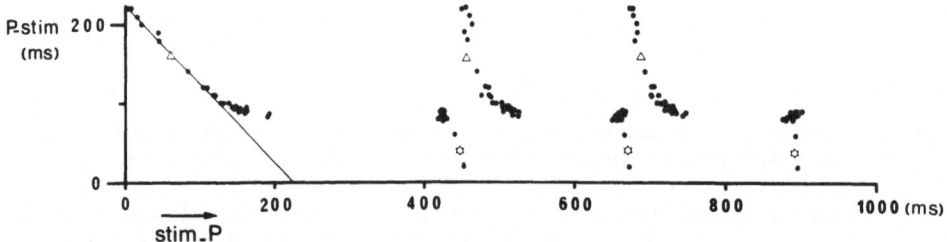

Fig. 2. Strong rescheduling of sino-atrial node induced by one short-lasting stimulus burst to the vagus nerve (see Figure 1 for explanation). Open stars indicate the effects on three consecutive P-waves caused by one stimulus early in the cycle, open triangles were obtained by stimulation late in the cycle.

A number of peculiarities is to be observed in Figure 2:

a) Only stimuli applied in the first 100 ms of the cycle will have their effect on <u>that cycle</u>, stimuli arriving 120 ms or less before the next P-wave are unable to alter its moment of occurrence. This is explained further in Figure 2 by the "open star" symbols, which represent three successive cycles after stimulation early in the cycle, versus the three "open triangle" symbols, where stimulation was applied late in the cycle.

b) The pattern is clearly one of strong rescheduling. The transition between no (or little) effect and maximal effect on the next P-wave is found on stimulation somewhere in the middle of the cycle. This is due to the 120 ms delay between vagus nerve activity and the effect on the sino-atrial node.

c) In the transitional phase of the cycle a large amount of data points was gathered, as evidenced by the density of the plot. Still, we were unable to fill the "gap" between all and none in terms of effect on the first P-wave after the stimulus.

In the next type of experiment the vagus nerve was stimulated with one burst per interval, coupled to the last P-wave. This is supposed to mimic the physiological situation where the vagal activity, apart from tonic over long periods, is observed in bursts per heart beat (cf. Kunze, 1972). The burst was shifted through the interval, in the same way as in the previous experiment. Figure 3 shows the histograms of stimulus to P-wave distributions of 60 consecutive intervals in steady state for a specific coupling time between P-wave and next stimulus burst. We were unable to scan the whole cycle, because if the burst were delivered too late after a specific P-wave, the next P-wave might have occurred before the stimulus. The resting period of this preparation, without vagus nerve stimulation, was about 290 ms.

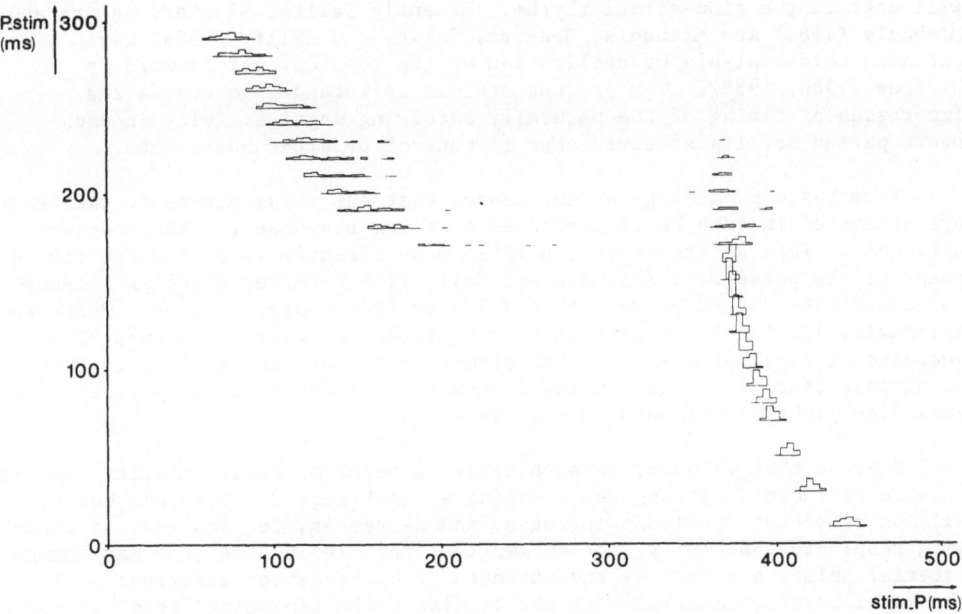

Fig. 3. Rescheduling of sino-atrial node induced by a stimulus burst in
each interval at a delay setting after the last P-wave as marked
on the orindate (P-stim). The abscissa denotes the moment of the
next P-wave after each stimulus; histograms of 60 consecutive
intervals have been assembled at each P-stim setting.

Figure 3 shows, basically, the same characteristics as Figure 2:

a) Only stimuli early in the cycle are able to induce immediate
strong rescheduling, as evidenced by the almost constant stimulus to next
P-time, while P-to stimulus time was changed from 0 - 150 ms. Stimuli
occurring late in the cycle do have an effect on the basic interval (it is
prolonged to roughly 350 ms); however, this cannot be ascribed to the
effect on the same interval where the stimulus was delivered, but on subsequent intervals.

b) There is a transitional phase in the cycle, where the observed
heart rate signal is completely random (as evidenced in the serial auto-
correlate - not shown). In the histograms the interval is seen to jump
between two states, although intervening intervals do occur. The stimulus
burst that was used in the experiment of Figure 3 was, by itself, unable to
induce strong rescheduling as the (much stronger) stimulus did in Figure 2.

DISCUSSION

Relation of the Present Experiments to the Understanding of Heart Rate
Variability

The above described experiments are not new; the fact that the effectiveness of a stimulus to the vagus depends on its timing in the cardiac
cycle was first established by Donders in 1868. In 1934, Brown and Eccles
published their classic analysis of the case. Repeated vagus nerve stimulation has been performed by Levy and co-workers (1969, 1972, 1978). To
date, however, the analysis of the phenomena has focussed on the entrainment problem, i.e., how repeated vagus nerve activity at a certain rate

will entrain the sino-atrial rhythm. Recently Jalife, Slenter, Salata and Michaels (1983) and Michaels, Slenter, Salata and Jalife (1983) have extended this analysis by application of the topology put forward by Winfree (1980, 1983). The present article is intended to stress the importance of timing of the naturally occurring vagal activity in each heart period for its effectiveness to control or alter heart rate.

From basic physiology we may expect that the vagus nerves to the heart are activated in each heart period as a reflex response to baroreceptor afference. This afference is generated most effectively during the rising phase of the pulse wave (Heymans and Neil, 1954). After a reflex latency, where estimates range between 50 and 350 ms (for a discussion see Borst and Karemaker, 1983) this activity may be expected to emerge as a burst-like increase of vagal efference to the sino-atrial node (Kunze, 1972). Pursuing this line of thought in the framework of heart rate variability, the reasoning might be extended as follows:

Suppose that we have, in each cycle, a burst of vagal activity that is capable of inducing strong rescheduling as in Figure 3. Now this burst will be subject to periodic increases and decreases, for instance in phase with respiratory activity (not to mention other influences that may change arterial pulses and thereby the strength of baroreceptor afference). If the vagal burst occurs early in the cardiac cycle (inducing "true" strong rescheduling - Figure 3), we may expect that changes in the strength of the burst will be clearly reflected in changes of the ensuing heart periods. This effect will be stronger when the burst occurs closer to the unstable phase of the cycle. The effect may seem dramatically amplified if the vagal burst occurs in the unstable phase itself. Even in the absence of changes in within-burst activity we may, then, observe a large beat-to-beat variability of heart periods. If the burst occurs late in the heart period, where the effect is no longer on the immediately following P-wave, but on subsequent ones, we may expect heart rate variability to diminish. This reasoning suggests that the same changes in vagus nerve activity may lead to different heart rate variability amplitudes; the more so, within one person, if the activity of the sympathetic system is changing, thereby changing the basic heart period, or, between persons, if the intrinsic heart rates are different. Under those circumstances the timing in the cycle will change. This effect might be even more dramatic if the bursts of vagal activity not only diminish in strength (number of nerve fibers active and/or firing rate of the active fibers) but change their timing in the cardiac cycle as well.

We are now in the process of gathering experimental proof for the former hypothesis. Thus far the experiments support the theory set forth above. The suggestion that the reflex time from baroreceptor afference to vagal efference is not constant but subject to changes under physiological circumstances is, evidently, hard to prove experimentally.

In conclusion it may be stated that heart rate variability should be used very cautiously as a measure of parasympathetic activity. Even if its amplitude changes in one person it may be erroneous to conclude that the modulation of vagal activity is changing. The problem becomes even more difficult if we want to compare heart rate variability between different persons, where we have no prior knowledge on such fundamental parameters as intrinsic heart rate.

Acknowledgements

The author gratefully acknowledges the many discussions with Roel de Boer, M.Sc., on the subject of strong rescheduling of the sino-atrial node.

REFERENCES

Borst, C., and Karemaker, J. M., 1983, Time delays in the human baroreceptor reflex, J. Auton. Nervous Sys., 9:399-409.

Brown, G. L., and Eccles, J. C., 1934, The action of a single vagal volley
on the rhythm of the heart beat, J. Physiol. (London), 82:211-241.

Donders, F. C., 1868, Zur Physiologie des Nervus vagus, Pfluegers Arch.
ges. Physiol., 1:331-361.

Eckberg, D. L., 1983, Human sinus arrhythmia as an index of vagal cardiac
outflow, J. Appl. Physiol., 54:961-966.

Heymans, C., and Neil, E., 1954, "Reflexogenic Areas of the Cardiovascular
System", Churchill, London.

Jalife, J., Slenter, V. A. J., Salata, J. J., and Michaels, D. C., 1983,
Dynamic control of pacemaker activity in the mammalian sinoatrial
node, Circ. Res., 52:642-656.

Koepchen, H. P., Wagner, P.-H., and Lux, H. D., 1961, Ueber die
Zusammenhaenge zwischen zentrale Erregbarkeit, reflektorischen Tonus
und Atemrhythmus bei der nervoesen Steuerung des Herzfrequenz,
Pfluegers Arch. ges. Physiol., 273:443-465.

Koizumi, K., and Brooks, C. M., 1980, The autonomic system and its role in
controlling body functions, Chapter 33 in: "Medical Physiology",
14th edition, V. B. Mountcastle, ed., C. V. Mosby Comp., St. Louis.

Kunze, D. L., 1972, Reflex discharge patterns of cardiac vagal efferent
fibres, J. Physiol. (London), 222:1-15.

Levy, M. N., Martin, P. J., Iano, T., and Zieske, H., 1969, Paradoxical
effect of vagus nerve stimulation on heart rate in dogs, Circ. Res.,
25:303-314.

Levy, M. N., Iano, T., and Zieske, H., 1972, Effects of repetitive bursts
of vagal activity on heart rate, Circ. Res., 30:186-195.

Levy, M. N., Wexberg, S., Eckel, C., and Zieske, H., 1978, The effect of
changing interpulse intervals on the negative chronotropic response
to repetitive bursts of vagal stimuli in the dog, Circ. Res.,
43:570-576.

Michaels, D. C., Slenter, V. A. J., Salata, J. J., and Jalife, J., 1983, A
model of dynamic vagus-sinoatrial node interactions, Am. J.
Physiol., 245:H1043-H1053.

Winfree, A. T., 1980, "The Geometry of Biological Time", Springer Verlag,
New York.

Winfree, A. T., 1983, Sudden cardiac death: a problem in topology, Sci.
Amer., 248:118-131.

QUANTIFICATION AND VALIDATION OF MODELS

INVESTIGATING HEART RATE VARIABILITY:

PROBLEMS AND PITFALLS

Otto Rompelman

Information Theory Laboratory
Department of Electrical Engineering
Delft University of Technology

1 INTRODUCTION

In this Chapter we will discuss the sometimes tedious path that leads
from the electrocardiogram to useful heart rate variability (HRV) information. Investigators in the psychophysiological field are usually not
very familiar with the rather mathematical area the road is running
through; therefore, this Chapter has a somewhat pretentious objective, i.e.
to serve as a guide along this interesting road. It should be of some help
in finding the path in areas where it might be covered with dust (or noise
as it is termed in that area), it might prevent the traveller from taking
an inferior route or even a wrong turn; on the other hand, it will
occasionally indicate an interesting by-pass. Finally, we hope it will be
of some help in repairing small overlooked damages that might have occurred
on the way. Also, this Chapter may facilitate defining the actual goal of
the trip.

The Chapter is organized in six sections:

1. Introduction
2. From ECG to cardiac event series
3. Sampling the event series
4. Conversion of the event series to an HRV-signal
5. Spectral analysis of HRV; why and how?
6. Some final remarks

Some mathematical details are worked out in three separate Appendices.

2 FROM ECG TO EVENT SERIES

The first step in the analysis of HRV is the conversion of the ECG
into what is called an event process. An event process is a process which
is only characterized by the times of occurrence of a number of identical
events. As such it is a mathematical abstration which can be very useful
because it can be employed as a model of a wide range of real processes
(e.g. the arrival times of patients at the emergency room or the points of
occurrence of action potentials generated by a neuron). Furthermore, a set
of mathmetical tools has been developed to treat event processes. In the
case of the ECG, it is not completely clear how to define the "cardiac

event" since one complete ECG-cycle takes about 550 msec, which is rather long compared to the average interbeat interval. We should, therefore, strive to be more specific.

In many studies HRV is derived from the QRS-complexes. This is an improvement since the average duration of the QRS-complex is about 90 msec. Before going further, it is important to ask ourselves, what is the event we are interested in when studying HRV? In fact, it appears that we are usually not interested in the heart itself: we hope to derive some useful information from the points in time that the electrical heart cycle begins, since it is assumed that neural influences on the sino-atrial (SA) node are largely responsible for the fact that heart rate deviates from strict regularity. In other words, we need to try to identify an event in the ECG which is related directly to the SA nodal firing moment. If this is not possible (and in fact it is not), we should use another event, bearing in mind that this practice is not completely correct. The nearest we can get is to define the onset of the P-wave as the SA-nodal-firing moment. However, this point is a very hard one to define in the ECG.

We usually choose another event, e.g. the P-wave or the QRS-complex. This choice leads directly to the problem which is usually referred to as P-wave or QRS-detection. It has been discussed elsewhere (Koeleman et al., 1984, Rompelman et al., 1986) that it is more correct to treat this problem as a two-stage process, viz., first, detection (did the waveform of interest occur at all?) and, second, estimation (if it occurred, at what time exactly?). These steps refer to the characteristics of reliability and accuracy, respectively. A detailed discussion of these steps and their practical realizations is given in the above-mentioned work. We will confine ourselves here to the following remarks when addressing the question as to which waveform (P-wave or QRS-complex) should be used for HRV studies:

P-Wave:

Good representation of the SA-nodal firing moment, reliable detection cumbersome but possible if use is made of the fact that the P-wave always precedes a much easier to detect QRS-complex; accuracy inferior to QRS-complex since it is slower and of much lower amplitude; maximum obtainable accuracy 1.2 msec.

QRS-Complex:

Poorer representation of the SA-nodal firing moment (due to AV and His-bundle conduction-time (about 60 msec); moreover, this time is subject to beat-to-beat fluctuations of up to 10 msec); reliable detection usually not difficult; accuracy far better than for the P-wave; maximum obtainable accuracy 0.1 msec.

In most cases a trade-off between the features involved still leads to the choice of the usual QRS-detection procedure. However, an important conclusion which remains if we use the QRS-complex occurrence times as estimates for the SA-firing moments is that this estimate has both a bias and a variance. If, for example, the R-peak is used, the bias is about 220 msec. If the R-peak estimation accuracy is 1 msec and the fluctuations in AV and His-bundle conduction time are not excessive, the variance is about 10 msec (Figure 1). The bias is only important if we relate HRV to other physiologic processes. In those cases we should correct for this delay! In the case that only HRV is studied or that HRV is related to much slower processes, this bias is of no importance. The variance should be treated as measurement error. As usual these types of error will give rise to noise. This noise becomes more important, the weaker the underlying process is. This means that we will suffer more from this measurement

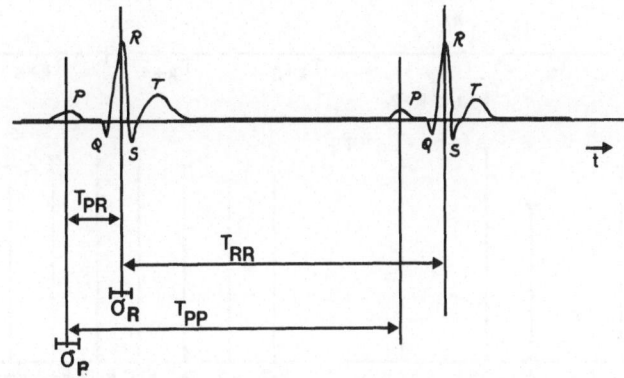

Fig. 1. The ECG with events, intervals and variances.

error as the fluctuations in heart rate become less. This can cause
serious problems in cases where the HRV is very low as with autonomic
neuropathy (Rompelman, 1986).

Despite all precautions, it may happen that we have made errors in the
detection procedure. In particular in the ambulatory recorded ECG, the
signal may suffer from sudden level changes and/or bursts of noise. Though
there is no better detector than the human observer, we do not recommend
the human observer as a detector. However, it should be emphasized that
the difference between the human observer and a computer can be characterized as the following: the human being is a poor calculator and has a
rather global and poor memory, but is a superior pattern recognizer; in
contrast, the computer is a very good and fast calculator with an exact
memory, but is a poor pattern recognizer. What is the impact of this
rather philosophical statement on the situation at issue? We could pass
the ECG through a detector-estimator procedure and display the result to a
human observer (i.e. in the form of an interval tachogram). The observer
has to decide which intervals are most likely due to either missed waveforms or spuriously detected artifacts. After having identified these, it
is perfectly reasonable to allow the computer to make corrections by means
of an interpolation algorithm.

We give two simple examples, the cases of one erroneous detection and
of one missed waveform. Let T_i be the interval between the detected events
at t_{i-1} and t_i. The corrected intervals will be denoted by T'_i.

First the erroneously detected event. In Figure 2 the measured interval tachogram is shown. We assume that the event at t_k is the incorrect
one giving raise to two incorrect intervals, viz., T_k and T_{k+1}. The
correction scheme is now quite simple. The correct intervals can be found
as follows:

$$
\begin{aligned}
\hat{T}_j &= T_j & \text{if } j \leq k-1 \\
\hat{T}_k &= T_k + T_{k+1} \\
\hat{T}_j &= T_{j+1} & \text{if } j \geq k+1
\end{aligned}
\qquad (2.1)
$$

Finally, the corrected event occurrence times t_i can be easily found from

$$
\hat{t}_j = \sum_{j=1}^{i} \hat{T}_j
\qquad (2.2)
$$

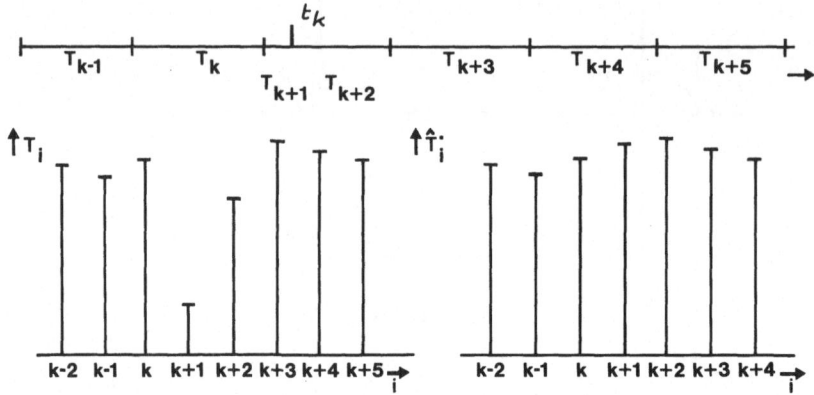

Fig. 2. Tachogram correction in the case of an erroneously detected event.

The case of a missed event is much more complicated. In this case, two intervals have been concatenated resulting in one (long) interval. We therefore should try to <u>estimate</u> the length of the two original intervals. In Appendix A, a possible procedure for this estimation is discussed; it is shown that it is, indeed, possible to restore the original intervals with an error which is less than a few percent.

3 SAMPLING THE EVENT SERIES

In the previous Section, the derivation of an event series from the ECG was discussed. Though due to the practical implementation of the detection/estimation procedure discussed in the previous Section, we have obtained a time-discretized event series; a discussion of the problem of sampling an event series may be useful for a better understanding of the analysis of HRV.

We introduce a mathematical description of the event series $x(t)$:

$$x(t) = \sum_{i=-\infty}^{\infty} \delta(t-t_i) \qquad (3.1)$$

$$t_i : i^{th} \text{ event occurrence time}$$

From sampling theory it is known that the frequency of sampling of a signal should be at least twice the maximum frequency present in the signal. On the other hand it is known that due to the properties of the δ-function, any series of δ-functions has an infinite bandwidth. Hence we are faced with a conflicting situation. We may, however, overcome this conflict by remembering that the event series $x(t)$ is, in fact, a mathematical abstraction of a physical process; so we should attempt to incorporate some prior knowledge. A very basic primary assumption is the band-limited character of the underlying physiological process. In particular it is assumed that the cyclic fluctuations in heart rate do not surpass one Hz. This means that we may replace the original event series $x(t)$ by a signal $\tilde{x}(t)$ under the condition that the low-frequency properties of $\tilde{x}(t)$ are identical (or nearly identical) to the low-frequency properties pf $x(t)$. The question to answer now is, what kind of signal will $\tilde{x}(t)$ be? One obvious solution is the application of a low-pass filter procedure to $x(t)$, since the low-frequency properties of a signal are not affected if this signal passes a low-pass filter. An interesting procedure following this approach was discussed by French and Holden (1971).

Another procedure is the so-called regularization method, which means that all events are shifted such that they will occur at multiples of a fixed interval Δt; in other words $x(t)$ is replaced by

$$\tilde{x}(k.\Delta t) = \sum_{i=-\infty}^{\infty} \delta[(k-n_i).\Delta t] \qquad (3.2)$$

$n_i.\Delta t$ occurrence time of the regularized event at t_i

It has been shown that, if $\frac{1}{\Delta t}$ is much higher than the highest frequency to be expected in HRV, the low-frequency properties of $\tilde{x}(k.\Delta t)$ are, indeed, nearly identical to those of $x(t)$ (Rompelman et al., 1982). Moreover, sampling of $\tilde{x}(k.\Delta t)$ is now very straightforward if we choose the sampling times to coincide with $k.\Delta t$ (in other words, the sampling rate is $\frac{1}{\Delta t}$). In practice we will choose Δt in agreement with the accuracy of the event estimation as discussed previously. For the QRS-complex this accuracy is about 1 msec; hence the (inherent) sampling rate of the event process is 1 kHz. The conclusion is that the problem of sampling the cardiac event series can be solved by a simple regularization process.

4   CONVERSION OF THE EVENT SERIES INTO A SIGNAL

Heart rate variability is often studied as a time-dependent phenomenon. This means that one wishes to convert the cardiac event series into a time signal. In the literature a number of procedures are used. We will shortly summarize the four most common methods.

a   The Interval Tachogram (IT) (Figure 3a)

The intervals between the events are given as function of the interval number:

$$Y(i) = [t_i - t_{i-1}] \qquad (4.1)$$

t_i: event occurrence times

This is a very easy to obtain plot since an event process is usually stored in the form of its intervals. Caution should be taken when this function is subjected to spectral analysis. Since $Y(i)$ in (4.1) is a function of the interval number rather than time we will obtain an interval spectrum, the independent variable (abcissa) being expressed in cycles/interval rather than cycles per second (or Hertz).

b   The Interval Function (IF) (Figure 3b)

The intervals between the events are given as a function of time:

$$Y(t) = \sum_{i=-\infty}^{\infty} (t_i - t_{i-1}) \cdot \delta(t - t_i) \qquad (4.2)$$

The IF can be considered as an irregularly sampled waveform. In order to make analysis possible, one usually applies a kind of interpolation in order to render a signal suitable for continuous sampling.

c   The Instantaneous Heart Rate (IHR) (Figure 3c)

This is the reciprocal of the IF, if the instantaneous heart rate is defined as the reciprocal of the cardiac event interval. Thus:

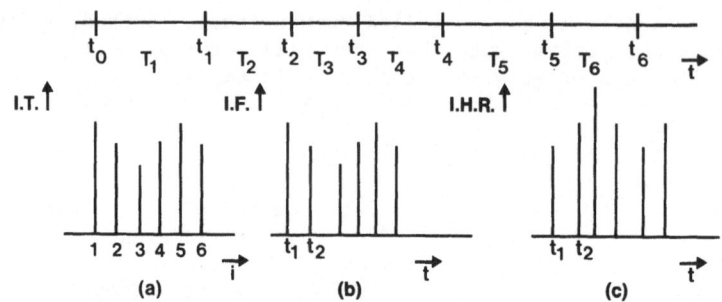

Fig. 3. Three ways of obtaining an HRV signal: (a) Interval Tachogram
(IT); (b) Interval Function (IF); (c) Instantaneous Heart Rate
(IHR).

$$Y(t) = \sum_{i=-\infty}^{\infty} \frac{1}{t_i - t_{i-1}} \cdot \delta(t - t_i). \tag{4.3}$$

If this signal is passed through a so-called zero-order hold circuit, one
obtains the signal which is produced by the well-known cardiotachometer
Figure 3c). Some practical consequences of both the IF- and the IHR-
approach will be discussed later.

d The Low Pass Filtered Event Series (LPFES)

This method is based on a model of the neural influence of the SA-node
as will be discussed later.

The question is, which method is to be preferred? Before directly
addressing this question it is important to note that whatever method we
use, it will be based (implicitly or explicitly) on a model. This model
accounts for the total neural influence on the SA-node resulting in fluctuations in heart rate. Hyndman and Mohn (1973) were the first to base the
analysis of HRV on a model of the natural pacemaker, including the neurally
induced variations in firing rate. This model, the Integral Pulse Frequency Modulator (IPFM) is shown in Figure 4. The input signal m(t), which
is supposed to represent the net vagal and sympathetic activity, is integrated, yielding y(t): when y(t) reaches a fixed reference level R, a pulse
is emitted, and the integrator is reset to zero where upon the cycle starts
again. The sequence of emitted pulses represents the cardiac event series
x(t). Earlier work of Bayly (1968) had shown that the modulating signal
m(t) can be regained by means of a low pass filter operation applied to the
event series. Since the origin of fluctuations in the rate of occurrence
of the events was explained in terms of a modulation, the low-pass filtering operation may also be called demodulation. More details are to be
found in Appendix B.

Hyndman's LPFES is, therefore, based on this model. It has been
shown, however, that the other methods mentioned can be thought to be based
on modifications of this model (Rompelman et al., 1977). The next question
is, how do we, in practice, perform this filtering (or demodulation)? As
will be discussed in more detail in Appendix B, this procedure is in fact
rather simple and can be carried out by means of a simple computer program
or by a special-purpose hardware device. An important feature of the
demodulator is the impulse response of the filter applied. We will not
discuss filter theory here but only remind the reader that filters with a
symmetrical impulse response do not affect the phase relations within the
signal. However, a symmetrical impulse response can only be realized off-
line. Off-line processing is usually carried out with a digital computer.

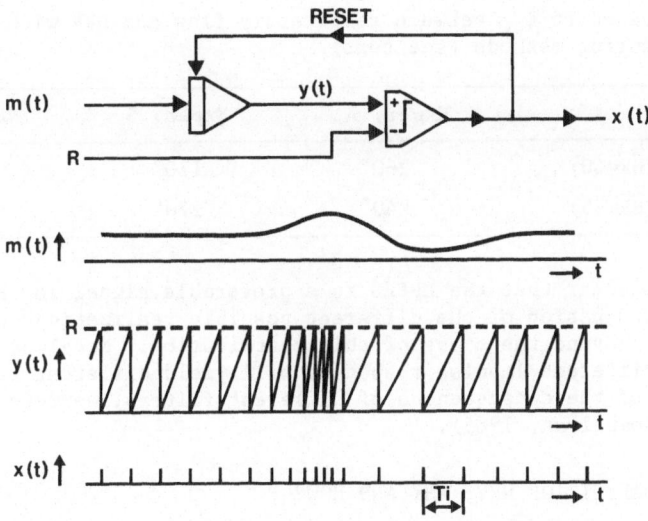

Fig. 4.   The Integral Pulse Frequency Modulator (IPFM) as a model for
autonomous pacemaker activity and rate modulation.

        If a filter with a symmetrical impulse response is used, we do not
introduce a time delay (or a fixed time delay if HRV is measured on-line
with a digital filter).   The IHR is a signal similar to the LPFES.   However, this signal is lagging with respect to the underlying process.   This
lag is dependent on the way the IHR is treated (and the same holds for the
IF).   If we use the rather jumping signal produced by the cardiotachometer,
this lag is equal to one cardiac interval duration. However, if we smooth
this signal in order to remove the jumps an additional lag is introduced.
If an off-line smoothing is carried out we can reduce the lag because a
symmetrical impulse response can be applied.   So recapitulating, if the
output of the cardiotachometer is used as an HRV-signal we have a lag with
respect to the underlying process, this lag lying in between about 0.5 T
and 1.5 T (T being the average cardiac interval), depending on how this
signal is processed.   Moreover, and this is more serious, the amount of lag
is not constant but varies with the interval duration or, in other words,
with the heart rate.   If we are only interested in the HRV information this
is of minor importance.   However, if we want to relate HRV to other physiological processes this becomes very important.

        As an example, suppose that we want to relate HRV to respiration and
that the mean heart rate during the experiment is 75 beats/min.   A cardiotachometer is used for the measurement of HRV.   The lag is then 800 msec.
Note that if the instrument is triggered from the QRS-complexes, we have to
add an additional delay of about 220 msec as was discussed in Section 1.

        Let us expand this example a bit more and introduce three exper-
imenters: "A" uses a QRS triggered cardiotachometer, "B" uses a QRS trigger
delay compensated low pass filter and "C" uses the same instrument and
compensates for the SA-QRS delay.   All three want to measure the phase
shift between respiratory flow and HRV of two subjects breathing at a
constant rate of 15 breaths/min (i.e. 0.25 Hz).   Subject I has a mean heart
rate of 60 beats/min and subject II has a mean heart rate of 75 beats/min.
The different results are summarized in Table 1.   It is obvious that a
scientific discussion between A, B and C on the physiological processes
underlying respiratory sinus arrhythmia will not be very enlightening if
the measuring conditions are not taken into account!

Table 1. Phase shift ϕ_{rh} between respiratory flow and HRV with different
measuring methods (see text).

	Exper. A	Exper. B	Exper. C
Subject I ($\overline{\overline{HR}}=60$)	260°	170°	150°
Subject II ($\overline{\overline{HR}}=75$)	240°	170°	150°

It may be clear that the LPFES is a preferable signal for HRV
analysis. A discussion of the different possible realizations of the low
pass filter is beyond the scope of this contribution. Needless to say,
filters with different impulse responses will yield different results. For
some examples of the consequences of different filters, we refer to another
publication (Rompelman, 1985).

5 SPECTRAL ANALYSIS OF HRV; WHY AND HOW?

In the preceding Section we have discussed the manner of arriving at a
signal which can be thought to be representative for HRV. The next question is, how do we analyse this signal? It is important to note that this
question, without accompanying information, is impossible to answer.
Signal analysis is not a goal in itself but rather a means of testing a
hypothesis. Hence, depending on the hypothesis we want to test, we have to
select a proper method from the, indeed, well stocked tool kit called
signal analysis. In order to shed some light on the possibilities of this
tool kit, it is useful to divide the methods in two groups. The first
group is meant to give some information on which data values actually occur
or, in more formal terms, first-order statistics. As examples, we can
think of the mean value or the variance. The statistical parameters may be
studied as (slowly) varying quantities, if such should be the case. The
second group gives information about the way the data is structured, i.e.
the interrelation between different data values; in formal terms these are
called second-order statistics. As examples, we mention the autocorrelation function and the power spectrum. The spectrum of a signal may give
an answer to the question of whether this signal comprises any, more or
less periodical components. Since biological systems often exhibit
periodical, or oscillatory, phenomena, it is not surprising that spectral
analysis is a wide-spread method in physiology. However, we should be
careful not to go for spectral analysis thoughtlessly: it should affirm a
hypothesis or refine the knowledge of underlying periodical phenomena.

It is beyond the scope of this contribution to give a thorough review
of spectral analysis. We will only point out some important aspects and
give some comments. For further details the reader is referred to e.g.
Bendat and Piersol (1971). First we should remember that spectral analysis
is usually based on Fourier analysis. We state the Fourier integral:

$$X(f) = \int_{-\infty}^{\infty} x(t) \cdot e^{-j2\pi ft} dt \qquad (5.1)$$

A practical problem immediately arises: we do not have an infinite time
series at our disposal. This problem has a large impact on spectral
analysis. Assume that we have only a data set ranging from 0-T sec. This
implies that we can rewrite (5.1) as follows:

$$X(f) = \int_{0}^{T} x(t) \cdot e^{-j \cdot 2\pi ft} \cdot \qquad (5.2)$$

Note that we have now written X(f) instead of X(f). This difference
indicates that X(f) is not the <u>true</u> spectrum of x(t) but an <u>estimate</u>, based
on the <u>sample</u> x(t), $0 \leq t \leq T$. As is usually the case, an estimation is
not the truth, but we do not have another choice!

A direct consequence of (5.2) is that we assume that x(t) is composed
of an (infinite) amount of harmonic functions (i.e. sine and/or cosine
functions), such that an entire number of periods is always comprised by
the sample duration T! Of course, this is not generally the case. There
are ways to reduce this problem. A well-known method is the application of
a tapering window. This means that we multiply the data with a function,
so that we get rid of the abrupt changes at the start and the end of the
data segment. Another problem arises from the so-called uncertainty principle in Fourier analysis. This is one of the many examples in nature
which, in fact, implies: "we cannot have two things at the same time". In
this case we mean resolution in time and resolution in frequency. The
spectral resolution is inversely proportional to the length of the data
segment. As an example assume that we have two sessions yielding two
segments of 1-minute data suitable for further analysis. The question is:
is there a 5% shift in frequency of the blood pressure oscillations (10-sec
rhythm) between the two sessions? Fourier analysis of a data segment of 1
minute yields a spectral resolution of 0.017 Hz. On the other hand a 5%
shift in frequency of the 10-sec rhythm would mean a shift of 0.005 Hz,
which is one-third of the spectral resolution. The conclusion is that we
will not be able to assess this shift on the basis of these measurements.
The only solution is to increase the duration of the measurement in order
to increase the spectral resolution.

Finally, we will shortly discuss the way we can obtain a HRV spectrum.
There are basically two ways, i.e. the indirect method and the direct
method. The indirect method consists of two steps: the generation of an
HRV signal as discussed in Section 4 of this Chapter and the Fourier
analysis of the thus obtained signal. The direct method has been introduced recently (Rompelman et al., 1982) and is, in fact, a spectral
analysis of the event process derived from the ECG as discussed in Section
2 of this Chapter. The advantage of this method is the possibility of
on-line processing since we do not need to derive a variability signal from
the event series. More details are given in Appendix C. The direct method
is easy to implement and can be used for on-line monitoring the HRV
spectrum during an experiment. An example of an HRV-spectrum is shown in

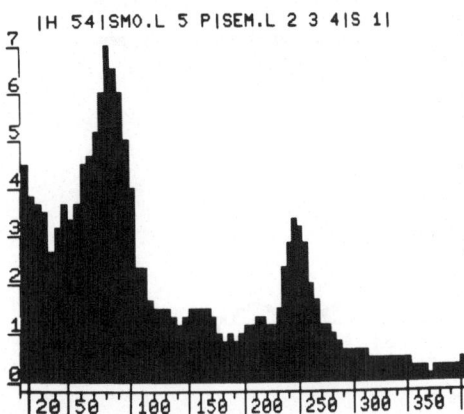

IH 54ISMO.L 5 PISEM.L 2 3 4IS 1I

Fig. 5. Example of an HRV spectrum obtained with the "direct" method (see
text): horizontal (frequency) axis in mHz (= 0.001 Hz).

(continued)

73

Figure 5. Both the respiratory arrhythmia (about 0.22 Hz) and the well-known blood pressure oscillations as reflected in HRV (10-sec rhythm, about 0.1 Hz) are clearly noticeable.

A few remarks should be made about applying spectral analysis to HRV. Though the direct method is very attractive, we do not obtain an HRV-signal which is consequently Fourier transformed. In a number of cases this information can be very useful, in particular in the case of possible errors in the generation of the event process and in the case of slow trends of considerable magnitude in the mean heart rate. Slow trends in a signal give rise to large contributions in the very low end of the spectrum, suppressing often all details at higher frequencies. Sometimes the situation may be improved by applying a high pass filter to the HRV-signal, prior to Fourier transformation. On the other hand, this may be very dangerous since this may introduce a peak at a low frequency which erroneously could, for example, be attributed to the 10-sec rhythm (Figure 6). An example of this situation has met the author's eyes, where it was claimed that under certain circumstances the 10-sec rhythm was shifted to a much lower frequency (i.e. 0.03 Hz). Later, after going back to the original data, it appeared that large trends had occurred and these were removed by a 18 dB/octave high pass filter with cut-off frequency of, indeed, 0.03 Hz.

There is no general solution to this sort of problem, as it is not always clear whether the trends in the data are part of the oscillations we want to study or just contamination of underlying phenomena. It is suggested, therefore, that experiments be carried out in such a way that possible trends are avoided. Should they still occur, then an interactive approach might be advised. As an example, we may suggest the usage of a computer with graphics and light pen facilities. After having displayed the HRV-signal we could "draw" a correction line through the data and subtract that line from the data. One should bear in mind, however, that any time domain procedure has its consequences in the frequency domain. Any linear method such as subtracting a polynomial fitted through the data, is, in fact, a high-pass filter operation.

We would like to conclude by mentioning the manner in which the spectrum is affected when different methods for the generation of an HRV signal are employed. All the real time domain methods (IF, IHR and LPFES)

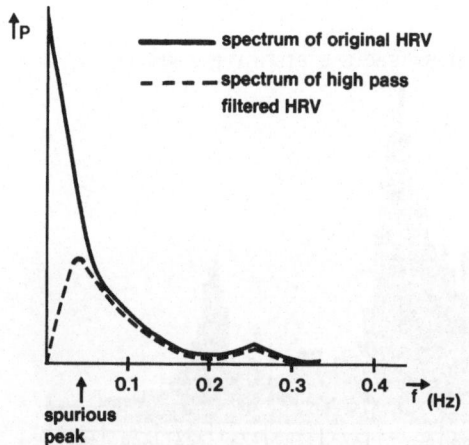

Fig. 6. The introduction of a spurious spectral peak if the HRV signal is passed through a high pass filter in order to reduce slow trends.

use filters. It is obvious that the resultant spectra will also reflect the frequency characteristics of the applied filter, as is discussed elsewhere (Rompelman, 1985). This is another reason why one should be most careful when trying to make a quantitative comparison between spectra generated by different investigators.

6 SOME FINAL REMARKS

It is customary to conclude a chapter by summing up the main points made. We will diverge somewhat from this practice, however, by stating first what was not envisaged. This Chapter has not aimed at demonstrating the usefulness of HRV in any specific field nor does it claim to present any evidence of a relation between HRV and physiological or psychological processes: many examples of this are certainly discussed in other chapters. We think that the analysis of HRV can be regarded as providing a window into the autonomic nervous system. It is hoped that this contribution will be of some help in preventing this window from becoming steamed or blurred.

REFERENCES

Bayly, E. J., 1968, Spectral analysis of pulse frequency modulation in the nervous system, IEEE Transact. on Biomed. Eng., BME-15:257-265.

Bendat, J. S., and Piersol, A. G.,1971, Random data: analysis and measurement procedures, John Wiley & Sons, New York.

French, A. S., and Holden, A. V., 1971, Alias-free sampling of neuronal spike trains, Kybernetik, 5:165-191.

Hyndman, B. W., and Mohn, R. K., 1973, A pulse modulator model for pacemaker activity, in: "Digest of the Tenth Int. Conf. on Med. & Biol. Eng.", p. 223, Dresden.

Koeleman, A. S. M., Akker, T. J. van den, Ros, H. H., Janssen, R. J., and Rompelman, O., 1984, Estimation accuracy of P-wave and QRS-complex occurrence times in the ECG: the accuracy for simplified theoretical and computer simulated waveforms, Signal Processing, 7:389-405.

Rompelman, O., Coenen, A. J. R. M., and Kitney, R. I., 1977, Measurement of heart rate variability: Part 1 - Comparative study of heart rate variability analysis methods, Med. & Biol. Eng. & Comp., 15:233-239.

Rompelman, O., Snijders, J. B. I. M., and Spronsen, C. J. van, 1982, The measurement of heart rate variability with the help of a personal computer, IEEE Transact. on Biomed. Eng., BME-29:503-510.

Rompelman, O., 1985, Spectral analysis of heart rate variability, in: "The Psychophysiology of Cardiovascular Control", J. F. Orlebeke, G. Mulder and L. J. P. van Doornen, eds., Plenum New York.

Rompelman, O., 1986, Accuracy aspects in ECG-preprocessing for the study of heart rate variability, in: "The Beat-by-Beat Investigation of Cardiovascular Function", R. I. Kitney and O. Rompelamn, eds., Clarendon Press, Oxford.

Rompelman, O., Janssen, R. J., Koeleman, A. S. M., Akker, T. J. van den, and Ros, H. H., 1986, Practical limitations for the estimation of P-wave and QRS-complex occurrence times, Automedica, 6:269-284.

APPENDIX A

Restoration of the event series in the case of one missed event

Assume that in the conversion of the ECG signal into an event series one event has been missed (detection failure). We want to estimate the time at which the missed event has occurred. A possible method will be discussed with the help of Figure A1. Assume that the kth event occurring at t_k has not been detected (Figure A1). The resultant tachogram T'_i (i.e. the series of cardiac event intervals) is shown in Figure A1b. The interval T'_k is incorrect and, in fact, is equal to the sum of the two original intervals T_k and T_{k+1}. Estimating the location of event t_k is the same as estimating the interval between the event at t_{k-1} and the event at t_k; in other words, we can try to create an estimate of the correct tachogram. This "corrected" tachogram will be denoted by $\hat{T}_i$. It should be clear that for most intervals there is a very simple relation between the measured tachogram and the corrected tachogram.

$$\hat{T}_j = T'_j \qquad \text{if } j \leq k-1$$
$$\hat{T}_j = T'_{j-1} \qquad \text{if } j \geq k+2 \tag{A1}$$

Hence (obviously) $\hat{T}_k$ and $\hat{T}_{k+1}$ are the intervals to be estimated. We know, however, that

$$\hat{T}_k + \hat{T}_{k+1} = T'_k \tag{A2}$$

The proposed estimation will be based on both a forward extrapolation from the intervals preceding T'_k (viz., T'_{k-2} and T'_{k-1}) and a backward extrapolation from the intervals following T'_k (viz., T'_{k+1} and T'_{k+2}). A preliminary estimation will then be:

$$\tilde{T}_k = \alpha \cdot (2 T'_{k-1} - T'_{k-2}) + (1-\alpha)(3 T'_{k+1} - 2 T'_{k+2})$$
$$\tilde{T}_{k+1} = \alpha (2 T'_{k+1} - T'_{k+2}) + (1-\alpha)(3 T'_{k-1} - 2 T'_{k-2}) \tag{A3}$$

with α a factor, which can be regarded as the balance between influence of the past versus the future on the estimated intervals. In this preliminary estimation we have not taken into account the condition as formulated in (A2). Therefore, we introduce a correction factor c:

$$c = \frac{T'_k}{\tilde{T}_k + \tilde{T}_{k+1}} = \frac{T'_k}{(3-\alpha)(T'_{k-1} + T'_{k+1}) - (2-\alpha)(T'_{k-2} + T'_{k+2})} \tag{A4}$$

Hence, the final estimates will be:

$$\hat{T}_k = c \cdot \tilde{T}_k$$
$$\hat{T}_{k+1} = c \cdot \tilde{T}_{k+1} \tag{A5}$$

In Table A.1 we show an example of the results obtained with this method. Starting from a set of events we found a set of intervals. Consequently, we assumed that one event was missed. The factor α was 1. After having estimated the missed intervals, the event occurrence times t_i were formed with the help of

$$t_i = \sum_{j=1}^{i} \hat{T}_j \tag{A6}$$

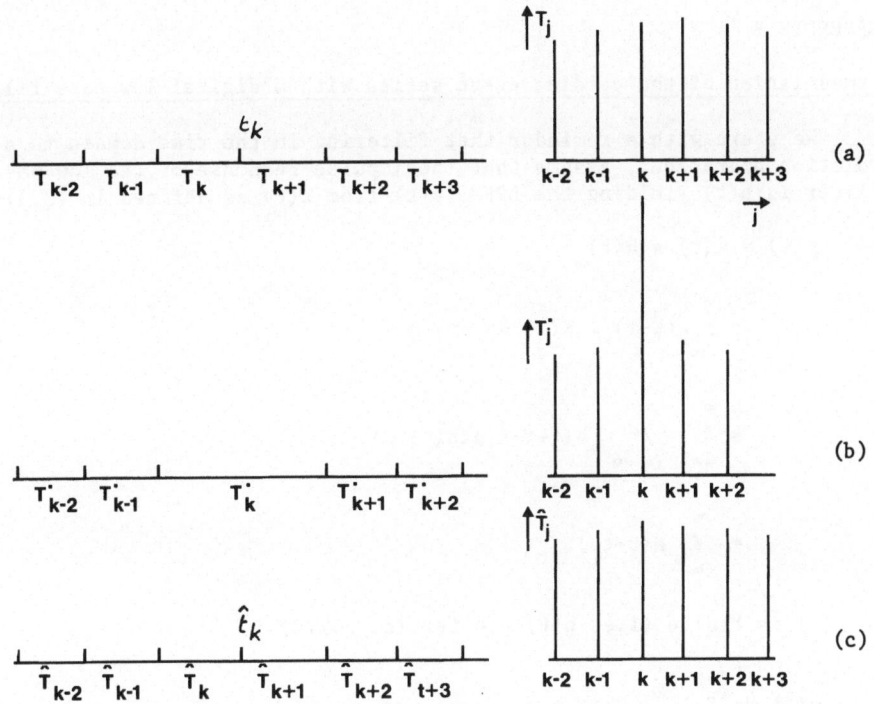

Fig. A1. (a) Example of an event series and its tachogram. (b) The event series of Figure A1(a) with one missed event and its tachogram. (c) The reconstructed event series and its tachogram.

Table A1. Restoration of RR-interval tachogram in the case of one missed event at t_k [$\alpha = 1$].

true intervals		measured intervals		corrected intervals			
					prelim.val.	final value	error
j	T_j (ms)	j	T'_j (ms)	j	$\tilde{T}_j$ (ms)	$\hat{T}_j$ (ms)	(%)
.							
.							
.							
k-2	800	k-2	800	k-2			
k-1	870	k-1	870	k-1			
k	920	k	1880	k	940	930.1	+1.1
k+k	960			k+1	960	949.1	-1.1
k+2	910	k+1	910	k+2			
k+3	860	k+2	860	k+3			
.							
.							
.							

APPENDIX B

Demodulation of the cardiac event series with a digital low pass filter

We start with a reminder that filtering in the time domain is a convolution operation. Assume that the impulse response of the low pass
filter is h(t) yielding the LPFES y(t) from x(t) as defined in (3.1):

$$y(t) = x(t) * h(t)$$

$$= \int_{-\infty}^{\infty} x(t-\tau) \cdot h(\tau) \, d\tau$$

$$= \int_{-\infty}^{\infty} \sum_{i=-\infty}^{\infty} \delta(t-\tau-t_i) \cdot h(\tau) \, d\tau$$

$$= \sum_{i=-\infty}^{\infty} h(t-t_i). \tag{B.1}$$

If h(t) is finite (i.e. h(t) = 0 for $|t| > T/2$)

$$y(t) = \sum_{t_i=t-\frac{T}{2}}^{t_i=t+\frac{T}{2}} h(t-t_i) \tag{B.2}$$

and after regularization ($h(m.\Delta t) = 0$ for $|m| > \frac{T}{2.\Delta t}$)

$$\hat{y}(k.\Delta t) = \sum_{n_i=k-\frac{T}{2\Delta t}}^{k+\frac{T}{2\Delta t}} h[(k-n_i)\Delta t] \tag{B.3}$$

or simply

$$\hat{y}(k) = \sum_{n_i=k-\frac{N}{2}}^{k+\frac{N}{2}} h(k-n_i) \qquad\qquad N = \frac{T}{\Delta t} \tag{B.4}$$

$\hat{y}(k)$ is the (discrete) low pass filtered signal; the sampling rate of y(t)
[viz $\frac{1}{\Delta t}$] may be much too high!! If the cut-off frequency of the filter is
f_0, we only need a sampling rate for y(t) of $2.f_0$.

Let $\alpha = \frac{1}{2f_0\Delta t}$, it will then be sufficient to compute samples of y(t) with

distance $\alpha.\Delta t$:

$$\hat{y}(\alpha k) = \sum_{n_i=k-\frac{N}{2}}^{k+\frac{N}{2}} h(\alpha k-n_i) \tag{B.5}$$

Example: if Δt = 1 ms

and f_0 = 0.5 Hz

then: $\alpha = \dfrac{1}{2f_0\Delta t} = \dfrac{1}{2 \times 0.5 \times 10^{-3}} = 1000.$

This is the principle of the stepwise convolution procedure as discussed by Coenen et al. (1977).

REFERENCE

B.1 A.J.R.M. Coenen, O. Rompelman and R.I. Kitney, Measurement of heart rate variability: Part II - Hardware digital device for the assessment of heart rate variability. Med. & Biol. Eng. & Comp., 15: 423-430 (1977).

APPENDIX C

The direct method for HRV spectral analysis

In section 4 it was mentioned that the LPFES method for generating an HRV-signal is based on the IPFM model (Figure 5). Bayly (1968) derived an expression for the event series x(t) generated by the model, if the input signal m(t) is given by:

$$m(t) = M_0 + M_1 \cos (2\pi f_m t + \emptyset) \qquad (C.1)$$

viz.:

$$x(t) = \frac{I}{R}\left\{[M_0 + M_1 \cos (2\pi f_m t + \emptyset)] + 2M_0 \sum_{k=1}^{\infty} \sum_{n=-\infty}^{\infty} c_{n,k} \cos[2\pi(kf_0 + nf_m) + \theta_{n,k}]\right\}$$
$$(C.2)$$

with: I : impulse content

$f_0 = \dfrac{M_0}{R}$: the unmodulated (average) pulse repetition frequency

$c_{n,k}$ and $\theta_{n,k}$: constants; only dependent on n and k.

An example of the amplitude spectrum $|X(f)|$ of x(t) is shown in Figure C1. From section 5 we recall that spectral analysis involves the Fourier transform of a signal. First, however, we must have a closer look at eq. (C2) and Fig. C1. It was concluded that the so-called modulating signal m(t) (i.e. the underlying HRV information) could be created by low-pass filtering of the event series. The spectrum of this signal is, in fact, identical to the very low frequency part of the event spectrum as shown in Figure C1. Hence it must be possible to obtain the HRV-spectrum by calculating only a relatively small number of spectral components of the event series.

The Fourier transform of a signal x(t), leading to the complex spectrum $\bar{X}(f)$, is defined by (the bar over X indicates that X is a complex variable):

$$\bar{X}(f) = \int_{-\infty}^{\infty} x(t) \cdot e^{-j2\pi ft} dt \qquad (C.3)$$

If we denote the cardiac event series x(t) according to (3.1) we find:

$$\bar{X}(f) = \int_{-\infty}^{\infty} \sum_{i=-\infty}^{\infty} \delta(t - t_i) \cdot e^{-j2\pi ft} dt$$

$$= \sum_{i=-\infty}^{\infty} e^{-j2\pi f.t_i} \qquad t_i: \text{ event occurrence times} \qquad (C.4)$$

We will shortly summarize 5 aspects when trying to make a practical implementation:

-a   Regularization
-b   Frequency-sampling (i.e. the generation of a discrete spectrum)
-c   Truncation (i.e. analysis of a finite segment of x(t))
-d   Conversion of the complex spectrum into a power spectrum
-e   Leakage reduction.

Ad a) At the end of section 3 we have discussed the necessary regularization.

This modifies eq. (C.4) into:

$$\bar{X}_1(f) = \sum_{i=-\infty}^{\infty} e^{-j2\pi fn_i.\Delta t} \qquad (C.5)$$

$$n_i.\Delta t: \text{ approximated event occurrence times.}$$

Ad b) Though the righthand side of eq. (C.5) is based on discrete time, the lefthand side is a function of continuous frequency. For practical implementation it is also necessary to calculate the spectrum for discrete frequency values. The conversion of the continuous spectrum $\bar{X}_1(f)$ into the discrete spectrum $\bar{X}_1(m.\Delta f)$ follows from:

$$\bar{X}_1(m.\Delta f) = \sum_{i=-\infty}^{\infty} e^{-j2\pi n_i m\Delta t.\Delta f}$$

The way Δf can be chosen is discussed next.

Ad c) Up till now we have assumed that we analyze an infinite signal. In practice of course we have a finite segment. Assume that the duration of this segment is $T = N.\Delta t$. The event process after this truncation is:

$$x_f(k.\Delta t) = \sum_{i=1}^{M} \delta(k-n_i)\Delta t \qquad (C.7)$$

$$0 < n_i \leq N$$
$$M: \text{ number of events in } T=N.\Delta t$$

Hence:

$$\bar{X}_f(m.\Delta f) = \sum_{i=1}^{M} e^{-j2\pi n_i m\Delta t\Delta f} \qquad (C.8)$$

Usually we choose:

$$\Delta f = \frac{1}{T} \qquad (C.9)$$

so that

$$\bar{X}_f(m) = \sum_{i=1}^{M} e^{-\frac{j2\pi mn_i}{N}} \qquad (C.10)$$

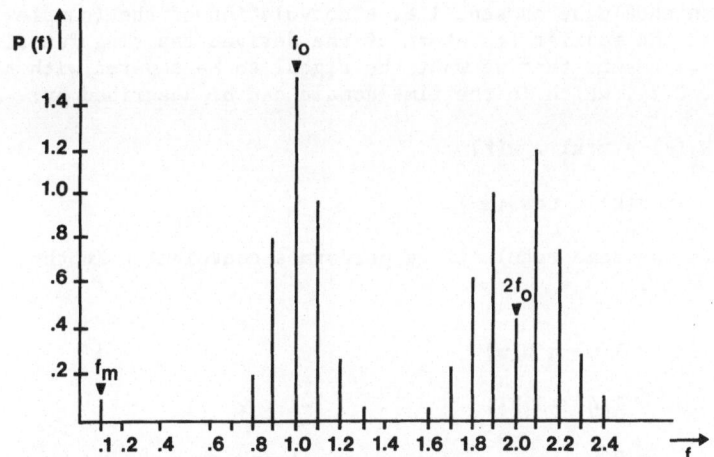

Fig. C1.   An example of the spectrum of the pulse series generated by the
IPFM if modulated with a single harmonic: mean rate, f_0 = 1 Hz;
modulation frequency, f_m = 0.1 Hz.

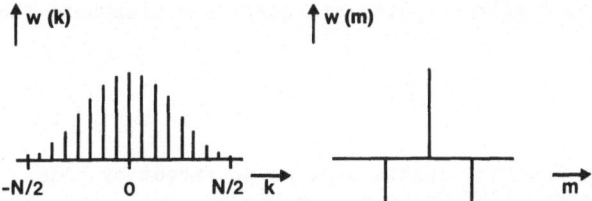

Fig. C2.   Time and frequency representation of the Hann-widow as a tapering
function.

As an example assume T = 200 s; then Δf = 0.005 Hz.   If the maximum frequency of interest in the HRV is 0.5 Hz, it follows that $1 \leq m \leq 100$.   In
other words: only 100 frequency components are to be calculated according
to eq. (C.10).

Ad d) The power spectrum S(m) is simply obtained from the complex spectrum
$\bar{\bar{X}}_f(m)$ by

$$
\begin{aligned}
S(m) &= \left| \bar{\bar{X}}_f(m) \right|^2 \\
&= \left(\sum_{i=1}^{M} \cos \frac{2\pi m n_i}{N} \right)^2 + \left(\sum_{i=1}^{M} \sin \frac{2\pi m n_i}{N} \right)^2
\end{aligned}
\qquad (C.11)
$$

Ad e)   Under c, the truncation (i.e. going from an infinite series to a
finite segment) was discussed.   This operation can be looked upon as a
multiplication of the original signal with a rectangular (or: boxcar-)
function.   It is well-known that the result in the frequency domain is a
convolution of the true spectrum with the Fourier transform of the boxcar
function (i.e. a sinc-function), causing serious leakage of spectral values
to incorrect frequencies (see e.g. Bendat and Piersol, 1971).   The traditional solution of the problem is the so-called tapering of the data,
i.e. multiplication by a window function changing from zero more smoothly
than the boxcar function.   In our case, however, this is not favored since
we would miss the binary character of the signal.   Therefore the alterna-

tive solution should be chosen, i.e. a convolution of the (complex) spectrum with the Fourier transform of the derived tapering function. As an example, we assume that we want the signal to be tapered with the Hann-window (Fig. C.2), which in the time domain can be described by:

$$\tilde{x}_f(k) = x(k) \cdot w(k)$$

$$= x(k) \cdot \cos^2(\frac{k\pi}{N}) \tag{C.12}$$

We can obtain the same result if we perform a convolution in the frequency domain with $W(m)$:

$$\tilde{\tilde{X}}(m) = X(m) * W(m) \tag{C.13}$$

with

$$W(m) = 1/4(2-3|k|) \qquad\qquad -1 \leq k \leq 1$$

$$= 0 \qquad\qquad\qquad \text{elsewhere} \tag{C.14}$$

Both from equations (C.13 and (C.14) and Fig. C.2 it is clear that the computational effort of this convolution is reasonable. (On the other hand this tapering function is not optimal in terms of leakage reduction).

Further details of the described method as well as a description of an implementation on a microcomputer are described elsewhere (Rompelman et al., (1982).

REFERENCES

C.1 E.J. Bayly, Spectral analysis of pulse frequency modulation in the nervous system. IEEE Transact. on Biomed. Eng., BME-15:257-265 (1968).
C.2 J. S. Bendat and A. G. Piersol, 1971, Random data: analysis and measurement procedures, John Wiley and Sons, New York.
C.3 O. Rompelman, J. B. I. M. Snyijers, C. J. van Spronsen, 1982, The measurement of heart rate variability with the help of a personal computer, IEEE Transact. on Biomed. Eng., BME-29:503-510.

HEART RATE VARIABILITY IN NORMAL ADULTS

R. I. Kitney

Engineering in Medicine Laboratory
Department of Electrical Engineering
Imperial College, London SW7, UK

INTRODUCTION

With the development of Cybernetics, Weiner (1948) showed that there
was considerable potential in the application to the study of biological
systems of techniques of analysis normally employed in the physical
sciences. Within the broad range of physiological oscillations is a subgroup which occurs in physiological systems involved in homeostasis. Such
systems have the potential for oscillatory behavior because their distributed nature allows the existence of significant time delays in reflex
arcs. Physiological systems of this type can be considered as a number of
different elements linked together, typically by neural pathways, to give
the negative feedback necessary for homeostasis. Often such systems behave
as spontaneous oscillators (Hyndman, Kitney and Sayers, 1971), the frequency of oscillation being determined by the characteristics of the
system. A change in these characteristics can be considered to be equivalent to changing the setting of an oscillator so that it takes up a new
and normally stable oscillatory mode. It is possible to envisage the human
body as containing a number of systems which frequently oscillate. There
is also evidence that biological systems which oscillate at frequencies
higher than that consistent with the 24-hour day interact with each other,
e.g. the interaction between the heart rate control and the respiration.

Historically, there have been a number of different theories relating
the nature of biological rhythms. The current consensus appears to be that
biological systems which exhibit oscillations can be divided into autonomous or endogenous systems (i.e. systems which are self-sustaining), which
usually oscillate at frequencies of less than 1 hour, and non-autonomous or
exogenous systems (systems which require external stimulation).

OSCILLATORY SYSTEMS

(a) Autonomous Systems

Systems or phenomena are called autonomous if time (t) does not appear
explicitly in the describing differential equation. The simplest case of
free (autonomous) oscillations is simple harmonic motion, which is
described by the differential equation:

$$\frac{d^2y}{dt^2} + w^2y = 0$$

The solution to this equation is:

$$y = A \cos wt + B \sin wt$$

where A and B are constants and w is the natural frequency of oscillation. In practical terms this type of oscillation is not self-sustaining, because of energy losses.

(b) Self-Sustaining Oscillations

If the energy dissipated per cycle is restored in some unspecified manner from a non-periodic source of energy, the oscillation is still autonomous. In biological terms this type of oscillation would be described as endogenous. The spectrum of endogenous oscillations varies from sinusoidal at one end to relaxation at the other.

The question of self-sustained biological oscillations was discussed by Wever (1965). Wever suggested endogenous oscillations are characterized by the amount of energy exchanged between the oscillator and the environment. At one end of the spectrum such oscillations emanate from small energy transfer systems which exhibit simple harmonic motion, while the other extreme is typified by large energy transfer systems which produce relaxation oscillations.

An alternative approach is to consider the oscillatory behavior of physiological systems in terms of their structure; for example, does oscillatory activity arise from a system in which the nonlinearity is purely due to the limitations of the dynamics of the system, or is the system working within the limits of its response but has within its structure discrete nonlinear elements? Minorsky (1962) discussed nonlinear oscillatory systems of this second type in some detail. An important phenomenon in such systems is "frequency entrainment". When two linear oscillatory systems are coupled but operate at different frequencies, beating occurs. The output of the combined linear systems contains only terms corresponding to the modes of oscillation of the individual systems. However, when the oscillators are nonlinear, the coupling causes the two oscillators to lock into a common frequency when the frequency difference is small. Minorsky described the series of events which occur in a non-linear physical system which is oscillating spontaneously at w_o, when a periodic external stimulus is applied. As the difference between the natural and stimulus frequencies is decreased, a point is reached where although the frequency difference is significant, the system output suddenly consists of only a single dominant component at the stimulus frequency w_s. This phenomenon is called frequency selective entrainment.

Although Minorsky (1962) was primarily discussing physical systems, the principle nevertheless holds for physiological systems. Kitney (1974) showed that it was possible to entrain finger blood flow involved in thermal vasomotor activity by periodic thermal stimulation of the contralateral hand. Research in this area over the last decade has shown that entrainment phenomena in physiological systems are rather more complex than is generally the case with physical systems. In the Minorsky model, there is a defined range of stimulus frequency (symmetrical about w_o) where entrainment occurs. In physiological systems, this range of stable entrainment is still present but is surrounded by other regions of interaction which exhibit more complicated interaction phenomena, e.g. modulation (Kitney et al., 1982), frequency pulling (Linkens, 1979), destructive interference (Davies and Neilson, 1967), chaotic behavior, sub- and ultra-harmonic entrainment.

In the study of physiological systems behavior, for example in a stimulation/response experiment, other spontaneous periodic variations may interfere with the primary synchronization, resulting in an unstable state where a system may fluctuate between stable and unstable entrainment. Figure 1 illustrates an example of the phenomenon using a segment of finger blood flow recording taken during the application of a stable periodic thermal stimulus of ten seconds period. The spectra a-f are sequential Fast-Fourier Transform (FFT) amplitude spectra (256-point data window, with 25% overlap). It is clear from the Figure that although theoretically the response should be constant, in practice the system response fluctuates between stable and unstable entrainment. The next section will consider the theoretical basis of spectral analysis techniques which are frequently employed in time series analysis of physiological data. Two techniques are discussed, the FFT and autoregressive spectral analysis.

SPECTRAL ESTIMATION OF BIOLOGICAL OSCILLATIONS

As illustrated by Figure 1, the analysis of data obtained from physio-logical oscillations often requires that the records are short-duration time series. As a general rule Fourier spectral analysis requires a minimum of approximately five cycles of the fundamental frequency for reasonable resolution (Bergland, 1969). With Fourier methods, the spectral content of the waveform can only be defined at harmonics of the fundamental frequency; hence if a true component lies between two harmonics, its power will be divided.

Autoregressive spectra have a number of important potential advan-tages, the principal among these being that reasonable spectral estimates

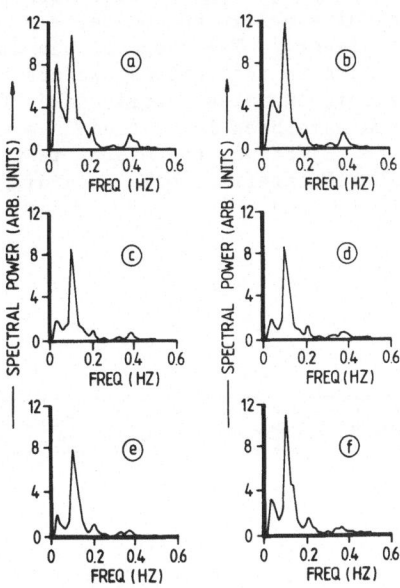

Fig. 1. Example of the entrainment taken from a section of finger blood flow recording during the application of a stable periodic thermal stimulus of ten seconds period. The spectra a-f are sequential FFT amplitude spectra (256-point data window, with 25% overlap).

can be obtained with as little as one cycle of the fundamental frequency (Ulrych, 1972) and the autoregressive spectrum is continuous.

The improvements in spectral estimation which can be obtained from autoregressive methods are associated with the fact that a particular model will be more parsimonious, provided certain criteria are satisfied, than the equivalent Fourier description. The main criterion which is discussed in the literature is that of model order (Ulrych and Bishop, 1975; Kay, 1979; Kay and Marple, 1981). Ulrych and Bishop (1975) suggest that as a rule of thumb the model order can be taken as lying in the range $1/3 \, N < p < 1/2 \, N$, where p is the model order and N the number of points. An alternative approach is to use the Final Prediction Error or Akaike Information Criterion developed by Akaike (1969). A second important factor is sampling rate (Kitney and Giddens, 1982).

ENTRAINMENT PHENOMENA

A number of physiological systems have been identified as exhibiting nonlinear oscillatory interaction phenomena; these include the SA node (Winfree, 1967), the respiratory system (Bradley et al., 1975), synchronization of nonlinear biochemical oscillators (Torre, 1975), coupling in embryonic heart cells (Ypres et al., 1979), and digestive track motility. Although these physiological systems clearly perform different functions, in all cases underlying their dynamic behavior is the concept of synchronization or entrainment. In general the study of such systems has traditionally involved a linear dynamic approach. However, many of the phenomena which have been observed cannot be identified as arising from linear dynamics. An alternative nonlinear approach has therefore been employed. The basic ideas associated with the stable entrainment were discussed in the introductory section of the chapter; entrainment phenomena in biological systems are rather more .complex. Figure 2 illustrates the range of phenomena which can be observed in a biological system as the frequency of an external stimulus is increased from zero to w_o, where w_o is the natural frequency of the system. Associated with the various regions of the Figure are a number of specific phenomena, e.g. nonlinear modulation and frequency pulling (see later). The range of phenomena observed in physiological data in relation to the various sectors of the Figure will be discussed in terms of specific examples largely taken from our own work, although the same phenomena have been identified in a number of other physiological systems. The objective, therefore, is to concentrate on a specific phenomenon of general interest while providing limited background physiology.

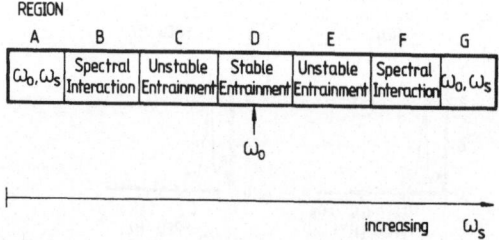

Fig. 2. The range of phenomena which can be observed in a biological system as the frequency of an external stimulus is increased from zero to w_o, where w_o, is the natural frequency of the system (w_s, frequency of external stimulus).

STABLE ENTRAINMENT

Stable entrainment is observed when either a naturally occurring stimulus or an applied stimulus causes the spontaneous oscillations associated with a physiological system to synchronize or entrain. Figure 3 illustrates the types of results which are obtained when finger blood flow is recorded from a photoelectric plethysmogram attached to the small finger of the right hand with and without a 20 second thermal stimulus applied to the left hand for a period of 15 minutes (Kitney, 1974). An examination of the power spectra of these waveforms (Figure 3c) illustrates that under spontaneous conditions the spectrum consists of a number of frequency components spread throughout the thermal range of 0.01-0.06 Hz (Burton and Taylor, 1940). Figure 3d is markedly different and comprises a single large component at the stimulus frequency. Stable entrainment, of which this is an example, is identified by the existence of a stable component at the stimulus frequency. As discussed by Hayashi et al. (1960), stable entrainment is a function of both stimulus amplitude and frequency, i.e. the range of entrainment around the center frequency (w_o) is a nonlinear function of the stimulus amplitude.

COMPUTER MODELLING

Outside the range of stable entrainment the situation becomes more complex. Therefore, in order to investigate these regions of the entrainment diagram, it is often useful to resort to computer modelling of the system being studied. In early studies of nonlinear oscillatory phenomena associated with biological systems, van der Pol oscillator models were

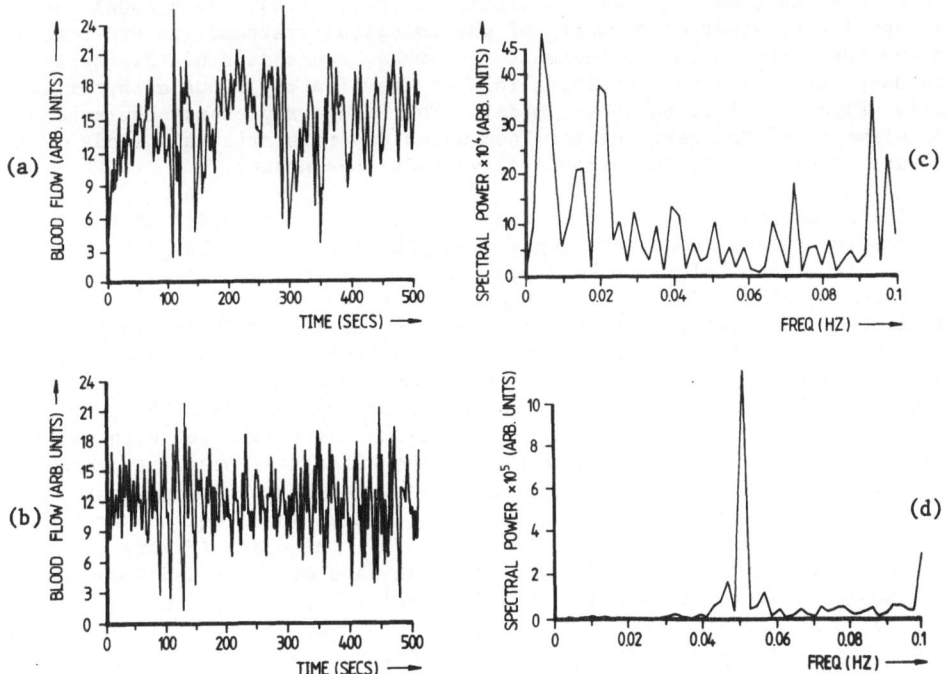

Fig. 3. Types of results which are obtained when finger blood flow is recorded from a photoelectric plethysmogram attached to the small finger of the right hand with (b) and without (a) a 20-second thermal stimulus applied to the left hand for a period of 15 minutes. (c) and (d) are the power spectal density functions of waveforms a and b.

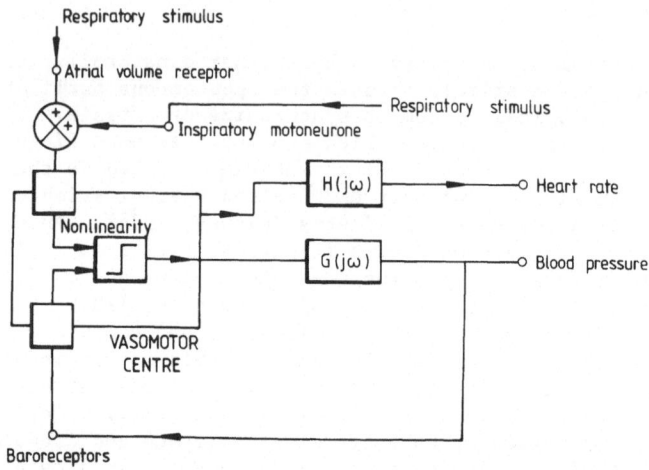

Fig. 4. Block diagram of the computer model used in the study. See text
for details.

often used (Hayashi, 1964; Wever, 1965). However, van der Pol models
suffer from the disadvantage that it is difficult to relate the analytical
results to physiology. An alternative model which contains the essential
elements of a number of physiological systems was introduced by Hyndman et
al. (1971). The basic model consists of a single unity feedback loop and a
forward loop comprising a nonlinear element, a linear filter and a pure
time delay. In order to achieve stable oscillations only the nonlinear
element and the time delay are essential (Kitney, 1979). This model has
been applied to study of a number of physiological systems. In order to
examine the more complex entrainment phenomena, two models of this type
were used, the first was developed to study respiratory sinus arrhythmia
(RSA). Figure 4 illustrates the model. The Figure represents the essential elements of the baroreceptor loop which controls arterial blood
pressure by changes in the peripheral vascular resistance.

The model was developed from the observed characteristics of the
baroreceptor reflex (Scher and Young, 1963; Grodins, 1963; Levison, Barnett
and Jackson, 1966; Spickler, Kezdi and Geller, 1967; Hatakeyama, 1967;
Rosenbaum and Rice, 1968). These papers are cited because they contain
quantitative data relating to the baroreceptor reflex which are suitable
for incorporation into a computer model. The frequency response of the
vasomotor response of the baroreceptor reflex has been studied on several
occasions (Scher and Young, 1963; Grodins, 1963; Hatakeyama, 1967). Similar methods were used whereby the carotid sinus was stimulated with square
wave and sinusoidal pressure pulses while the effects of other baroreceptor
areas were excluded and the response of the systemic arterial pressure, or
the peripheral vascular resistance, was monitored. The frequency response
characteristics were similar in all studies. In the model (Figure 4) the
characteristics of $G(j\omega)$ are derived from the data of Scher and Young by a
least-squares fitting technique. The time delay, or latency, of the vasomotor response has been estimated as between 2.0 and 4.5 seconds (Scher and
Young, 1963; Hatakeyama, 1967). This time delay is distinct from the time
delay of 1.5 seconds between the respiration and its effect on HRV which
has been demonstrated (Selman et al., 1982). More recently it was shown
(Ninomiya, Nisimaru and Irisawa, 1971) that the delay in provoking peripheral sympathetic nerve discharge was only 200 msec., while the neuro-
effector delay was estimated as 2 or 3 seconds. This order of delay
appears to be generally accepted (Kirchheim, 1976). The time delay is,
therefore, predominantly in the periphery and reflects the rate of release

of noradrenaline, the local rate of destruction and removal, and the functional characteristics of arteriolar smooth muscle. The incorporation of a time delay into the linear transfer function creates the conditions for oscillation, but it is only with the addition of the third essential feature of the model - the nonlinear element - that a stable and sustained oscillation can be achieved (Kitney, 1979). The physiological identity of the nonlinear element is not as definite as the time delay. The sigmoid response of individual baroreceptors is nonlinear because of the coupling of the receptor with the arterial wall (Brown, 1980) and because they have a threshold and a saturation level. The nonlinear element in the model represents the central integration in the mid-brain of the afferent baroreceptor activity. While the major part of the nonlinear element is considered to be the centrally integrated effect of all active baroreceptors, it may also lump together other nonlinearities.

FREQUENCY PULLING AND NONLINEAR MODULATION

The results obtained from driving a linear model with an external periodic stimulus show that, as the stimulus amplitude is increased, the self-oscillation and stimulus continue to add and the result is two separate spectral components in the frequency domain. However, using the model described in the previous section, it is possible to show that the situation is fundamentally different with a nonlinear model. If the nonlinear model is set to oscillate at a natural frequency of 0.1 Hz, then the oscillation frequency is mainly, but not entirely, a linear function of the loop time delay (Kitney, 1979). In the simulation results which will be presented, the model is driven with a constant-frequency external stimulus and the amplitude is varied. Figure 5a shows the response of the model before the application of the stimulus. The amplitude spectrum consists of a large component at the stimulus frequency (0.1 Hz) together with its third harmonic; the attenuation of the third harmonic being due to the effect of the low-pass filter in the efferent pathway of the model. Figure 5b illustrates the amplitude spectrum obtained when the stimulus amplitude has been increased to a value large enough to produce full entrainment. The spectrum now comprises a dominant stimulus component at 0.17 Hz together with its third and fifth harmonics. The model has been stably entrained by the stimulus. When stimulus amplitudes between these two extremes are applied, a number of specific phenomena occur.

(a) Frequency Pulling

Frequency pulling was described by Linkens (1977). The phenomenon arises when the amplitude of the stimulus is insufficient to cause full entrainment but is capable of displacing or pulling the natural or self component. Linkens discussed frequency pulling in relation to electromyographic signals recorded from the human gut. We have observed the same phenomenon in the effect of respiration on heart rate. Figures 6a-6c illustrate an example of the response in heart rate to steady state breathing at a constant frequency of 0.17 Hz (ten breaths per min.) for tidal volumes of 1200, 1000 and 800 ml., respectively. The data was recorded from a healthy young male subject (Selman et al., 1982). Figure 6a shows full entrainment with the dominant component in the spectrum at 0.17 Hz. Comparing this result to those of Figures 6b and 6c, it can be seen that the largest component in the spectrum is pulled in frequency as the tidal volume is increased. Similar results occur in the model as shown in the equivalent diagrams (Figures 6d-6f).

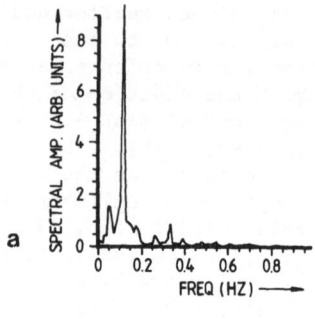

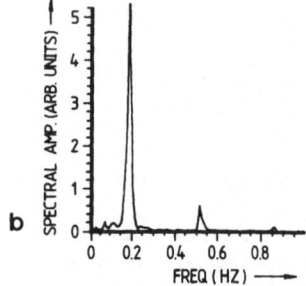

Fig. 5. (a) Shows the response of the computer model before the application of a stimulus. The amplitude spectrum consists of a large component at the stimulus frequency (0.1 Hz) together with its 3rd harmonic. (b) Illustrates the amplitude spectrum obtained when the stimulus amplitude has been increased to a value large enough to produce full entrainment. The spectrum now comprises a dominant stimulus component at 0.17 Hz together with its 3rd and 5th harmonics.

(b) Nonlinear Modulation

In addition to frequency pulling, two modulation phenomena have been identified in the unstable region prior to full entrainment. Figures 7a and 7b are examples of Mode 1 and Mode 2 modulation. The phenomena occur in this order prior to full entrainment. If the stimulus frequency is f_s and the self frequency f_o, Mode 1 modulation produces frequency components at:

$$f_k = f_s + k\Delta f$$

where k = 1, 2, 3, etc. and $f = f_s - f_o$.

Referring to Figure 7a, f_o = 0.08 Hz, f_s = 0.17 Hz, hence if f = 0.09 Hz, the other frequency components occur at, for example, 0.26 and 0.35 Hz.

Mode 1 modulation changes to Mode 2 as the stimulus amplitude increases. It can be seen from the Figure that in Mode 2 modulation the frequency structure of the signal breaks down into clusters of components. The frequency positions of Mode 2 modulation are defined by the relationship:

$$f_k = kf_s \pm \Delta f$$

where the terms of the equation are as previously defined. Hence the frequency components in Figure 7b occur as sidebands around harmonics of the stimulus frequency. Figure 8a is an example of Mode 2 modulation in

90

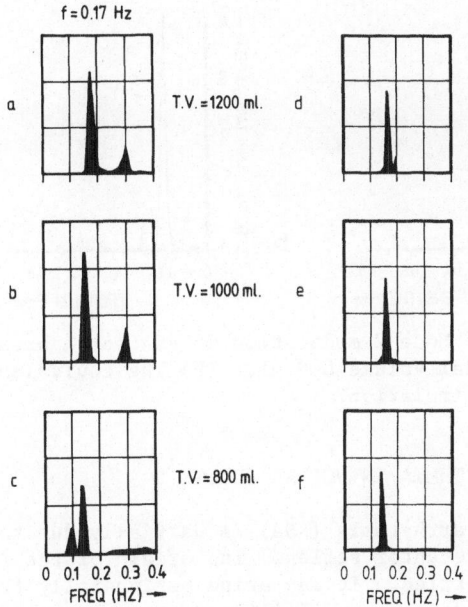

Fig. 6.   a–c illustrate an example of the response in heart rate to steady
          state breathing at a constant frequency of 0.17 Hz (10 breaths per
          min) for tidal volumes of 1200, 1000 and 800 ml., respectively.
          Similar results occur in the model as shown in the equivalent
          diagrams (d, e and f).

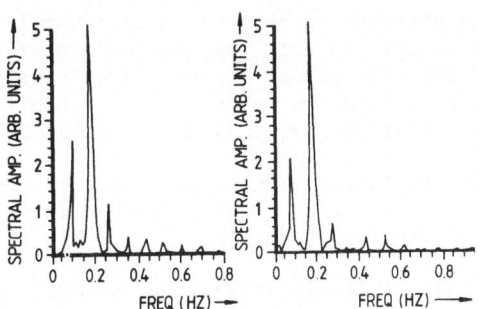

Fig. 7.   Examples of Mode 1 and Mode 2 modulation.

RSA for a breathing frequency of 0.2 Hz, tidal volume 800 ml. Figure 8b is
the equivalent obtained from the computer simulation. Mode 1 and Mode 2
modulations appear to be related in that Mode 2 is a multicarrier version
of Mode 1 with less sidebands. Hence for Mode 1 the signal may be
described by:

$$f(t) = F_o \cos w_s t + F_1 \{\cos(w_s + \Delta w)\, t\}$$
$$+ F_2 \{\cos(w_s + 2\Delta w)\, t\} \text{ etc.}$$

where F_o, F_1, F_2 are amplitude factors which are functions of the system
nonlinearity and low pass filter.

91

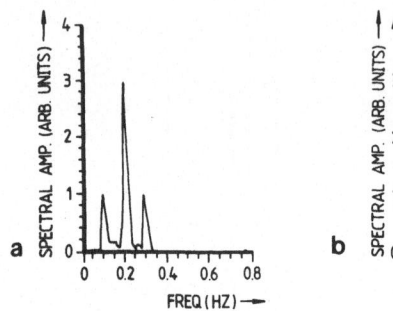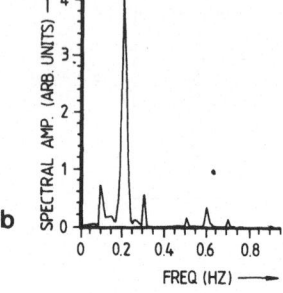

Fig. 8.   (a) Example of Mode 2 modulation in RSA for a breathing frequency
          of 0.2 Hz, tidal volume 800 ml.   (b) The equivalent obtained from
          the computer simulation.

RESPIRATORY SINUS ARRHYTHMIA IN NORMAL ADULTS

     Respiratory sinus arrhythmia (RSA) is partially due to respiratory
modulation of the baroreceptor reflex.   The origin of the respiratory
modulation remains unsettled.   It may arise peripherally from intrathoracic
pressure changes causing increased filling of the heart and stimulation of
thoracic stretch receptors and low-pressure receptors in the atria.   Alternatively, a direct inhibition arising from the central respiratory rhythm
may be the cause.   Indeed, both types of mechanisms might play a role
depending on the experimental circumstances, thus resolving some of the
experimental contradictions discussed in the literature.   Selman et al.
(1982) carried out an experimental study in which the effect of tidal
volume and respiratory frequency on RSA was documented over a wide range of
steady states.   It was shown that the interaction was highly nonlinear;
there was a time delay between respiration and heart rate variability of
about 1.5 seconds; the efferent pathway was almost completely by way of the
vagal branches to the heart.   In this chapter, a hypothesis will be discussed which proposes that RSA can be considered as arising from the interaction of two nonlinear oscillatory systems which exhibit the phenomenon of
frequency entrainment (Minorsky, 1962; Winfree, 1980).   The concept that
physiological systems oscillate as an inherent feature of their control
function has been used to study the human thermoregulatory system (Kitney,
1974; Kitney, 1975).   The nonlinear model described earlier forms the basis
of the computer model of the study of RSA.

     In the original model (Kitney, 1979), the external interacting
stimulus was shown as entering the control loop at point "A" (Figure 4).
This would imply that the external stimulus, in this case respiration, was
sensed by the vasomotor center via baroreceptors.   Such a peripheral modulation (Davies and Neilson, 1967) seems unlikely (Freyschuss and Melcher,
1976), and it is now proposed that atrial pressure receptors transmit
afferent information to the brainstem, or the external stimulus arises in
the brainstem.   The present model, therefore, suggests that the external
stimulus affects the blood pressure control loop at the vasomotor center
(Figure 4).   This is an important change in reconciling the model with
known physiology.

     The effect of atropine in vitrually abolishing RSA justifies the
notion of a single efferent pathway of the vagus to the sino-atrial node
(Selman et al., 1982).

     The control theory analysis of RSA and the entrainment analysis of the
model (Kitney et al., 1982) lead to some important conclusions which will
be used in the detailed comparison of physiological and simulation results.

First, parameter sensitivity trials on the model showed that the oscillation frequency is a function of the time delay round the loop. Second, the similarity between the gain characteristics of the nonlinear element and those of the complete model indicate that the specific entrainment conditions for RSA may primarily be a function of the vasomotor non-linearity. Third, as with other physiological systems, the observed entrainment can be stable or unstable. Consequently, for the nonlinear hypothesis to be correct, both the physiological and simulation results should exhibit the specific phenomena associated with these types of entrainment such as modulation and frequency pulling. These specific phenomena occur in the transition zone between no entrainment and stable entrainment. For the case of nonlinear oscillatory systems, the modulation observed will not be of the simple sum and difference type seen in linear systems. The interaction produces more complicated terms, e.g. the reflection of one component around the other. To recapitulate, frequency pulling occurs when the stimulus is unable to entrain the self component but has sufficient effect to displace or "pull" the frequency of the self component towards the stimulus frequency. Fourth, the amplitude of the RSA response should be a function of the frequency characteristic G(jw) which is effectively a low pass filter.

SIMULATION OF THE EFFECT OF TIDAL VOLUME ON RSA

In order to study the influence of respiration on heart rate in detail, a second, more comprehensive, set of simulations were undertaken. In these, the frequencies of the two oscillators were set, 0.1 Hz for the blood pressure oscillator and 0.25 Hz for the respiratory stimulus. The protocol was designed to cover the entire range of entrainment for these frequencies. Preliminary results established that the entire range could be encompassed by a stimulus amplitude range of 0.1-3.6, unity amplitude corresponding to the amplitude of the unstimulated blood pressure oscillation. For each stimulus amplitude the main oscillator (the baroreceptor loop) was allowed to run freely for 100 seconds and the stimulus switched in for the remainder of the record (412 seconds).

COMPARISON OF THE SIMULATION AND EXPERIMENTAL RESULTS

(a) Modulation and Other Entrainment Phenomena

Figures 9a-9e illustrate the results obtained from the computer simulation of the effect of tidal volume on RSA. Each plot illustrates different observed phenomena. The original set from which these examples are drawn comprises 36 simulations in the range 0.1-3.6, the inter-simulation increment being 0.1 and the stimulus frequency 0.25 Hz (constant).

When the stimulus amplitude is 0.4 (Figure 9a) the stimulus has only a minor effect on the time domain waveform, and is reflected in the amplitude spectrum which comprises the fundamental self component (0.1 Hz) plus its third harmonic. At a stimulus amplitude of 1.3 (Figure 9b) the stimulus is evident in the time domain waveform while its exact effects can be more clearly seen in the spectrum. The self component (0.1 Hz) is produced by modulation of the two main components, i.e. their difference reflected around the stimulus. This phenomenon is more evident in Figure 9c where the stimulus is 1.9. The relative amplitudes of the stimulus and reflected components are now larger in relation to the self component. Of particular interest (Figure 9d) is the existence of the third harmonic of the stimulus at 0.75 Hz and its upper and lower sidebands of 0.9 and 0.6 Hz, respectively. This illustrates that the system is not only capable of harmonic

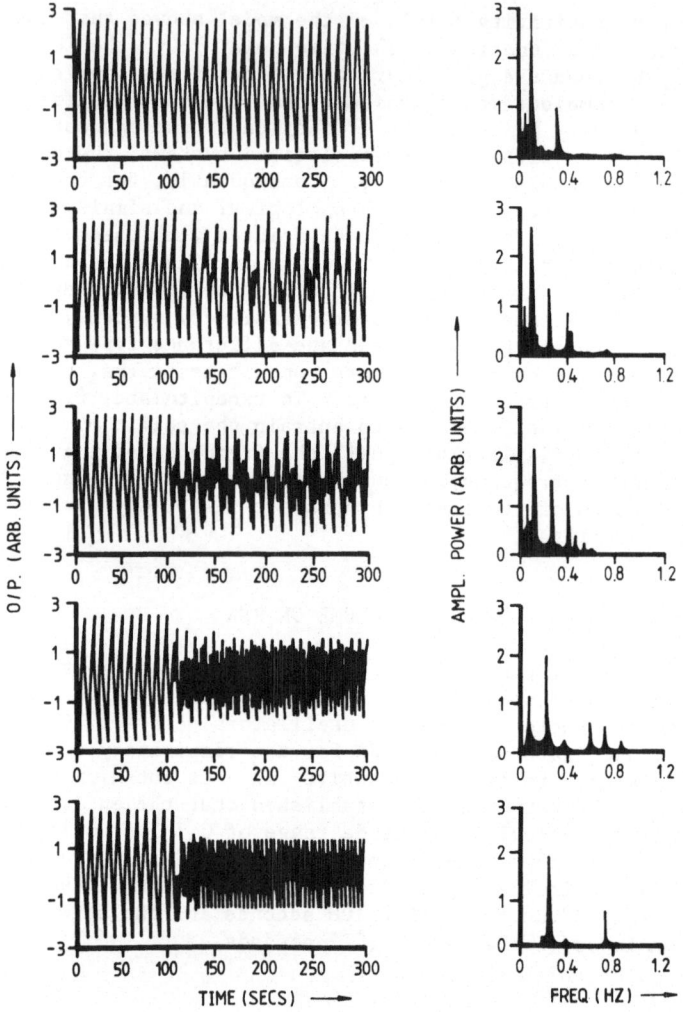

Fig. 9.   Results obtained from the computer simulation of the effect of
          tidal volume on RSA.   Each plot illustrates different observed
          phenomena.   See text for details.   O/P, oscillating peak
          amplitudes in arbitrary units.

entrainment but is also susceptible to modulation.   With a large stimulus
(Figure 9e), the system has completely entrained, there is no evidence of
the self component and its output comprises solely the stimulus together
with its third harmonic.

(b) Comparison of Spectral Maps

     A direct comparison between experimental results and the computer
model can be achieved by calculating a spectral map for the experimental
results and comparing it to the map for the simulation (Figures 10 and 11).
The effect of respiration on heart rate is seen as both a function of
respiratory stimulus amplitude (tidal volume) and frequency.   The central
region of respiratory entrainment of heart rate, i.e. RSA, occurs for
frequencies of breathing at 0.2 and 0.17 Hz, and for tidal volumes at 600
and 1200 ml; the equivalent to this range of tidal volumes for the model is
an input amplitude range of 0.8 to 1.2.

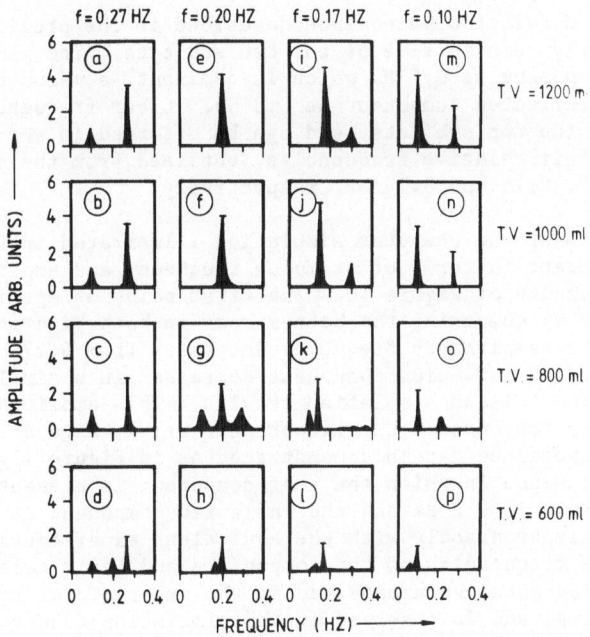

Fig. 10. Amplitude spectra of HRV signals (experimental results) for a range of tidal volumes and frequencies of breathing.

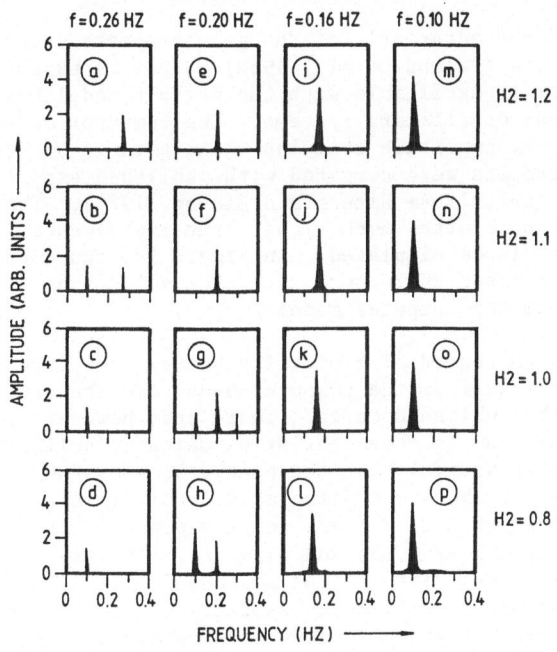

Fig. 11. Simulation results for the range covered by the experimental data of Figure 10.

In the experimental data (Figure 10), for tidal volumes of 1000–1200 ml. and frequencies of 0.27–0.17 Hz., there is evidence of a strong respiratory component in the HRV signals. Rows beginning b and d illustrate the transition from non-entrainment to entrainment. For example, comparing Figures 10f and 10h, there is a factor of two difference in the magnitude in the respiratory effect on the HRV. Figure 10g is a good

95

example of the modulation phenomenon described in the previous section, which was clearly seen in five of the ten subjects. The plot comprises a respiratory component at 0.2 Hz which is dominant, a vasomotor component at 0.1 Hz, and a reflected component at 0.3 Hz. Clear frequency pulling was seen in six of the ten subjects, and can be observed in the Figures 10i, 10j and 10k; their relative frequencies (obtained from the original larger plots) are 0.17, 0.16 and 0.14 Hz, respectively.

The results of the computer simulation illustrated in Figure 11 are directly equivalent in terms of stimulus frequency and amplitude to the experimental results of Figure 10. The first point of specific similarity can be observed by comparing the bottom rows in both Figures. It can be seen that as the respiratory frequency decreases from 0.27 Hz to 0.1 Hz, the amplitude of the stimulus component decreases in a similar manner for both the experimental and simulation results. This amplitude change is due to the frequency response of the linear part $G(jw)$, Figure 1. Further specific correspondence can be demonstrated as in Figure 11g which shows a modulation phenomenon in which the self component is present at 0.1 Hz, the stimulus component at 0.2 Hz and the reflected component at 0.3 Hz. This result agrees almost exactly with the equivalent experimental results both in terms of the frequencies of the components and their relative magnitudes. The third phenomenon observed in the experimental results was frequency pulling, and is observed in the simulation results at the same frequency (0.16 Hz), by comparing Figure 11l and 11j; the frequencies are 0.14 Hz and 0.16 Hz, respectively.

(c) Comparison of Input-Output Characteristics

The M-shaped characteristic of the gain response demonstrated in the experimental results (Selman et al., 1982) cannot be explained by a linear control system but is explicable with the present model based on the interaction of nonlinear oscillatory systems. The computer model was set for a constant, mid-range, amplitude stimulus while a range of frequencies was simulated. The results were compared with published experimental data (Angelone and Coulter, 1964; Hirsch and Bishop, 1981). The resolution of computer simulation is often much higher than experimental results as many intermediate data can be simulated. In Figure 12, the dotted line shows the unsmoothed published characteristic. The solid line is the characteristic obtained from the computer model.

There is a high degree of similarity between the overall shape of the characteristic derived from the computer model and the true characteristic which underlies the published curve. There are, however, four specific phenomena contained in the characteristics which underline the significance of the match. These are (a) that the peak values of the experimental and model characteristics, both occurring at 0.1 Hz; (b) the second peak in the model characteristic at 0.15 Hz; and (c) the peaks in the experimental and model data at 0.33, 0.5 and 0.35 and 0.54, respectively. All these phenomena are specifically explained by the hypothesis that RSA results from the interaction of nonlinear oscillatory systems. The peaks at 0.1 Hz are due to the self component of the baroreceptor loop and the other peaks are explicable as examples of harmonic entrainment, 3/2 (the 0.15 Hz peak), a third harmonic (the 0.33 and 0.35 Hz peaks) and a fifth harmonic (the 0.5 and 0.55 Hz peaks).

DISCUSSION

In the previous experimental study (Selman et al., 1982), it was shown that the effect of respiration on heart rate was highly nonlinear. These results suggest inadequacies of earlier models (Clynes, 1960; Womack,

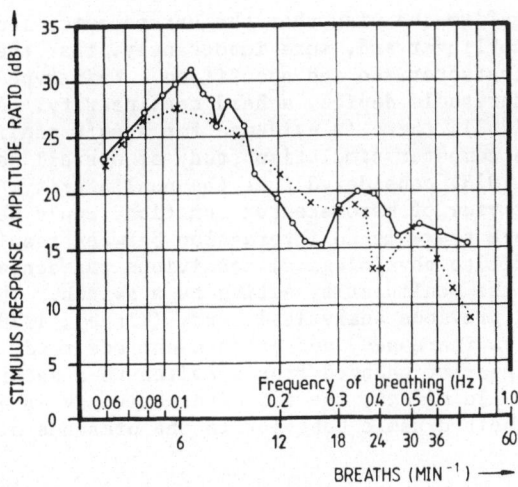

Fig. 12. Stimulus/response characteristics for experimental (Angelone and Coulter, 1964) and simulation data. Dashed characteristic experimental data; solid line-experimental results.

1971), which could only be applied over a restricted range of function. Based on the experimental findings, a hypothesis is proposed that suggested that RSA could be considered as the interaction of two nonlinear systems exhibiting frequency entrainment. The main oscillator in the models consists of the vasomotor response of the baroreceptor loop, with respiration acting as the second oscillator, the external stimulus. As with all computer models of physiological systems, identification of the elements of the system is incomplete, but the model outlined in this study is consistent not only with our own experimental data (Selman et al., 1982) but also with previous studies of RSA (Angelone and Coulter, 1969; Eckberg, 1980; Melcher, 1980). There would appear to be general agreement that RSA results from central reflex interaction. There is, however, no evidence which would distinguish between the respiratory modulation of the sensitivity of the baroreflex being due to irradiation from the respiratory motoneurones or due to a central input from afferents arising from receptors, possibly in the heart or lungs. The model allows for both options, even that each may contribute to the respiratory stimulus to the baroreflex loop.

The comparison between the results of the experimental data and the computer simulation shows good general agreement. More convincing with regard to the validity of the model is the demonstration that specific phenomena, modulation and frequency pulling which would occur from the interaction of two nonlinear oscillatory systems exhibiting frequency entrainment (Davies and Nielson, 1967; Linkens, 1979b), can be found in the experimental data. The modulation and frequency pulling observed in both experiments and simulation studies occur in the unstable transition zone between non-entrainment and entrainment. As a result, it would not be expected that they would be seen in all subjects. Nor would they be expected to occur at the same frequency in all individuals. However, most subjects exhibited one phenomenon and a number showed both. There is also close agreement between the input-output characteristics of the computer simulation and the unsmoothed experimental data of Angelone and Coulter (1964). In both cases the primary peak of 0.1 Hz and both other characteristics showed third and fifth harmonic entrainment at approximately 0.3 Hz and 0.5 Hz.

The results confirm the view that the baroreceptor loop being considered is highly nonlinear and, more importantly, that the nonlinearity may be adequately characterized and quantified. This type of response is consistent with a threshold device, a hard nonlinearity. Alternatively (Scher and Young, 1963), there is evidence for a soft nonlinearity of the saturation type. A computer simulation study of overall cardiovascular function (Hyndman, 1973) considered that the nonlinearity, which is implicit in current view of baroreceptor function, could be altered by varying sigma. Where there is no interaction between respiration and heart rate, the closest fit to physiological conditions was achieved if sigma was zero, that is with the nonlinearity acting as a switch. The results of the present study and a previous analytical study (Kitney, 1979) showed that as the external stimulus increased, and entrainment occurred, the dynamic nature of the nonlinearity changed from a switch to a saturation element, a sigmoidal response. In effect, the two alternative types of nonlinearity merge in terms of their dynamic behavior in the presence of an external stimulus.

The three principle elements of the model influence it in different ways. The character of the nonlinearity determines the specific nature of the entrainment with regard to the gain characteristics and its range. The time delay, principally related to the neuro-effector delay, determines the oscillation frequency and the characteristics of the vascular resistance; the linear transfer function, the amplitude of the response.

The concordance achieved between the experimental and simulated results supports strongly the proposed nonlinear hypothesis. Conventional physiological analysis tends to simplify and linearize the system under study (Garfinkel, 1980), but this is almost certainly inappropriate with complex biological systems. Nonlinear analysis with computer simulation permits the effective study of complicated feedback systems without excessive simplification.

REFERENCES

Akaike, H., 1969, Fitting autoregressive models for prediction, Ann. Inst. of Statis. Math., 21:243-247.
Angelone, A., and Coulter, N. A., 1964, Respiratory sinus arrhythmia: a frequency dependent phenomenon, J. Appl. Physiol., 19:479-482.
Bergland, G. D., 1969, A guided tour of the fast Fourier transforms, IEEE Spectrum, 6:41-52.
Bradley, G. W., Euler, C. von, Martilla, I., and Roos, B., 1975, Biol. Cybernetics, 19:105.
Brown, A. M., 1980, Receptors under pressure: an update on baroreceptros, Circ. Res., 46:1-10.
Burton, A. C., and Taylor, D., 1940, A study of the adjustment of peripheral vascular tone to the requirements of body temperature, Am. J. Physiol., 129:565-577.
Clynes, M., 1960, Respiratory sinus arrhythmia: laws derived from computer simulation, J. Appl. Physiol., 15:863-874.
Davies, C. T. M., and Neilson, J. M. M., 1967, Sinus arrhythmia in man at rest, J. Appl. Physiol., 22:947-955.
Freyschuss, U., and Melcher, A., 1976, Respiratory sinus arrhythmia in man: relation to cardiovascular pressures, Scand. J. Clin. Invest., 36:221-229.
Grodins, F., 1963, Control theory and biological systems, Columbia Univ. Press, NY.
Hayashi, C., 1964, Nonlinear oscillations in physical systems, McGraw Hill, New York.

Hayashi, C., Shibayama, H., and Nishikawa, Y., 1960, Frequency entrainment in a self-oscillatory system with external force, IRE Trans. Circuit Theory, 413–422.

Hatakegama, I., 1967, Analysis of the baroreceptor control of the circulation, in: "The Physical Basis of Circualtory Transport: Regulation and Exchange", A. C. Guyton and E. B. Reeve, eds., Pub. Saunders.

Hirsh, J. A., and Bishop, B., 1981, Respiratory sinus arrhythmia in humans: how breathing pattern modulates heart rate, Am. J. Physiol., 241: H620–629.

Hyndman, B. W., Kitney, R. I., and Sayers, B. McA., 1971, Spontaneous rhythms in physiological control systems, Nature, 233:339–341.

Kay, S. M., 1979, The effects of noise on the autoregressive spectral estimator, IEEE Trans.. ASSP., 5:478–485.

Kircheim, H. R., 1976, Baroreceptor reflexes, Physiol. Rev., 56:100–176.

Kitney, R. I., 1974, The analysis and simulation of the human thermoregulator control system, Medical & Biological Engineering, Jan. 57–65.

Kitney, R. I., 1975, An analysis of the nonlinear behavior of the human thermal control system, J. Theoretical Biol., 52:231–248.

Kitney, R. I., 1979, A nonlinear model for studying oscillations in the blood pressure control system, J. Biomedical Engineering, 1:89–99.

Kitney, R. I., and Giddens, D. P., 1982, Extraction and characterization of underlying velocity waveforms in post stenotic flow, IEE Proc., 129:651–662.

Kitney, R. I., Linkens, D. A., Selman, A. C., and McDonald, A. H., 1982, The interaction between heart rate and respiration: Part 2 – nonlinear analysis on computer modelling, Automedica, 4:141–153.

Levison, W. H., Barnet, G. O., and Jackson, W. D., 1966, Nonlinear analysis of baroreceptor reflex system, Circ. Res., 18:673.

Linkens, D. A., 1977, The stability of entrainment conditions for RLC coupled van der Pol Oscillators used as a model for intestinal electrical rhythms, Bull. Math. Biol., 39:359–372.

Melcher, A., 1980, Carotid baroreflex heart rate control during the active and the assisted breathing cycle in man, Acta. Physiol. Scand., 108:165–171.

Minorsky, N., 1962, Nonlinear Oscillations, Van Nostrand, London and New York.

Ninomiya, I., Nisimaru, N., and Irisawa, H., 1971, Sympathetic nerve activity to the spleen, kidney and heart in response to baroreceptor input, Am. J. Physiol., 221:1346–1351.

Rosenbaum, M., and Rice, D., 1968, Frequency response characteristics of the vascular resistance vessels, Am. J. Physiol., 315:1397.

Scher, A. M., and Young, A. C., 1970, Reflex carotid sinus regulation of heart rate unanaesthetized dogs, Am. J. Physiol., 218:780–789.

Selman, A. C., McDonald, A. H., Kitney, R. I., and Linkens, D. A., 1982, The interaction between heart rate and respiration: Part 1 – Experimental studies in man, Automedica, 4:131–139.

Spickler, J. W., Kezdi, P., and Geller, E., 1967, Transfer characteristics of the carotid sinus pressure control system, in: "Baroreceptors and Hypertension", P. Kedzi, ed., Pergamon Press, Oxford.

Torre, V., 1975, Synchronization of nonlinear biochemical oscillators coupled by diffusion, Biol. Cybernetics, 17:137–144.

Ulrych, T. J., 1972, Maximum entropy power spectrum of truncated sinusoids, J. Geophys. Res., 77:1396–1400.

Ulrych, T. F., and Bishop, T. N., 1975, Maximum entropy spectral analysis and autoregressive decomposition, Rev. Geophys. and Space Physics., 13:138–300.

Weiner, N., 1948, Cybernetics, J. Wiley & Sons, New York.

Wever, R., 1965, in: "Circadian Clocks", J. Aschoff, ed., North Holland, Amsterdam.

Winfree, A. T., 1980, The geometry of biological time, Van Nostrand, Amsterdam.

Womack, B. F., 1971, The analysis of respiratory sinus arrhythmia using spectral analysis methods, IEEE Trans. Bio-med Eng., BME-18 162:399-409.

Ypres, D. L., Clapham, D. E., and De Haan, R. L., 1979, Development of electrical coupling and action potential synchrony between paired aggregates of embryonic heart cells, Membrane Biol., 51:75-96.

RESPIRATORY SINUS ARRHYTHMIA: PHYSIOLOGICAL BASIS,

QUANTITATIVE METHODS, AND CLINICAL IMPLICATIONS*

Stephen W. Porges

Department of Psychology
University of Illinois at Urbana-Champaign

Of the many observable physiological oscillations, the oscillations in
the heart rate pattern associated with respiration (i.e. respiratory sinus
arrhythmia) are the most relevant to psychophysiological research. The use
of respiratory sinus arrhythmia in psychophysiological research may be
justified by the facts that: (1) neurophysiology justifies the measurement
of the amplitude of respiratory sinus arrhythmia as an index of cardiac
vagal tone; (2) the amplitude of respiratory sinus arrhythmia indexes
general central nervous system status; and (3) the changing amplitude of
respiratory sinus arrhythmia parallels psychological constructs often used
in psychophysiological paradigms such as sustained attention and stress.

Although respiratory sinus arrhythmia has been a well documented
phenomenon for about 100 years, it has only recently become the focus of
psychophysiological research. The Chapter will discuss three points: (1)
the physiological basis justifying the use of the amplitude of respiratory
sinus arrhythmia as a measure of cardiac vagal tone; (2) a description of a
unique quantitative approach to accurately extract the amplitude of respiratory sinus arrhythmia from the complex heart rate pattern; and (3) the
sensitivity of the amplitude of respiratory sinus arrhythmia to central
nervous system status.

REASONS FOR LIMITED RESEARCH ON RESPIRATORY SINUS ARRHYTHMIA

Respiratory sinus arrhythmia is one of many oscillations which are
manifested in the heart rate pattern. It is, however, one of the few

* Preparation of this manuscript and portions of the research described
  have been supported, in part, by Research Scientist Development Award
  K02-MH-0054 from the National Institute of Mental Health and research
  grant HD 15968 from the National Institutes of Health. The contributions
  of Dr. Robert E. Bohrer on the development of the time-series methods
  described in this Chapter are gratefully acknowledged. Present address
  is Institute for Child Study/Department of Human Development, University
  of Maryland, College Park, Maryland 20742.

physiological oscillations which may be directly linked to a specific physiological mechanism. It is possible to provide empirical evidence that the amplitude of respiratory sinus arrhythmia accurately maps into the efferent influence of the vagus on the heart. In surveying the literature in psychophysiology and cardiovascular physiology, the study of respiratory sinus arrhythmia has been neglected.

Respiratory-cardiac interactions are seldom discussed on either a functional or anatomical level. Although texts on the neuroanatomy of the autonomic nervous system describe the importance of the vagus in the maintenance of respiratory and cardiac function, there is seldom any discussion of the interaction of these two systems. Reasons for this functional dichotomy have been determined, in part, by the traditional distinction in physiology between the respiratory and the cardiac systems. This is confounded by the focus on the structural components of anatomy (i.e. morphology) rather than on the functional aspects. Respiratory sinus arrhythmia is a functional manifestation of the interaction between respiratory and cardiac control systems neuroanatomically located in the brainstem. Physiological theories have not emphasized the mechanisms and manifestations of respiratory-cardiac rate interactions.

The research preparations used by cardiovascular physiologists tend to involve drug treatments, anesthesia, and other manipulations which depress the central nervous system mechanisms which mediate the respiratory-cardiac interactions. Thus, the basic research preparations used by cardiovascular physiologists markedly attenuate the amplitude of respiratory sinus arrhythmia and other spontaneous oscillations in the heart period pattern.

The methods of measurement have not provided the precision to detect small deviations in heart period. In many instances the magnitude of heart period changes which characterize respiratory sinus arrhythmia is small. The amplitude of respiratory sinus arrhythmia may at times be only a few msec. The ability to observe these small changes are a function of the sensitivity of the recording devices which evaluate the interbeat intervals. If the interbeat intervals are not timed to the nearest msec, the ability to quantify and evaluate individual differences and situational influences on the amplitude of respiratory sinus arrhythmia will be greatly compromised. Today, modern computers are able to accurately measure slight changes in sequential heart periods which would have been imperceptible from polygraph recordings or with the method of ausculation used in clinical practice.

Observations derived from new technologies do not always conform to the traditions of a research area. In the past, the study of small amplitude oscillations in the heart period pattern was not a valid research question. Even today, many cardiovascular physiologists and psychophysiologists contend that the central nervous system has negligible impact on heart rate. Given the methods and experimental procedures that these scientists employ, such conclusions are consistent with their observed data.

The view that the heart period reflects solely the metabolic needs of the organism evolved during the years prior to the advent of the new computer and statistical technologies. Similarly, theoretical constructs, such as homeostasis, instead of emphasizing the range of plasticity of the heart period response pattern, emphasized the notion of a "set-point" or a constant level. These views contributed to a belief that the heart period pattern reflected the "vegetative" state of the organism instead of mapping directly into the neural control systems mediated by the central nervous system. Thus, most physiologists and psychophysiologists have not found compelling reasons to study periodic heart period activity.

It is generally accepted by those who study the heart period rhythmicity (e.g. Sayers, 1973; Chess, Tam, and Calaresu, 1975; Kitney and Rompelman, 1980; Akselrod, Gordon, Ubel, Shannon, Barger, and Cohen, 1981; Porges, McCabe, and Yongue, 1982) that there are at least two periodic processes encoded in the heart period pattern: a fast oscillation at the dominant respiratory frequency (i.e. respiratory sinus arrhythmia); and a slower oscillation with a periodicity of approximately 10 to 15 seconds a cycle. The slower oscillation has been implicated in blood pressure control and hypothesized to be associated with the duration of the baro-receptor feedback loop (see Kitney, Byrne, Edmonds, Watkins, and Roberts, 1982) and has been labeled the Traube-Hering-Mayer wave. The literature on the Traube-Hering-Mayer wave is scant, and, in particular, there is little experimental evidence demonstrating its mediating mechanisms.

Once the oscillations in heart period are observed, there are two questions that need to be addressed: (1) what are the physiological mechan-isms mediating the oscillations; and (2) is the periodic process sensitive to physiological and behavioral state. Since, at present, the mechanisms underlying the Traube-Hering-Mayer wave are unknown and the emphasis of this volume is on cardiovascular-respiratory interactions, this Chapter will focus on respiratory sinus arrhythmia.

Respiratory sinus arrhythmia was first described by Ludwig in 1847 (see Anrep, Pascual, and Rossler, 1936a). One of the earliest references to respiratory sinus arrhythmia in psychology may be found in Wundt's (1902) classic Principles of Physiological Psychology. Wundt stated that "...the movements of the lungs: their inflation accelerates, their collapse reduces the frequency of heart beat. The respiratory movements are there-fore regularly accompanied by fluctuations of the pulse, whose rapidity increases in inspiration and decreases in expiration".

The functional relation between the amplitude of respiratory sinus arrhythmia and cardiac vagal function was clearly stated by H. E. Hering (1910). Hering reported that breathing provided a functional test of the vagal control of the heart. Hering stated that "... it is known with breathing that a demonstrable lowering of heart rate ... is indicative of the function of the vagi".

A relation between vagal tone and behavior was proposed by Eppinger and Hess (1915). They were, perhaps, the first to relate the construct of vagal tone to the amplitude of respiratory sinus arrhythmia. They noted that "... clinical facts, such as respiratory arrhythmia, habitual brady-cardia, etc., have furnished the means of drawing our attention to the variations in the tonus of the vagal system in man". Subsequently, Anrep, Pascual, and Rossler (1936a, 1936b) examined respiratory influences on the heart in detail.

Thus, the scientific literature published over 70 years ago supports three of the major points of this Chapter: (1) that respiratory sinus arrhythmia is mediated by the vagus; (2) that the amplitude of respiratory sinus arrhythmia is related to the functional status of the cardiac vagi (i.e. cardiac vagal tone); and (3) that an individual with pronounced respiratory sinus arrhythmia has specific behavioral characteristics.

It has been proposed that respiration, either by a central mechanism or via a peripheral feedback loop to medullary areas, phasically inhibits, or "gates" the source nuclei of the vagal cardio-inhibitory fibers (Lopes and Palmer, 1976). Although the concept of a respiratory "gate" (i.e. either on or off) on vagal influences to the heart is not universally accepted, it has been established that respiration does influence phasic modulation of vagal influences to the heart; maximal inhibition of vagal efferent output occurs during the mid to late inspiratory phase and maximal vagal efferent output occurs during the expiratory phase.

Recordings from cardiac vagal efferents have indicated that firing in these fibers is inhibited during inspiration and released from inhibition during expiration (Iriuchjima and Kumada, 1964; Jewett, 1964; Katona, Poitras, Barnet, and Terry, 1970; Kunze, 1971). Moreover, during expiration, baroreceptor and chemoreceptor stimuli elicit a prompt bradycardia whereas during inspiration these responses are blocked or attenuated (Angell-James and Daly, 1978; Davidson, Goldner, and McCloskey, 1976; Davis, McCloskey, and Potter, 1977; Haymet and McCloskey, 1975; Lopes and Palmer, 1976).

Recent research on neural pathways of vagal cardio-inhibitory neurons has demonstrated that the vagal cardio-inhibitory neurons show a respiratory-related pattern of discharge with the primary efferent action on the heart occurring during expiration. This has been demonstrated in the cat (Gilbey, Jordan, Richter, and Spyer, 1983) and in the rabbit (Jordan, Khalid, Schneiderman, and Spyer, 1982). Data from electrophysiological studies have been so consistent that functional properties including bradycardia to neural stimulation, pulse rhythm, and firing primarily during expiration have been used to determine when a neuron is a vagal cardio-inhibitory neuron (Jordan et al., 1982).

Given the above characteristics of vagal cardio-inhibitory neurons, a strong argument may be made that quantification of the amplitude of respiratory sinus arrhythmia provides an accurate index of cardiac vagal tone. Since the vagal cardio-inhibitory neurons, by definition, slow the heart rate and exhibit a respiratory frequency, the impact on heart rate should be manifest as a slowing of heart rate during the expiratory phase of respiration. The greater the vagal efferent output to the heart, the greater the slowing of heart rate during expiration. Thus, respiratory sinus arrhythmia is a peripheral manifestation of the influence of the vagal cardio-inhibitory neurons on the heart (i.e. cardiac vagal tone).

To further establish that the amplitude of respiratory sinus arrhythmia is a sensitive estimate of vagal tone (as first shown by Katona and Jih, 1975), we conducted a series of studies in which vagal activity was manipulated with pharmacological treatments and electrical stimulation. In our research we label the amplitude of respiratory sinus arrhythmia, $\hat{V}$, to emphasize that it is an estimate of vagal tone. Our research demonstrated that stimulation of the aortic depressor nerve in the rabbit increased the amplitude of respiratory sinus arrhythmia (McCabe, Yongue, Porges, and Ackles, 1984). Stimulation of the aortic depressor nerve produces a baroreceptor reflex characterized by increased vagal inhibitory action on the heart. Vagal blockade with atropine removed the effect. Propranolol, a beta-adrenergic blocker, did not alter the magnitude of the evoked increase in respiratory sinus arrhythmia. Respiratory sinus arrhythmia was evaluated during manipulations of the baroreceptor reflex in anesthetized cats (McCabe, Yongue, Ackles, and Porges, 1985). Hypertension, induced via phenylephrine infusion was used to increase vagal tone. Hypotension, induced by infusion of nitroprusside was used to inhibit vagal tone. The manipulations effectively produced state changes in blood pressure and reflexively influenced the cardio-inhibitory influence on the heart (i.e. vagal tone). Hypertension produced an increase in respiratory sinus arrhythmia amplitude. Hypotension produced a decrease in respiratory sinus arrhythmia amplitude. Specific autonomic contributions were assessed with administration of practolol (a beta-adrenergic blocker) and atropine.

104

Although the above studies were conducted in anesthetized preparations, we also have conducted research with alert and moving preparations. In a study with rats, phenylephrine increased, atropine
abolished, and saline had no effect on the amplitude of respiratory sinus
arrhythmia (Yongue et al., 1982).

We have evaluated the amplitude of respiratory sinus arrhythmia in
conscious human adults during various doses of atropine sulfate (Dellinger
and Porges, 1984). The atropine manipulation blocks vagal efferent
activity and was used as an attempt to validate the use of the amplitude of
respiratory sinus arrhythmia as an index of cardiac vagal tone in conscious
human adults. In most cardiovascular research with atropine, the change in
heart period in response to the atropine is used as the criterion measure
of vagal tone. If atropine produces a large decrease in heart period, it
is assumed that vagal tone is high. If atropine does not change heart
period or decreases it slightly, then it is assumed that the vagal tone is
low. Since respiratory sinus arrhythmia reflects the dynamic interaction
between respiration and the heart, two other variables were evaluated: (1)
the weighted coherence (Cw) between heart period and respiration (Porges et
al., 1980); and (2) respiration frequency. These variables were selected
because the weighted coherence has been hypothesized by the author (Porges,
1976) as an index of central parasympathetic or cholinergic control, and
respiration has been empirically related to the amplitude of respiratory
sinus arrhythmia (Grossman et al., 1984; Hirsch and Bishop, 1981).

Five doses of atropine sulfate were used (0.0 mg/75 kg, 0.5 mg/75 kg,
1.0 mg/75 kg, 2.0 mg/75 kg, 4.0 mg/75 kg). The data demonstrated that the
vagal blockade was monotonically manifested in the amplitude of respiratory
sinus arrhythmia. The sensitivity of the amplitude of respiratory sinus
arrhythmia to the atropine manipulation was compared with heart period.
This comparison was conducted on two levels. First, the changes as a
function of drug dose were tested with an analysis of variance. Second,
the magnitude of the treatment effect was calculated for each dose in
contrast with the 0.0 mg/75 kg control treatment. The magnitude of the
treatment effect evaluates the amount of variance of the dependent variable
which may be accounted for by any specific effect or interaction. Thus, if
the respiratory sinus arrhythmia is more sensitive to vagal blockade than
heart period, a higher percentage of the variance would be accounted for by
the treatment effect for the various atropine contrasts.

As illustrated in Figure 1, heart period exhibited a paradoxical
effect with the low dose of atropine, while the amplitude of respiratory
sinus arrhythmia (i.e. $\hat{V}$) was unaffected. The paradoxical effect of low
doses of atropine on heart period is well-known and assumed to be related
to the differential effect of atropine on peripheral and central sites.
Thus, although both heart period and amplitude of respiratory sinus
arrhythmia are significantly influenced by atropine, the amplitude of
respiratory sinus arrhythmia is not paradoxically increased with low doses
of atropine and is monotonically attenuated with higher doses. When the
magnitude of treatment effects on heart period and the amplitude of respiratory sinus arrhythmia (i.e. $\hat{V}$) are compared, as illustrated in Figure 2,
the treatment effects consistently account for a higher percent of the
variance of $\hat{V}$.

The weighted coherence was also sensitive to the atropine manipulations. However, as illustrated in Figure 1, the direction of the
response was not predicted by the hypothesis that the weighted coherence is
a manifestation of central parasympathetic tone (Porges, 1976). With the
exception of the low dose which decreased the weighted coherence below the
control level, the weighted coherence monotonically increased with increasing doses of atropine. However, when the magnitude of treatment effects on

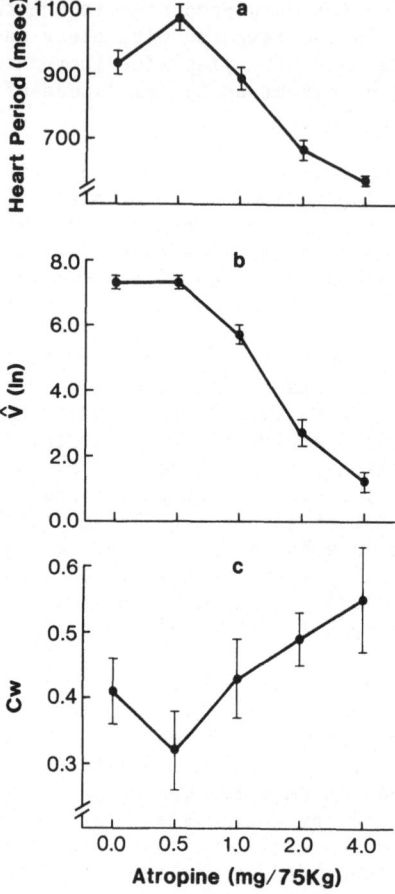

Fig. 1. (a) Heart period as a function of atropine sulfate. (b) The amplitude of respiratory sinus arrhythmia ($\hat{V}$) as a function of atropine sulfate. (c) The weighted coherence (Cw) as a function of atropine sulfate.

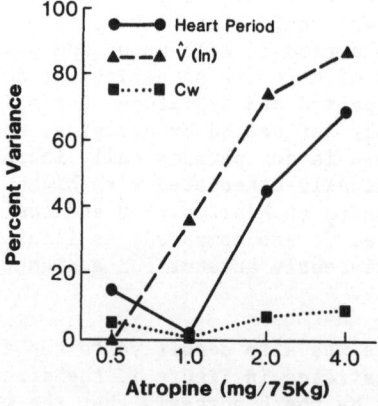

Fig. 2. The magnitude of treatment effects for heart period, $\hat{V}$, and Cw. Percent of variance was calculated from the analysis of variance summary tables for each contrast with the control condition (i.e. SS DOSE/SS TOTAL).

Cw are evaluated, the effects are very small relative to the robust influences on heart period and $\bar{V}$. Respiration frequency was unaffected by
atropine. Even on an individual difference level, the frequency of spontaneous breathing tended not to be related to the amplitude of respiratory
sinus arrhythmia under atropine.

The Dellinger and Porges study clearly demonstrated that: (1) the
amplitude of respiratory sinus arrhythmia was extremely sensitive to
manipulations of cardiac vagal tone; (2) the amplitude of respiratory sinus
arrhythmia may be more sensitive to vagalytic manipulations than heart
period; (3) the changes in amplitude of respiratory sinus arrhythmia under
atropine were independent of changes in respiratory frequency; and (4) the
weighted coherence may be sensitive to neurophysiological mechanisms which
do not directly map into the construct of central or peripheral vagal tone.

In summary, the amplitude of respiratory sinus arrhythmia is physiologically determined by the modulation of vagal efferents to the heart.
Based upon the above physiological arguments and empirical data, it appears
justified to suggest that the amplitude of respiratory sinus arrhythmia may
be an important criterion variable of cardiac vagal tone.

METHODS OF QUANTIFICATION

a. Sampling Heart Period as a Point Process

Many physiological processes are, by their nature, events which may be
characterized as point processes (i.e. categorized as "occurring" or "not
occurring"). For example, the beating of the heart may be operationalized
as a point process detected by the occurrence of the R-wave. Similarly,
single-unit activity in the central nervous system is characterized by
"spikes" and "inter-spike intervals". Although there are methods for
performing spectral analysis on the "interval" characteristic of point
processes (e.g. Bartlett, 1966), these methods are not applicable for the
study of heart period patterns. The Barlett method precludes the application of time domain filters and assumes a constant baselevel. Since time
domain filters are needed to detrend the heart period data, it is necessary
to sample heart period at equal time intervals.

Point processes create a statistical problem when attempts are made to
sample point processes at equal time intervals (e.g. second by second).
Time series texts (e.g. Gottman, 1981) deal virtually exclusively with
equal time sampling of continuous processes. Although this is not problematic for many physiological processes (e.g. respiration, EEG, and electrodermal activity), it is a quantitative problem for all cardiovascular
events which are dependent upon the beating of the heart. For example,
although blood pressure changes are time locked to the beating of the
heart, is it legitimate to view blood pressure as a continuous process and
sample at equal time intervals? Moreover, how would one estimate the
duration of any specific cardiac cycle component (e.g. P-R interval)
indexed across time? These questions have never been adequately discussed
in the psychophysiological literature.

There are a variety of methods that may be used to generate an
estimate of a point process at equal time intervals, such as interpolation,
weighting, and sampling. Each method has its own unique characteristics.
An important requirement is to make the "time window" short enough to map
into the temporal variability of the process. If the time window is longer
than twice the shortest inter-event interval, then the time window may
smooth or alias a component of the variance of the process. In the case of
heart period, it is necessary to estimate the heart period at sequential

intervals of approximately one-half the duration of the shortest heart
period. This sampling procedure will preserve the variance of the original
heart period process in the transformed data set. Moreover, the transformed data will be amenable to time-domain detrending and filtering techniques. The methods that I employ, either weighting (see Cheung and
Porges, 1977) or sampling (i.e. probing the heart period in progress)
provide an instantaneous estimate. These methods provide an estimate which
is not offset by a time delay (e.g. tachometer) and allow time indexed
comparisons with other physiological response systems and between subjects

b. Detrending and the Partitioning Variance

In most situations the heart period pattern is composed of rhythmic
activity such as respiratory sinus arrhythmia superimposed on a complex
baseline trend. In many situations the baseline trend accounts for most of
the variance of the heart period process. Relationships between average
heart period (i.e. trend) and oxygen consumption are commonly cited in the
literature (e.g. Brener, Philips, and Connally, 1980; Woodson, Field, and
Greenberg, 1983). The rhythmic activity superimposed on the trend tends to
be neurally mediated. Often there are numerous mediating factors determining these rhythmic adjustments.

It is difficult to estimate accurately the amplitude of a periodic
process when it is superimposed on a complex baseline trend. Most statistical procedures that have been used to assess the amplitude of respiratory sinus arrhythmia include procedures to detrend, filter, and describe
residual variance. The detrending and filtering procedures produce a
processed signal by removing linear or low order polynomial trends. The
high-passed signal may then be decomposed through spectral analysis into
constituent frequencies. Although these methods are commonly employed,
most detrending techniques inadequately remove the complex baseline trend
and alter the amplitude of the periodic process being evaluated. These
methods, however, function adequately if the periodic signal of interest is
large relative to the instability of the baseline or the baseline trend has
virtually no variance in the frequency band of the periodic signal (e.g.
unit recordings).

If the baseline trend is a complex function that cannot be mathemat-
ically described by a linear or a low-order polynomial trend or by a sum of
sine waves slower than the frequencies characteristic of respiratory sinus
arrhythmia, the spectral composition of the baseline trend will include
faster frequency components. The higher frequencies associated with the
trend will "leak" through the detrending techniques and be superimposed on
the spectral representation of the amplitude of respiratory sinus
arrhythmia. Since the amplitudes of the faster frequency components of the
baseline trend are not known a priori and cannot be estimated a posterior
from the spectrum because they change over time when the baseline is not
constant (i.e. nonstationary), high-pass filters do not eliminate all of
the variance of baseline trend; a traditional high-pass filter cannot
discriminate between the high frequency component of the trend and the
frequency of respiratory sinus arrhythmia.

The baseline trend in heart period tends to exhibit large shifts over
time (relative to the amplitude of respiratory sinus arrhythmia). This
shift in mean and variance over time violates a basic assumption underlying
many forms of time series analyses. This assumption has been labeled
stationarity. A weakly stationary time series has certain properties
including a mean and variance which are independent of time and an auto-
covariance function which is dependent only on lag (Chatfield, 1975).
Spectral analysis provides reliable and interpretable estimators of the
amplitude of a periodic oscillation only if the data are at least weakly

stationary. Thus, unless the data set is stationary, spectral analysis is inappropriate for describing the amplitude of respiratory sinus arrhythmia.

There are problems in accurately quantifying the amplitude of respiratory sinus arrhythmia. First, the time series of heart period activity is usually not stationary. Second, the traditional methods for detrending and filtering do not effectively remove the variance of the baseline trend to make the transformed heart period data stationary. The error caused by the above constraints may make the estimate of vagal tone from respiratory sinus arrhythmia unreliable.

These points focus on the problems in applying spectral technology to describe rhythmic heart period processes. In some situations it may be possible to minimize the impact of a complex baseline trend on the periodic activity by analyzing relatively short epochs. This approach is based on the assumption that a complex trend may be approximated by a series of adjacent linear trends. This method will be effective only if the trend component in each epoch is primarily linear. It is, however, possible to model the complex aperiodic baseline with a series of localized polynomials (see Bohrer and Porges, 1982). These short-duration polynomials may be stepped through the data set. The moving polynomial procedure smooths the data set by conforming to the shifting levels of the baseline. When the smoothed baseline is subtracted from the raw data, the residual time series is free from the influence of the baseline.

Figure 3 illustrates how the moving polynomial procedure functions. The top panel illustrates 60 seconds of heart period data sampled every 500 msec. The data were collected from a healthy adult. Note the rhythmic oscillations occurring approximately 20 times within the 60 second data set. This oscillation is respiratory sinus arrhythmia. A graph of simultaneously recorded respiration would reflect the same periodicity.

The heart period data were collected while the subject was seated quietly and not involved in any experimental task. However, the pattern of the heart period data, even during these conditions, exhibited a complex trend which included contributions of slower periodic activity (e.g. Traube-Hering-Mayer wave) and aperiodic activity (e.g. acceleratory trend). A simple way of estimating the relative contributions of the variance components to the total variance of the heart period pattern is to approximate the amplitude of each component. In the example plotted in Figure 3, respiratory sinus arrhythmia has an amplitude of about 50 msec, the Traube-Hering-Mayer wave has an amplitude of about 50 msec, and the trend has an amplitude of about 100 msec. Thus, even in an example in which respiratory sinus arrhythmia is visually apparent, respiratory sinus arrhythmia contributes far less than 50% of the total variance of the time series. There are situations, such as with the fetus, when heart period oscillations in the respiratory frequencies account for less than 1% of the total heart period variance (Donchin, Caton, and Porges, 1984).

The complex trend cannot be fit accurately with a linear regression over the entire data set (i.e. the most common method of detrending). Moreover, the Traube-Hering-Mayer wave cannot be fit with a perfect sine wave. Thus, if spectral analysis were used to describe respiratory sinus arrhythmia, the amplitude of respiratory sinus arrhythmia may be inflated because linear detrending and frequency domain filtering would pass variance unrelated to respiratory sinus arrhythmia into the respiratory frequency band. Thus, traditional filtering strategies will inflate respiratory sinus arrhythmia amplitude. This presents the possibility that estimates of respiratory sinus arrhythmia amplitude derived from spectral analyses may be modulated, not by changes in cardio-vagal tone mediated by respiration, but by changes in trend and Traube-Hering-Mayer wave profile.

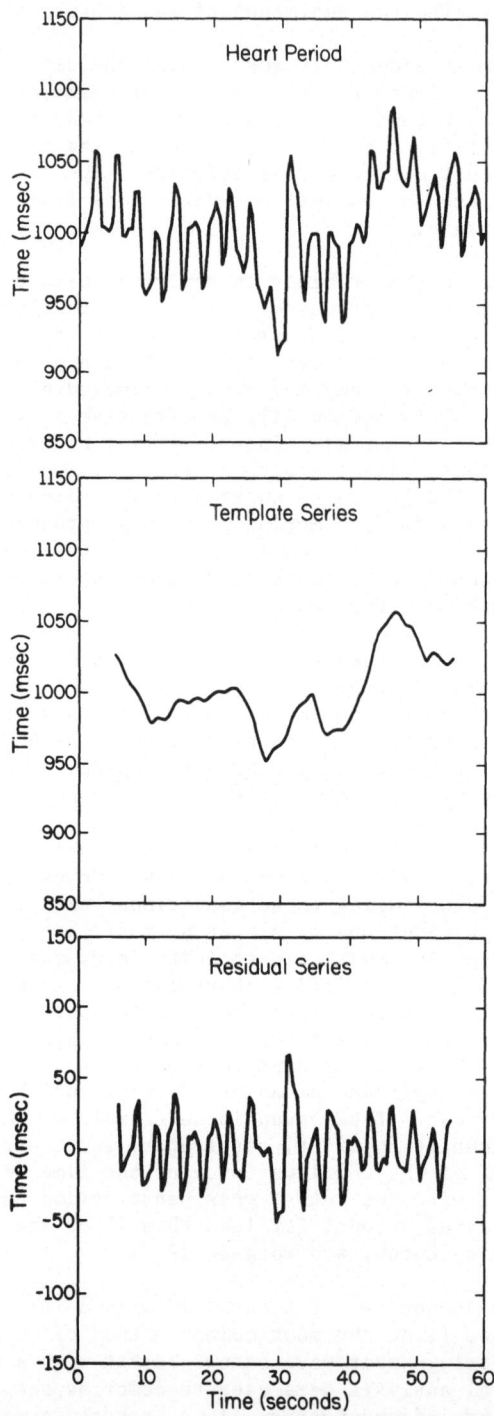

Fig. 3. Moving polynomial filter procedure: top panel is the unfiltered heart period series; middle panel is the smoothed template series which is fit to the changing baseline and slow periodic processes; bottom panel is the filtered heart period series illustrating respiratory sinus arrhythmia.

The moving polynomial procedure functions as a high pass filter and partitions the time series into two uncorrelated components: a smoothed template series (see middle panel) containing the slow periodic and aperiodic activity (i.e. trends) that occur at frequencies slower than breathing; and a residual series (see bottom panel) generated by subtracting the template series from the unfiltered data that conforms to the requirements of weak stationarity. Note how effectively the template series fits the complex aperiodic baseline and the quasi-periodic Traube-Hering-Mayer wave. The residual series clearly and accurately passes the frequency components associated with respiratory sinus arrhythmia.

The moving polynomial procedure has unique performance characteristics as a filter, since it does not make specific assumptions regarding the spectral characteristics of the trend prior to detrending. The number of coefficients and order of the moving polynomial procedure are critical. In the example illustrated in Figure 1, a filter was designed to pass variance associated with frequencies above 0.1 Hz. With knowledge of the transfer function of the moving polynomial procedure and the sampling rate of the time series, it was possible to design a sensitive filter which dynamically fits the changing baselevel (Porges, 1985). The residual series may then be analyzed with spectral analysis to extract the variance associated with the respiratory frequency band.

Alternative methods have been employed to quantify the amplitude of respiratory sinus arrhythmia. One of the most common methods is the peak-to-trough measure (Katona and Jih, 1975; Hirsch and Bishop, 1981; Grossman et al., 1984; Grossman and Wientjes, this volume; Fouad et al., 1984). Although this method has been very successful in physiological studies demonstrating systematic changes in the amplitude and frequency of respiratory sinus arrhythmia due to breathing maneuvers and vagal manipulations, the method presents severe quantitative vulnerabilities.

The vulnerability of the peak-to-trough method becomes clear when one evaluates the statistical properties of the heart period time series. The primary problem is associated with the fact that heart period data are not stationary. Violations of the stationarity are known to influence the stability of the spectral densities (see above). Few researchers realize that the peak-to-trough measure suffers from the same problem.

In employing the peak-to-trough measure, the researcher measures the change in heart period from a point when the heart period starts to increase as a function of the initiation of exhalation to a point when the heart period reaches its longest duration within the same cycle. Or, the researcher may employ a trough-to-peak measure. In this case the change is evaluated during the "up-phase" of the cycle, rather than during the "down-phase" of the cycle. Both approaches evaluate the difference between a maximum and a minimum point. If the variability of the heart period activity were solely determined by respiratory sinus arrhythmia, measurement of either the "up-phase" or the "down-phase" would be identical and both methods would result in an accurate representation of the amplitude of respiratory sinus arrhythmia. However, it is obvious that heart period is not composed of one sinusoidal process superimposed on a constant mean.

Since the respiratory sinus arrhythmia is usually superimposed on a complex trend and other periodic processes which are not perfect sine waves (e.g. Traube-Hering-Mayer wave), the "up-phase" measurements will not be identical to the "down-phase" measurements. There are two critical features to this argument: (1) the impact of a complex trend; and (2) the impact of slower underlying periodic processes such as the Traube-Hering-Mayer wave. Although there are problems with many of the detrending methods used in the application of spectral analyses to the study of heart period oscillations, the literature on "peak-to-trough" measurements is devoid of attempts to remove trends. Even linear trends would greatly influence the quantification of minimum and maximum points of respiratory sinus arrhythmia. Similarly, since the slower periodicities are not perfect sine waves, the duration of the "up-phase" and "down-phase" of these processes are different. Thus, even if the trend did not exist, the shape of the Traube-Hering-Mayer wave and the thermo-regulatory influences on heart period would influence the number of samples of the amplitude of respiratory sinus arrhythmia which would be underestimated or over-estimated. Arguments that these differences "average out" are erroneous, since the argument would only be credible if the heart period process were stationary. This is not the case.

In special populations such as diabetics, head injury patients, and risk infants, the amplitude of respiratory sinus arrhythmia is very small and may account for a small percentage of the total heart period - variability. Thus, although it may be possible to use the peak-to-trough measure in controlled experiments with normal human subjects to understand some of the basic neurophysiological mechanisms, it is extremely difficult to evaluate, with any quantitative confidence, an accurate estimate of the amplitude of respiratory sinus arrhythmia.

CLINICAL IMPLICATIONS

An important justification for studying indices of cardio-vagal tone, is that the vagal control of the heart is directly influenced by the brain. Conceptually, this approach treats components of the heart period pattern (e.g. respiratory sinus arrhythmia) as indexing variables of underlying neurological function. Thus, the heart period pattern may provide critical information regarding the central nervous system.

Currently, we are conducting a large study evaluating the vagal tone of human neonates. The project is an attempt to relate neonatal measures of respiratory sinus arrhythmia amplitude to developmental outcome. We have tested approximately 500 neonates, many with risk factors, in an attempt to assess the predictive validity of the measure of respiratory sinus arrhythmia amplitude. At present, the distribution of respiratory sinus arrhythmia amplitude is very different for risk and healthy neonates. Risk neonates, as a population, have significantly lower respiratory sinus arrhythmia amplitude. Moreover, the outcome of the risk infants with normal respiratory sinus arrhythmia amplitude is good. For example, a subset of our risk infants were part of an apnea project. 90% of this subset of risk infants who had respiratory sinus arrhythmia amplitudes at least one standard score below the mean of the normal infants, had sub-sequent apnea problems. In contrast, if the risk infants had respiratory sinus arrhythmia amplitude in the normal range, only 20% had apnea problems.

In another study (Fox and Porges, 1985), respiratory sinus arrhythmia amplitude was quantified in neonates and correlated with the Bayley Mental Development Index at 8 and 12 months. The main finding in the study was that neonates who have "good" respiratory sinus arrhythmia amplitude (defined as being above the mean of a normal control group) always had a positive developmental outcome (i.e. over 100 on the Mental Development Index) at 8 and 12 months. Although infants with "low" respiratory sinus arrhythmia amplitude at 40 weeks conceptional age had varied outcomes, they were more likely to have a low Mental Development Index.

It is interesting to note that respiratory sinus arrhythmia amplitude appears to follow a developmental trend which parallels the development of

112

vagal control of the heart. In a pilot study (Porges, 1983), data were collected from term and preterm infants who were free from major clinical complications. The relationship between respiratory sinus arrhythmia amplitude and gestational age was calculated. The correlation was 0.82. This correlation is similar to the correlation of 0.74 between weeks of pregnancy and increase in fetal heart rate in response to atropine reported by Schifferli and Caldeyro-Barcia (1973). In a more recent analysis, based upon our large sample of risk infants, we confirmed the strong relationship between gestational age and respiratory sinus arrhythmia amplitude with correlations of about 0.7.

Convergent with the above developmental data is the research studying the morphology of the vagus in premature infants who have died from causes other than sudden infant death syndrome. Sachis, Armstrong, Becker, and Bryan (1982) have reported that the total myelinated vagus fibers increase in a linear fashion between the conceptional ages of 24 and 40 weeks. The slope of their data is extremely similar to our data relating respiratory sinus arrhythmia amplitude to conceptional age. These data support the assumption that respiratory sinus arrhythmia amplitude provides a sensitive noninvasive measure of vagal tone.

The ability to accurately measure respiratory sinus arrhythmia amplitude to estimate vagal control of the heart is important to biomedical researchers and clinicians. Since the vagal control of the heart is sensitive to central nervous system status, it provides one of the few available methods to assess the condition of the fetus during labor. Since neonatal vagal tone appears to be related to developmental outcome, it may provide a sensitive screening procedure to identify children who are risk for developmental disabilities. Research on senility and diabetes has also used measures of respiratory sinus arrhythmia to assess autonomic neuropathy. In our research, we have evaluated respiratory sinus arrhythmia amplitude during anesthesia and have found it to be a very sensitive index of level of anesthesia (Donchin, Feld, and Porges, 1985).

REFERENCES

Akelrod, S. D., Gordon, D., Ubel, F. A., Shannon, D. C., Barger, D. C., and Cohen, R. J., 1981, Power spectrum analysis of heart rate fluctuations: a quantitative probe of beat-to-beat cardiovascular control, Science, 213:220-222.

Angell-James, J. E., and Daly, M. D. B., 1978, The effects of artificial lung inflation on reflexly induced bradycardia associated with apnea in the dog, J. Physiol., 274:349-366.

Anrep, G. V., Pascual, W., and Rossler, R., 1936a, Respiratory variations of the heart rate: I - The reflex mechanism of respiratory arrhythmia, Proc. Roy. Soc., 119:191-217.

Anrep, G. V., Pascual, W., and Rossler, R., 1936b, Respiratory variations of the heart rate: II - The central mechanism of the respiratory arrhythmia and the interrations between the central and reflex mechanisms, Proc. Roy. Soc., 119:218-230.

Bartlett, 1966, An Introduction to Stochastic Process, 2nd ed., Cambridge University Press, Cambridge.

Bohrer, R., and Porges, S. W., 1982, The application of time-series statistics to psychological research: an introduction, in: "Statistical and Methodological Issues in Psychology and Social Sciences Research", G. Keren, ed., LEA, 309-345, Hillsdale, N.J.

Brener, J., Philips, K., and Connally, S. R., 1980, Oxygen consumption, heart rate and ambulation during shock avoidance conditioning of heart rate increases and ambulation in freely moving rats, Psychophysiology, 17:64-74.

Chatfield, C., 1975, The analysis of time series: theory and practice, Chapman & Hall, London.

Chess, G. F., Tam, M. K., and Calaresu, R. F., 1975, Influences of cardiac neural inputs on rhythmic variation of heart period in the cat, Am. J. Physiol., 228:775.

Cheung, M. N., and Porges, S. W., 1977, Respiratory influences on cardiac responses during attention, Physiol. Psychol., 5:53-57.

Davidson, N. S., Goldner, S., and McCloskey, D. I., 1976, Respiratory modulation of baroreceptor and chemoreceptor reflexes affecting heart rate and cardiac vagal efferent nerve activity, J. Physiol., 259:523-530.

Davis, A. L., McCloskey, D. I., and Potter, E. K., 1977, Respiratory modulation of baroreceptor and chemoreceptor reflexes affecting heart rate through the sympathetic nervous system, J. Physiol., 272:691-703.

Dellinger and Porges, 1984, The effect of atropine sulfate on the amplitude of respiratory sinus arrhythmia ($\hat{V}$) in humans, Abstract, Psychophysiology, 21:575.

Donchin, Y., Feld, J. M., and Porges, S. W., 1985, Respiratory sinus arrhythmia during recovery from isoflurane-nitrous oxide anaethesia, Anesthesia and Analgesia, 64:811-815.

Eppinger, H., and Hess, L., 1915, Vagotonia: a clinical study in vegetative neurology, J. Nervous & Mental Disease, Monograph Series, whole issue #20.

Fouad, F. M., Tarazi, R. C., Ferrario, C. M., Fighaly, S., and Alicandri, C., 1984, Assessment of parasympathetic control of heart rate by a noninvasive method, Am. J. Physiol., 246:H838-H842.

Fox, N. A., and Porges, S. W., 1985, The relation between neontal heart period patterns and developmental outcome, Child Development, 56:28-37.

Gilbey, M. P., Jordan, D., Richter, D. W., and Spyer, K. M., 1983, The inspiratory control of vagal cardio-inhibitory neurons in the cat, J. Physiol., 343:57-58.

Gottman, J. M., 1981, Time-Series Analysis, Cambridge University Press, New York.

Grossman, P., Wientjes, C., and Defares, P., 1984, Individual differences in cardiac parasympathetic control predicted by ventilatory parameters, Abstract, Psychophysiology, 21:579.

Haymet, B. T., and McCloskey, D. I., 1975, Baroreceptor and chemoreceptor influences on heart rate during the respiratory cycle in the dog, J. Physiol., 245:699-712.

Hering, H. E., 1910, A functional test of heart vagi in man, Munch. Medig. Woch., 57(2):1930-32.

Hirsch, J. A., and Bishop, B., 1981, Respiratory sinus arrhythmia in humans: how breathing pattern modulates heart rate, Am. J. Physiol., 241:H620-H629.

Iriuchjima, J., and Kumada, M., 1964, Activity of single vagal fibers efferent to the heart, Japanese J. Physiol., 14:479-487.

Jewett, D. L., 1964, Activity of single efferent fibers in the cervical vagus nerve of the dog, with special reference to possible cardio-inhibitory fibers, J.Physiol., 175:321-357.

Jordan, D., Khalid, M. E. M., Schneidnerman, N., and Spyer, K. M., 1982, The location and properties of preganglionic vagal cardiomotor neurones in the rabbit, Pflügers Arch., 395:244-250.

Katona, P. J., and Jih, F., 1975, Respiratory sinus arrhythmia: noninvasive measure of parasympathetic cardiac control, J. Appl. Physiol., 39:801-805.

Katona, P. G., Poitras, J. W., Barnett, G. O., and Terry, B. S., 1970, Cardiac vagal efferent activity and heart period in the carotid sinus reflex, Am.J. Physiol., 218:1030-1037.

Kitney, R. I., Byrne, S., Edmonds, M. E., Watkins, P. J., and Roberts, V. C., 1982, Heart rate variability in the assessment of autonomic diabetic neuropathy, Automedica, 4:155-167.

Kitney, R. I., and Rompelman, P., 1980, The Study of Heart Rate Variability, Oxford University Press, Oxford.

Kunze, D. L., 1972, Reflex discharge patterns of cardiac vagal afferent fibers, J. Physiol., 222:1-15.

Lopes, O. V., and Palmer, J. F., 1976, Proposed respiratory gating mechanism for cardiac slowing, Nature, 264:454-456.

McCabe, P. M., Yongue, B. G., Porges, S. W., and Ackles, P. K., 1984, Changes in heart period, heart period variability, and a spectral analysis estimate of respiratory sinus arrhythmia during aortic nerve stimulation in rabbits, Psychophysiology, 21:149-158.

McCabe, P. M., Yongue, B. G., Ackles, P. K., and Porges, S. W., 1985, Changes in heart period, heart-period variability and a spectral analysis estimate of respiratory sinus arrhythmia in response to pharmacological manipulations of the baroreceptor reflex in cats, Psychophysiology, 22:195-203.

Porges, S. W., 1976, Peripheral and neurochemical parallels of psychopathology: a psychophsyiological model relating autonomic imbalance to hyperactivity, psychopathy, and autism, in: "Advances in Child Development and Behavior", H. W. Reese, ed., pp. 35-65, Academic Press, New York.

Porges, S. W., Bohrer, R. E., Cheung, M. N., Drasgow, F., McCabe, P., and Keren, G., 1980, A new time-series statistic for detecting rhythmic co-occurrence in the frequency domain: the weighted coherence and its application to psychophysiological research, Psychol. Bull., 88:580-587.

Porges, S. W., 1982, Method and apparatus for evaluating rhythmic oscillations in aperiodic phsyiological response systems, Patent pending.

Porges, S. W., McCabe, P. M., and Yongue, B. G., 1982, Respiratory-heart-rate interactions: psychophysiological implications for pathophysiology and behavior, in: "Perspectives in Cardiovascular Psychophysiology", J. Cacioppo and R. Petty, eds., Guilford Press, New York.

Porges, S. W., 1983, Heart rate patterns in neonates: a potential diagnostic window to the brain, in: "Infants Born at Risk: Physiological, Perceptual, and Cognitive Processes", T. Field and A. Sostek, eds., pp. 3-22, Grune & Stratton, New York.

Sachis, P. N., Armstrong, D. L., Becker, L. E., and Bryan, A. C., 1982, Myelination of the human vagus nerve from 24 weeks postconceptional age to adolescence, J. Neuropath. & Exp. Neurol., 41:466-472.

Sayers, B. M., 1973, Analysis of heart rate variability, Ergonomics, 16:17-32.

Woodson, R., Field, T., and Greenberg, R., 1983, Estimating neonatal oxygen consumption from heart rate, Psychophysiology, 20:558-561.

Wundt, W., 1904, Principles of physiological psychology, The MacMillan Co., New York.

Yongue, B. G., McCabe, P. M., Porges, S. W., Rivera, M., Kelley, S. L., and Ackles, P. K., 1982, The effects of pharmacological manipulations that influence vagal control of the heart on heart period, heart-period variability and respiration in rats, Psychophysiology, 19:426-432.

RESPIRATORY SINUS ARRHYTHMIA AND PARASYMPATHETIC CARDIAC
CONTROL: SOME BASIC ISSUES CONCERNING QUANTIFICATION,
APPLICATIONS AND IMPLICATIONS

P. Grossman and K. Wientjes*

Institute for Stress Research;
*TNO-Institute for Perception, and
Free University of Amsterdam,
Department of Physiological Psychology

In recent years, increasing attention has been directed to the phenomenon of respiratory sinus arrhythmia (RSA) by physiologists and psychophysiologists (e.g. Fouad et al., 1984; Haddad et al., 1984; Porges, McCabe
and Yongue, 1982; Zemaityte, Varoneckas and Sokolov, 1984). This has
largely been a consequence of the finding that RSA magnitude is a sensitive
index of cardiac parasympathetic control under various conditions (first
shown by Katona and Jih, 1975). An easily obtainable noninvasive measure
of specific neural influences upon the heart is likely to generate much
enthusiasm, debate and discussion revolving around issues of the actual
validity of the index, the most appropriate RSA parameter to use for the
measure, the physiological mechanisms precisely underlying the phenomenon,
and potential research and clinical application areas. The purpose of the
present paper is to delve into these various aspects of RSA as cardiac
vagal index, not in terms of a comprehensive review of these issues, but
rather in an effort to point out certain misunderstood and overlooked
areas.

The approach we use will be to integrate our own relevant research
findings with the work of others where appropriate. We will not, however,
detail experimental procedures, except when specifically relevant. A brief
summary here of the following major points we shall cover may help to
quide the reader:

1.   What are the various RSA quantification procedures used to index
parasympathetic control of heart rate, and is there evidence concerning the
validity of different RSA measures as indices of vagal tone? There are a
number of RSA measures currently used to assess cardiac vagal tone, and
users of particular measures typically either tacitly assume or else boldly
claim that their measure is most closely associated with variations in
parasympathetic cardiac control (Eckberg, 1983; Fouad et al., 1984; Porges,
this volume; McCabe et al., 1985). We shall review the physiological
evidence for such claims and assumptions and discuss advantages and dis-
advantages of the main quantification techniques.

2.   Along a different line, respiratory sinus arrhythmia is a phenomenon
derived from the interaction of respiratory and cardiovascular processes.
Although much is known about how respiratory variations can profoundly
alter RSA parameters, the relevant research in this regard has largely been

carried out by investigators not directly concerned with its meaning for cardiac vagal processes (Angelone and Coulter, 1964; Clynes, 1960; Davies and Nielsen, 1967; Hirsch and Bishop, 1981). On the other hand, scientists primarily emphasizing RSA as a vagal index, in most cases, have overlooked the inherent respiratory contribution and have treated RSA as though it were a purely cardiovascular affair that just happens to occur around the respiratory frequency of the individual (Fouad et al., 1984; Katona and Jih, 1975; Porges, McCabe and Yongue, 1982). To our minds, much confusion has been generated concerning the role respiratory processes actually play in this context. Furthermore, our own and others' research concerning respiratory influences upon RSA and cardiac vagal control points toward a possible direct link between vagal control mechanisms and respiratory processes that could be of major importance for understanding vagal control (e.g. Eckberg, 1983; Grossman, Wientjes and Defares, 1984; 1985; Grossman and Wientjes, 1985). Hence, we should like to elaborate upon just these interactions between respiration, RSA and vagal processes, as well as to discuss what they may mean for the psychophysiology of cardiac control.

3.   Most of the psychophysiological research applications of RSA as vagal index have been oriented toward inferring aspects of central processes often among physically disordered populations (e.g. neurologically impaired infants and children with minimal brain dysfunction; Fox and Porges, 1985; Piggott et al., 1973; Porges, 1985 and this volume; Porges et al., 1981; Richards, 1984; 1985). However, there is compelling evidence that RSA ought only to be used to reflect peripheral vagal effects upon the heart, and under certain conditions may not at all mirror central processes (Katona, Lipson and Dauchot, 1977). Furthermore, little emphasis has been placed in the psychophysiological literature upon using RSA to infer aspects of cardiac competence across situations and among different populations that may vary for cardiovascular risk. Thus here we will consider the potential of this index as a purely cardiac measure and not as a window to central neural processes. Our interest in this section will be focussed upon how utilization of RSA, as cardiac vagal index, may contribute to an improved understanding of specific interactions between psychoenvironmental factors and neural influences upon the heart.

RSA AS INDEX OF CARDIAC PARASYMPATHETIC CONTROL: WHICH RSA
QUANTIFICATIONS INDEX VAGAL CONTROL BEST?

Various more and less sophisticated measures of RSA have emerged in the last years as putative indices of cardiac parasympathetic control (Coker et al., 1984; Eckberg, 1983; Fouad et al., 1984; Haddad et al., 1984; Harper et al., 1978; Katona and Jih, 1975; Porges et al., 1981). These include measures that can be simply and immediately derived from ECG or cardiotachometer recordings, as well as those measures requiring considerable computer processing and analysis of ECG data (e.g. spectral analytic and certain digital filtering techniques). The major quantification procedures for measuring RSA can thus be divided into the two following general sorts:

1.   The first method is often referred to as the peak-to-trough method (Fouad et al., 1984; Grossman, Wientjes and Defares, 1984; 1985; Katona and Jih, 1975). The unfiltered R-R interval series is used to assess maximal heart period (or heart rate) differences corresponding to the inspiratory and expiratory phases of consecutive respiratory cycles: heart period typically decreases with inspiration and increases with expiration, and the shortest R-R interval corresponding to inspiration is subtracted from the longest expiration-related interval. The breath-by-breath differences are then averaged across respiratory cycles for the measurement period (see Figure 1). Hence, for this quantification technique, it is necessary to monitor respiration simultaneously with the cardiac signal.

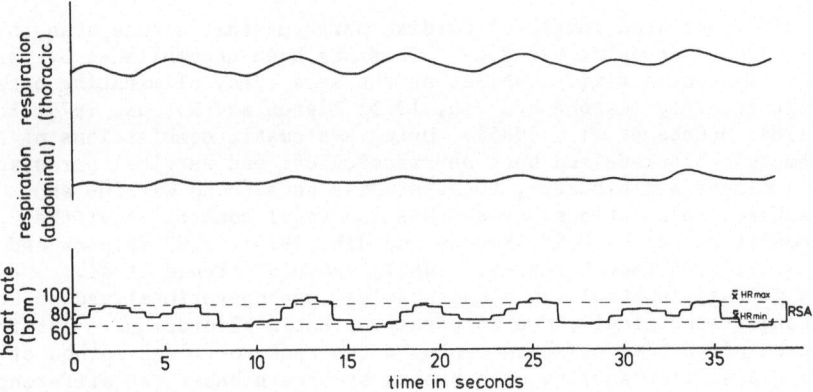

Fig. 1. Peak-to-trough method of quantifying respiratory sinus arrhythmia
(RSA). Top two tracings: respiration (abdominal and thoracic).
Bottom tracing: cardiotachogram showing RSA. RSA is scored in
maximal heart period differences within respiratory cycles.
Dotted lines indicate average differences across the measurement
period shown.

2. The second class of procedure is oriented toward derivation of an RSA
measure that is uncontaminated by nonrespiratory rhythmic and nonrhythmic
fluctuations in cardiac activity (De Boer, Karemaker and Strackee, 1985;
Harper et al., 1978; Kitney, this volume; Porges, McCabe and Yongue, 1982;
Richards, 1985). Consequently, various digital filtering and statistical
techniques (spectral analysis) are employed to isolate the respiratory
oscillations in the cardiac time series. This type of procedure frequently
requires considerable computer processing of the physiological signal and
can be used to yield an estimate of RSA that is <u>assumed</u> to reflect only
respiration-induced heart period fluctuations. Although respiratory
activity should probably also be simultaneously recorded, this is not
always in practice the case, since researchers often arbitrarily define a
band of frequencies as respiratory (usually approximately between 9 and 24
cycles per minute for human adults) and assess cardiac fluctuations only
within this bandwidth (e.g. Mulder, 1985; Mulder and Mulder, 1981; Porges,
McCabe and Yongue, 1982).

The information that each class of quantification technique yields is,
therefore, somewhat different, and there has yet to be a definitive
empirical comparison to determine just how closely related these indices
are to one another. Of primary concern to the researcher posed with the
problem of which to use, are at least three major issues: (1) which technique of assessing RSA provides the parameter most closely associated with
variations in cardiac vagal tone; (2) which RSA measure is most likely to
enable the researcher to extract the most detailed information concerning
RSA and its interactions with other experimental variables of interest; and
(3) which technique entails the most effective use of laboratory resources
(e.g. cost-effectiveness).

Regarding the first question, there are a number of studies that have
related individual measures of RSA to pharmacologically induced variations
in vagal tone. All of these studies, independent of the RSA measure used,
have found that vagal blockade (usually by atropine) produces marked
reduction or abolishment of RSA and elevation of heart rate (Coker et al.,
1984; Fouad et al., 1984; Katona and Jih, 1975; Lipson and Katona, 1979;
Porges, this volume; Selman et al., 1982; Wheeler and Watkins, 1973;
Zemaityte, Varoneckas and Sokolov, 1984). However, only a few investigations have examined the degree of correlation between variations in RSA

and more differentiated levels of cardiac parasympathetic tone than that obtained by total atropine blockade. This has been accomplished by varying the extent of vagal activity, while, at the same time, eliminating beta-sympathetic activity (Katona and Jih, 1975; Lipson and Katona, 1979; Fouad et al., 1984; McCabe et al., 1985). Using systematic combinations of beta-adrenergic blockade and both pharmacological and surgical parasympathetic stimulants and blockers, these studies have found within- and between-subject correlations between RSA and vagal control under the various conditions to be 0.97 (Katona and Jih, 1975), 0.83 (Lipson and Katona, 1979), 0.86 (McCabe et al., 1985), and 0.91 (Fouad et al., 1984); variation in vagal control, in these studies, was operationalized as heart period changes specifically due to parasympathetic alterations. Interestingly, three of four experiments employed the peak-to-trough method of quantifying RSA, i.e. scoring on a breath-by-breath basis the difference between the shortest heart period (HP) corresponding to inspiration and the longest HP corresponding to expiration, and averaging these scores across the number of breaths during the measurement period. The only equivalent evidence of sensitivity available for any other measure of RSA, including spectral analytic and digitally filtered indices, is that of Porges' vagal tone index (McCabe et al., 1985; see also Porges, this volume). In this regard, however, it is interesting to mention that Porges' digitally filtered estimate of RSA has been found to be insensitive to vagal changes induced by low-dose atropine administration (Porges, this volume), whereas the peak-to-trough quantification has proven to be sensitive to such alterations (Raczkowska, Eckberg and Ebert, 1983).

Spectral and other filtered RSA measures are often thought necessary in order to partition the respiratory component of cyclic heart rate fluctuations from other, possibly confounding nonrhythmic trends and non-respiratory rhythmic components (e.g. the rhythmic fluctuation occurring approximately every ten seconds, thought to be related to blood pressure control; see Mulder and Mulder, 1981). However, once again, there is no evidence that such filtered RSA parameters will yield more sensitive, or even as sensitive, indices of cardiac vagal tone as unfiltered peak-to-trough measures. Most spectral analysis and filtering techniques require extensive processing of the cardiac signal, often including such treatments as interpolation of the cardiac event series in order to make it equidistant or continuous, preliminary filtering of the data to provide a more-or-less stationary time series, choice of a spectral window with specific frequency-response characteristics that may vary over the range of the frequency band of interest, Fourier analysis, definition of frequency bandwidths for providing boundaries between respiratory and other components of cardiac variability and smoothing spectral values over adjacent frequencies (e.g. Bohrer and Porges, 1982). There are a number of choices which can be made for each of the steps. The resulting estimate of RSA may vary greatly, depending upon decisions taken at each stage of signal processing and data reduction. Exactly what the consequences of such decisions will be for indexing parasympathetic tone is impossible to say, without actually subjecting the specific analytic packages to rigorous tests of sensitivity to vagal changes. Furthermore, the fact that RSA magnitude will vary, depending upon the package chosen, of course, makes comparisons between studies out of different laboratories often difficult or impossible.

There are, additionally, a number of other problems with spectral analysis and other filtering procedures for deriving RSA estimates:

1. A basic statistical assumption of spectral analysis is that the mean and variance of the time series being analyzed remain constant from segment to segment (i.e. stationary), so that there are no slow drifts in the time series and the standard deviation does not fluctuate from, say, breath to breath. Whereas there appear to be adequate techniques for removing slow

nonstationary trends in the mean (Porges, this volume), there seems to be
no satisfactory way of handling nonstationary changes in variance over the
time series (Yuen & Fraser, 1979, p. 49). Since variations in RSA amplitude are large even at relatively constant respiration rates (see Figure
4), spectral analytic techniques for assessing RSA may yield incorrect
estimates.

2. Spectral estimates of RSA seem to be computationally unstable. One or
two missed R-waves in a 3- minute record can have large effects upon RSA
magnitude estimates, as illustrated in Figure 2.

3. On the basis of the spectral or filtered RSA estimate alone, it is not
possible to detect whether nonrespiratory phasic and nonphasic phenomena
(e.g. body-movement-related and task-related HP changes), occurring at a
frequency within the arbitrarily defined respiratory frequency band (but
not necessarily at the respiratory frequency itself), are included in the
RSA estimate. This indicates the potential for artifacts slipping into the
respiratory band.

4. In order to isolate the respiratory component from other contributors
to HP variation, the respiratory band of frequencies must be narrow enough
to prevent overlap with other rhythmic components of variability. Respiratory frequency, however, is often very variable within the individual and
between individuals, and a sizeable proportion of breathing cycles may
occur at the same frequencies as these other nonrespiratory components
(Grossman, 1983; Schaefer, 1958; White et al., 1983). In order to deal
with the problem, spectral and filtered estimates have usually opted for a
respiratory bandwidth approximately between 9 and 24 cycles per minute
(cpm) for adults, roughly corresponding to the range of average normal
resting respiration rates. Given these boundaries, this means that both
with spectral and other filtered estimates of RSA, RSA for respiratory
cycles slower than 9 cpm or faster than 24 cpm will be totally missed or
incorrectly attributed to other nonrespiratory HP rhythms. The result is
especially alarming when slower respiratory cycles are missed since RSA
amplitude is greatest at slower breathing frequencies (e.g. Hirsch and
Bishop, 1981). Furthermore, for digitally filtered estimates in which the

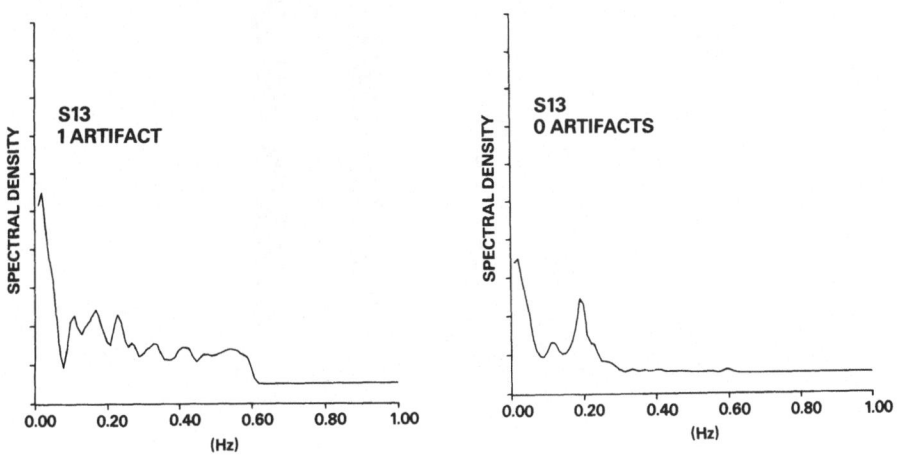

Fig. 2. Power spectrograms of a resting subject during the same period
         with and without a single heartbeat artifact (i.e. an R-peak that
         was missed in the calculations). Note that with the single
         artifact the total power is sizeably increased across the fre-
         quency band shown. Estimates of RSA from this record would be
         greatly distorted.

filters do not have ideal cut-off properties (e.g. see De Boer, Karemaker and Strackee, 1985), respiratory HP variations occurring close to the boundaries of the respiratory bandwidth will also be sizeably under-estimated (i.e. approximately between 9 to 11 and 22 to 24 cpm).

In order to assess the actual magnitude of this problem, we randomly selected the data records of 16 normal male student subjects from a larger pool. We examined all consecutive breaths for each subject during a five-minute rest period and during a mentally demanding five-minute reaction-time task. For each period, we computed the total number and percentage of respiratory cycles that would have been missed or misattributed to other components of HP variability using spectral analysis or digital filtering procedures with a respiratory bandwidth between 9 and 24 cpm. We addition-ally calculated the number of cycles that would likely be underestimated by digital filtering techniques (i.e. cycles between 9 to 11 and 22 to 24 cpm). Over 2350 breaths were examined. Figure 3 presents our fairly disturbing findings.

Both for the rest and mental task conditions, 24% of all breaths would be missed using these range of frequencies. During rest, almost all the missed breaths were slow ones, thus indicating a marked underestimation of RSA magnitude in the event of spectral analysis using this respiratory band. During the mental task condition, the missed breaths were over-whelmingly rapid ones, suggesting, in this case, a danger of overestimation of RSA with these procedures. An extra 15% of all breaths would probably be underestimated using certain digital filtering procedures. One must emphasize that these data come from normal healthy university students who

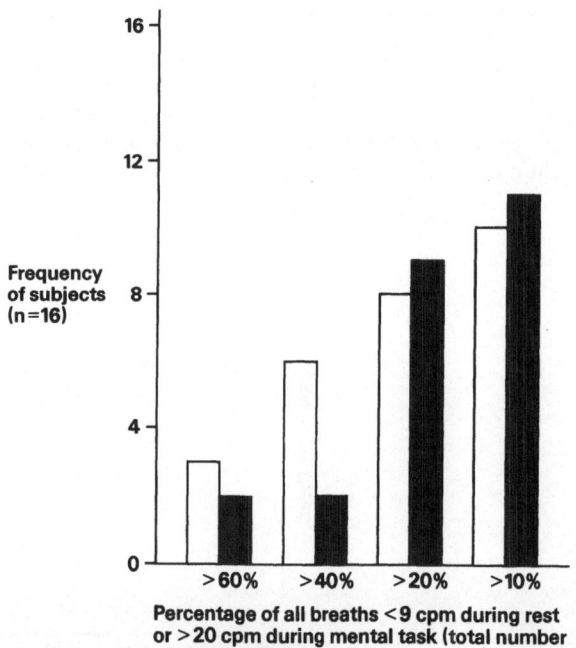

Fig. 3. Cumulative histogram illustrating the percentage of breaths that would have been missed in a group of sixteen subjects if using a frequency bandwidth between 9 and 20 cycles per min (cpm) for estimating RSA. Data are derived from two laboratory conditions, a rest period and a demanding memory-search reaction-time task. Dark bars represent percentage breaths < 9 cpm; light bars, per-centage breaths > 20 cpm.

were spontaneously breathing without intrusive respiratory closed-system devices (e.g. noseclips and mouthpieces). Since such a large proportion of the breaths occurred around the slower 10-second frequency, our results demonstrate that with many subjects, spectral analysis and other digital techniques for deriving RSA estimates are inadequate for disentangling the respiratory from the 10-second component of HP variability; the two cardiac rhythms are inherently confounded using these methods.

The major problem that is raised with peak-to-trough quantification of RSA is the potential contamination of this measure by slower nonrhythmic trends and other rhythmic cardiac oscillations. Such interference between respiratory and nonrespiratory fluctuations in heart period could possibly distort RSA estimation in either the direction of underestimation or over-estimation. However, it is presently unclear that this is actually the case, or if it is, that RSA quantification would be greatly compromised under most conditions. Peak-to-trough measures, with their supposed poten-tial for such contamination, have, nonetheless, consistently yielded precise estimates of cardiac vagal tone, capable of distinguishing between rather subtle levels of natural and experimentally induced variations in parasympathetic cardiac control among normal humans and animals (e.g. Eckberg, 1983; Eckberg, Kifle and Roberts, 1980; Haddad et al., 1984; Katona, Lipson and Dauchot, 1977; Raczkowska, Eckberg and Ebert, 1983; Zemaityte, Varoneckas and Sokolov, 1984); this measure has also been frequently and successfully used to assess differences in levels of cardiac vagal neuropathy among clinical groups (i.e. diabetics: Ewing et al., 1981; Hilsted and Jensen, 1979; Smith, 1982; Sundkvist, Almer and Lilja, 1979; Wheeler and Watkins, 1973; cardiovascular disorders: Bristow et al., 1969; Hinkle et al., 1972; Johnston, 1980; Schlomka, 1937; Zemaityte, Varoneckas and Sokolov, 1984a; asthma: Kallenbach et al., 1985). One would not expect such uniformity of findings across species, conditions, states, develop-mental phases and clinical groups, should this measure be highly vulnerable to nonvagal influences. Furthermore, the peak-to-trough method may itself be considered a type of filtering technique, one that utilizes the ongoing respiratory pattern as a frequency window in order to estimate correspond-ing cardiac oscillations; as respiratory frequency changes, so does the breadth of the filter window.

Although Porges (this volume) claims that this method will not average out nonrespiratory influences (because of nonstationary complex trends), his own data appear to contradict this claim: his Figure 3 shows a 1-minute period of cardiac activity, first with a complex trend (Figure 3a) and later with the trend filtered out (Figure 3c). Notice the sizeable trend in the first one-minute segment. In order to ascertain whether the filtered data would yield a significantly different RSA estimate than the raw data, we scored both segments using the peak-to-trough method. Should Porges be correct, one would expect considerably different RSA estimates for the two segments. In fact, this is not the case. The average RSA of the unfiltered series (Figure 3a) was 56.1 msecs (±21 msecs., S.D.), whereas mean RSA of the filtered segment (Figure 3c) was 53.4 (±18.4) msecs. Although the nonrespiratory fluctuations were substantial and the measurement period very brief, the difference between the filtered and unfiltered estimates was only 2.7 msecs., suggesting that filtering out· nonrespiratory variations may, in general, be unnecessary.

Considering the presently available evidence, then, it would seem that the peak-to-trough technique of RSA estimation provides the most sensitive and trustworthy index of cardiac parasympathetic control of all those measures currently employed. Detailed evaluation of alternative quantifi-cation procedures (which have been proposed as providing more accurate assessment of vagal tone) reveals an array of serious problems that, for the most part, can be circumvented by using the peak-to-trough method.

A second related question of importance concerns the type of results that are derived from the particular quantification technique used. Obviously a breath-by-breath analysis of RSA provides a continuous record of respiration-related HP or heart-rate (HR) changes over the measurement period of interest. Thus, any variable that can be quantified on a breath-by-breath basis can, in principle, be related to within-individual variations that take place during the measurement period (e.g. within-subject breath-by-breath correlations of RSA with respiratory parameters). Furthermore, one can either easily examine very short-term experimental effects upon RSA (e.g. attentional responses that take place within single breaths), or average RSA over the entire measurement period. On the other hand, most spectral analysis procedures require several minutes of measurement (3-5 minutes) in order to obtain a reliable RSA estimate, and thus shorter-term changes cannot be followed. Therefore, spectral analytic and digitally filtered results typically provide one summary estimate of RSA for the entire period analyzed, which gives information about the total amount of HP variability within the respiratory frequency band for that period. It is, however, possible to relate spectral estimates of RSA to other simultaneously oscillating variables (e.g. respiration and blood pressure) provided that these are also subjected to spectral analysis, although putative relationships are sometimes difficult to subject to tests of statistical probability (Orr and Naiton, 1976). Nevertheless, a clear advantage of spectral analysis is that possible relationships and interactions between respiratory and other rhythmic components of HP variability can be quantified, provided stringent conditions are met (e.g. equal frequency-response characteristics across bands of interest); thus, the relative contributions of respiratory versus other components (e.g. blood pressure) of HP variability can, in this manner, be assessed (e.g. De Boer, Karemaker and Strackee, 1985).

Given the state of uncertainty concerning the diverse techniques for assessing RSA, an additionally relevant question would seem to be, how to best utilize available laboratory resources when quantifying RSA. The obvious answer from the literature thus far is that the simpler the quantification procedure, the more certain one is of what is being quantified, and the more sure one is of a reliable index of vagal tone. An additional bonus of less complex quantification methods is that the techniques and results are able to be easily understood in terms of concrete parameters; data can be analyzed with conventional statistics as opposed to the more-difficult-to-grasp transformational parameters encountered with spectral analysis (e.g. coherence coefficients and transfer function parameters). Limitations of simple peak-to-trough quantification of RSA may possibly occur under special conditions where other rhythmic and non-rhythmic upon HP variability are so large that they may substantially interfere with RSA estimation in this manner (e.g. perhaps comparisons within certain clinical groups and ambulatory normal subjects). Under these circumstances, more sophisticated approaches to RSA quantification that decompose the total HP variance into specific components may be necessary. However, in our experience with normal and cardiac disorder patients, exposed to a variety of psychologically demanding tasks while in a stable position, relatively unconfounded peak-to-trough measures have been very easy to reliably obtain with all subjects.

In sum, both simple and complex methods of quantification of RSA are available. Parameters derived from simpler methods are easy to obtain, have been shown to be highly related to within- and across-individual variations in cardiac vagal control, can be statistically related within individuals to any other measures that are quantifiable on a breath-by-breath basis, and can be assessed for very short or very long measurement durations; peak-to-trough measures have the additional advantages that they can be subjected to comparison across studies, and they are easily understood by researchers not schooled in complex signal analysis and elaborate statistical techniques for handling time-series analyses. However, this type of RSA quantification may under special circumstances be susceptible to contamination by other rhythmic and nonrhythmic influences upon HP variability.

Spectral analytic and other digital filtering approaches for the quantification of RSA aim at partitioning respiratory HP rhythms from other potentially confounding cyclic and noncyclic fluctuations in cardiac signal variability. However, there is no available evidence that these techniques provide a superior vagal index to that provided by peak-to-trough measures of RSA. Another disadvantage of filtered and spectral measures of RSA is that there are a number of possibilities for processing the data at each step of the multistage analytic procedure, and it is not known which of these possibilities serves to contribute to a more sensitive index of parasympathetic control. Furthermore, since spectral RSA estimates may significantly differ according to the different choices made during these stages, comparability of findings across studies is often impossible. Spectral analysis provides one estimate of RSA for an entire period usually not shorter than three minutes. Thus, information concerning shorter-term changes in RSA is lost. The advantage of decomposing the respiratory component from other influences upon HP fluctuation may be largely offset by the facts that, on the one hand, nonrespiratory influences occurring within the respiratory band of frequencies may contaminate RSA estimates by inflating them, and, on the other hand, respiratory influences on HP variability will be wrongly estimated when some breaths occur at frequencies on the border of or beyond the arbitrarily defined RSA bandwidth of frequencies. Spectral analytic methods, if properly used, require much expertise in signal analysis and statistical procedures, and computer programming that usually represent a substantial investment for a research laboratory; the resulting RSA parameters and measures of association with other variables are difficult to interpret without such expertise, which often creates substantial confusion for less knowledgeable researchers.

For these various reasons, our own research program has, thus far, chosen primarily to quantify RSA by means of the peak-to-trough method. In the following section we will direct attention to recent findings, largely from our laboratory, that explore relations between respiratory parameters and RSA, in light of their significance for cardiac parasympathetic control.

RESPIRATION, RSA AND CARDIAC PARASYMPATHETIC CONTROL

We have relied upon certain findings of others in our own research concerned with respiratory influences upon RSA and cardiac vagal tone. These include the following: (1) RSA magnitude, in the manner that we measure it, is a sensitive index of variations in parasympathetic control of HR, both within- and across-individuals (e.g. Katona and Jih, 1975; Fouad et al., 1984); (2) respiratory parameters importantly influence the magnitude of RSA (e.g. Angelone and Coulter, 1984; Clynes, 1960); and (3) these relations between respiration and RSA are the same whether breathing parameters are consciously, voluntarily changed or are altered via spontaneous unconscious processes (Hirsch and Bishop, 1981). This last finding must be underlined, since it strongly suggests that respiratory and cardiac processes are not merely associative, but that respiratory processes have direct influence upon cardiac parasympathetic mechanisms: therefore, correlations between the two can be interpreted in a unidirectional causal model whereby respiration influences parasympathetic tone.

Within-Individual Respiratory-Cardiac Coupling

Given these lines of evidence, we have been interested in the extent to which both intra- and inter-individual differences in vagal tone can be explained by respiratory variations. We will first treat our within-individual findings. The data come from studies in which we examined healthy university students, during both resting and demanding mental-task conditions. In one investigation exploring cardiorespiratory relations, we chose to calculate, on a breath-by-breath basis, correlations between RSA magnitude, on the one hand, and respiratory rate (RR) and tidal volume (V_t), on the other. We specifically examined intra-individual correlations within five-minute task periods. The average number of observations per subject per period, varied, depending upon the number of respiratory cycles during a particular period; the range of observations was between 40 and 80 for the resting condition, between 55 and 114 for the mental task condition (a visual memory-comparison reaction-time task). All data were automatically scored by computer.

RR and V_t were each correlated with RSA magnitude for all individual subjects during the resting condition ($p < 0.05$; 17 subjects). The strength of the relationship between subjects varied greatly even during the resting period (r's = -0.23 to -0.65 for RR; 0.22 to 0.82 for V_t). The median r's were 0.53 and 0.42, respectively, for rest. During the reaction time task, the median r's were slightly lower for both sets of correlations, and the range of variations of the r's was slightly increased.

These findings then suggest that, within the individual, respiratory variables exert influences upon variations in the magnitude of RSA under resting and psychologically taxing conditions. Coupling between respiratory variables and RSA tended to be a bit tighter during resting conditions, although even during rest, the average amount of variance accounted for by the individual respiratory parameters was only on the order of 25%.

Within-Individual Respiratory Modulation of Vagal Outflow to the Heart

The absence of a stronger within-individual correlation between breath-by-breath RSA and respiratory variables would, at first glance, appear to contradict other reports showing very potent relations between RSA magnitude and respiratory rate and volume under controlled ventilatory conditions (i.e. where subjects were required to systematically alter RR and V_t; e.g. Angelone and Coulter, 1967; Hirsch and Bishop, 1981). However, scrutiny of these earlier studies reveals that subjects were paced at different breathing patterns for a minimum of several minutes per pattern; it was the average RSA magnitude per respiratory-pacing condition that turned out to be highly dependent upon breathing parameters, and not the breath-by-breath relation between variables.

At the more microscopic level of breath-to-breath variations, however, we have very consistently observed, among spontaneously breathing subjects, fluctuations in RSA amplitude <u>across consecutive breaths</u>, that appear to be independent of ventilatory parameters. That is to say, RSA magnitude would fluctuate from breath to breath, even when RR and V_t remained almost constant. An in-depth examination of these variations has made it clear that the breath-to-breath changes in RSA are not random but rather appear to be highly regular and rhythmic oscillations that each span typically three to four breaths (see Figure 4). Furthermore, both the amplitude and the frequency of these oscillations seem to be a function of RR, so that oscillations in RSA become smaller in amplitude and more rapid with more rapid respiration rate. We have now examined the data sets of twenty subjects, and each clearly reveals this phenomenon during regular breathing.

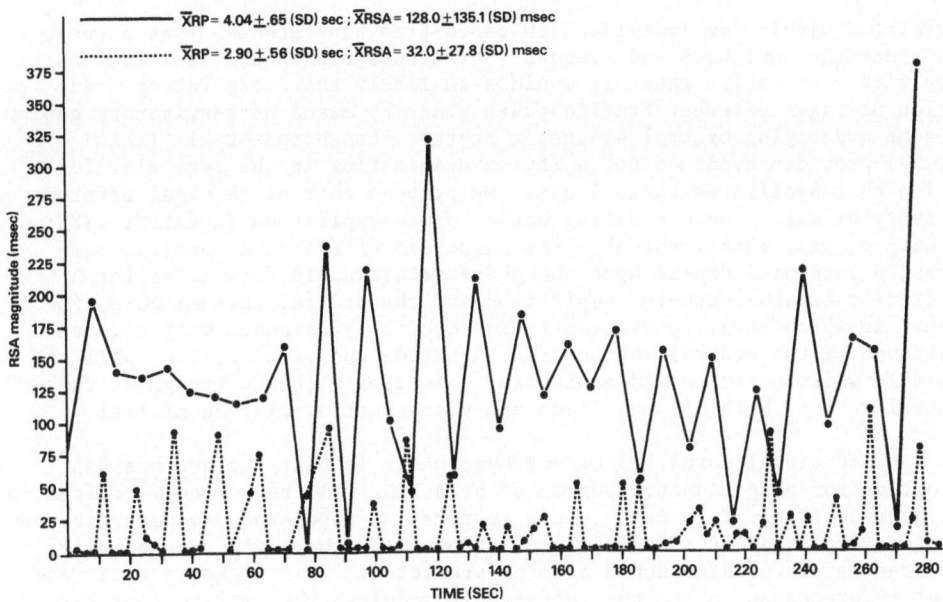

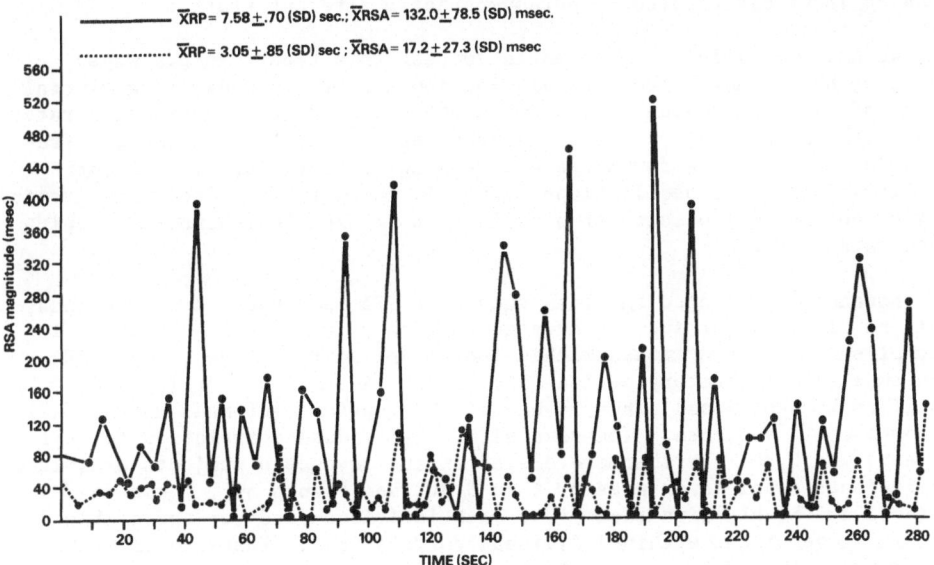

Fig. 4. Across-breath fluctuations in RSA magnitude (peak-to-trough estimation) during two conditions of 300 secs length. Every point is
the RSA amplitude for a single breath. Each chart represents an
individual subject. Subjects here illustrated were chosen for
their spontaneously regular respiratory period (RP) and tidal
volume (not shown) within the specific conditions. Thus, note the
rhythmicity of fluctuations within conditions that appears to be
independent of respiration. However, also note that within subjects, increasing respiratory period is associated with a higher
mean level of RSA magnitude.

These findings have led us to a specific hypothesis concerning
relations between respiration, RSA and cardiac vagal tone within the
healthy individual: since average RSA and respiratory parameters are highly

correlated within the individual in paced-breathing studies (see above), and since the amplitude and frequency of across-breath RSA oscillations vary with respiration rate, it would seem likely that respiratory modulation of vagal efferent traffic takes place by means of respiratory gating of some underlying central brainstem rhythm. Langhorst et al. (this volume) provides evidence for a rhythm originating in the reticular formation that oscillates up to 6 cpm. We propose that since vagal efferent activity primarily occurs during early to mid-expiration (Eckberg, 1983; Gilberg et al., 1984), the absolute magnitude of RSA at a specific respiration rate will depend upon the phase relationship (occurring for a particular breath) between respiration and the central rhythm: thus, for a breath in which early to mid-expiration occurs synchronous with the peak amplitude of the central rhythm, RSA magnitude and vagal outflow will be maximal; where early to mid-expiration coincides with the trough of the central rhythm, both RSA magnitude and vagal outflow will be minimal.

An additional corollary of our hypothesis is that the average RSA magnitude for a spontaneous period of breathing will be strongly related to the average respiratory rate, since respiration rate seems to determine the absolute amplitude of across-breath RSA oscillations, and, consequently, the mean levels of RSA should also be predicted. This suggests that respiratory processes in healthy individuals modulate the amplitude of the central rhythm that is expressed in vagal outflow to the heart, changes in RR being inversely related to parasympathetic efferent traffic.

We have preliminarily attempted to test this theory in two ways: first, we have constructed a simulation model where an underlying central rhythm of 6 cpm is proposed to be modulated by different respiration rates. We have found that the number of breaths per RSA oscillation and the frequency of oscillations for different RR's agree very closely with our empirical data; thus oscillations typically cover three to four respiratory cycles, and the periodicity of oscillations becomes lengthened as respiration rate slows.

Secondly, we tested the idea that mean RSA magnitude across periods would be highly determined by average RR within individual subjects. To accomplish this, we examined within-individual correlations between RSA magnitude and respiratory period (RP) across 14 5-minute resting and mental-task conditions. Thus we had 14 observations (of mean RSA and RP) for each of 17 subjects. The mean within-individual correlation for all subjects was 0.88. Furthermore eleven of the seventeen subjects exhibited coefficients equal to or greater than 0.90 (see Figure 5). These coefficients are highly significant for each individual and for the combined group average of the within-individual correlations. Inasmuch as it has been previously indicated that RSA magnitude under spontaneous breathing is largely determined by ventilatory parameters (Hirsch and Bishop, 1981), these results provide additional support for our theory that respiration mediates cardiac vagal tone by modulating the amplitude of a central rhythm from which vagal efferent traffic originates.

In sum, we have just presented evidence that, within the individual, the average amount of RSA, as well as the range of RSA fluctuations, may be largely a function of respiratory processes. Since RSA has previously been shown to be a sensitive index of cardiac vagal tone (e.g. Katona and Jih, 1975), our findings also suggest that variations in respiratory parameters may exert a major mediating influence upon cardiac vagal tone by their modulation of the peripheral expression of rhythmic alterations in central brainstem activity, often considerably slower than the respiratory cycle. To our knowledge, this is the first time that this relationship has been described or in any manner empirically documented. Of course, much additional research is needed to further substantiate our theoretical model.

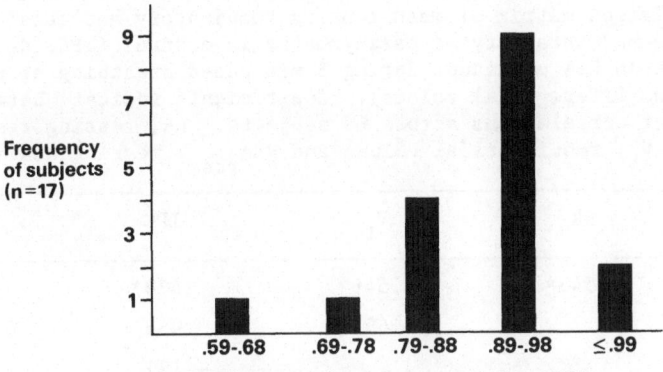

Fig. 5. Frequency histogram of within-individual coupling of respiratory period and RSA. Correlation coefficients were determined from the average levels of respiratory period and RSA across 14 five-min periods of rests and varying tasks for each of 17 subjects. Thus, for example, eleven subjects manifested correlation coefficients between RSA and RP beyond 0.89. All data was automatically scored by computer.

Respiratory-Vagal Coupling Across Individuals

    We have also been interested in the manner by which individual differences in cardiac vagal tone (as indexed by RSA) may be influenced by individual differences in respiratory pattern. It would seem justifiable for several reasons to assume that variations in cardiac parasympathetic control between individuals could at least partially be explained by differences in breathing patterns: (1) as already shown, there is convincing evidence that within-individual variations in vagal tone can be largely accounted for by changes in breathing parameters; (2) there are large differences between normal individuals in respiratory measures for specific situations (see Grossman, 1983; Schaefer, 1958); and (3) studies have found a close correspondence between RSA magnitude and parasympathetic tone across individuals, in spite of the fact that respiratory pattern was uncontrolled and is most certain to have varied greatly between individuals (Fouad et al., 1984; Katona and Jih, 1975). This last point, in combination with the former two, would then suggest that the variations in vagal tone in these last studies may rather importantly be due to individual differences in breathing pattern, since if all subjects had been required to breath at the same rate and volume, much different results might have been expected: for example, we have found, with 69 normal subjects, very modest correlations between spontaneous RSA and RSA under controlled slow breathing (see Table 1).

    There is another stream of research, on the other hand, which provides clear evidence of large individual differences in cardiac parasympathetic control among normal individuals when ventilatory parameters are, indeed, held constant across subjects (e.g. Smith, 1982; Wieling et al., 1982): for example, very sizeable individual differences in RSA magnitude may be observed when normal subjects breathe at a frequency of six cycles per minute and maximal volume. Since RSA magnitude under controlled respiration rate and tidal volume appears to be a sensitive index of the underlying status of cardiac parasympathetic control mechanisms, among both normals and clinical populations with cardiac vagal neuropathy (see previous section), we refer to it as a measure of parasympathetic integrity.

Table 1. Correlation matrix of mean resting respiratory and cardiac parameters and integrity of parasympathetic control (IPC; derived from mean RSA magnitude during 3-min paced breathing at six cpm and two liters tidal volume). Coefficients indicate between-subject correlations across 69 subjects. RR, resting respiration rate; V_t, resting tidal volume and RSA_{rest}, resting RSA magnitude.

	RR	V_t	IPC	$\bar{x}\ HR_{rest}$
RSA_{rest}	−.543*	.546*	.470*	−.320[+]
RR		−.695*	.054	−.045
V_t			−.171	.056
IPC				−.364[+]

[+] $p < .005$
* $p < .001$

These investigations then suggest that individual differences in the underlying integrity of parasympathetic control (IPC) may - independently of respiration - also significantly contribute to differences in cardiac vagal tone among normals.

Inasmuch as both respiratory pattern and nonrespiratory-related underlying parasympathetic control would, therefore, seem to influence individual differences in cardiac parasympathetic tone, we decided to examine the relative contributions of each for predicting variations in resting vagal tone among a group of 69 normal, 20 to 26 year-old male students (Grossman, Wientjes and Defares, 1984; 1985). We used mean RSA during three minutes of a ten-minute period of quiet sitting as our dependent measure of cardiac parasympathetic tone. As predictor variables, we employed mean resting respiration rate and mean resting tidal volume (scored from the same three-minute period as resting RSA), and an index of underlying parasympathetic integrity (IPC). IPC was operationalized as the average RSA magnitude during a three-minute period of voluntary, paced breathing at six cycles per minute and two liters tidal volume (this period occurring immediately after the rest period); we chose the rate of six cycles per minute because numerous studies have found it sensitive to variations in status of cardiac vagal efferent mechanisms (e.g. Eckberg, 1983; Johnston, 1980; Smith, 1982). RSA magnitude was quantified in the same manner as previously described.

Table 1 provides the across-individual simple Pearson product-moment intercorrelations between all measures (mean resting HR is also included). It is evident that IPC and respiratory measures are each related to individual variations in resting parasympathetic tone, although the separate respiratory measures account for a somewhat larger share of resting vagal tone variance.

We subsequently performed a multiple regression analysis in order to examine independent relative contributions, and joint influences of the three predictor variables in accounting for individual differences in resting vagal tone. Table 2 presents the results. Predictor variables were entered in a fixed, stepwise order into the regression analysis, on the basis of previous findings and our own experimental hypotheses. Each of the predictor variables made their own independent contribution to the total explained variance in vagal tone during rest. Additionally, there was also a significant interaction between tidal volume and IPC which

Table 2. Multiple regression summary table for resting RSA as dependent variable. Step number indicates the order that predictor variables entered the regression analysis. The stepwise entrance order was determined *a priori* on the basis of previously published evidence and our own experimental hypotheses. N = 69 subjects.

Step	Variable entered	F to enter	Signif.	Multiple R	R Square	R^2 change	Overall F Signif.
1	Respiration rate	24.67	.000	.5430	.2949	.2949	24.67 .000
2	Tidal volume	4.92	.031	.5916	.3500	.0551	15.61 .000
3	Integrity of parasymp. control (IPC)	50.65	.000	.8098	.6558	.3058	36.21 .000
4	V_t by IPC interaction	23.83	.000	.8710	.7586	.1027	43.99 .000

accounted for another ten percent of the total variance. Altogether, over
75% of the individual variation in resting parasympathetic tone was
accounted for in this analysis.

These findings indicate that variations among individuals in vagal
tone are determined jointly by respiratory processes and factors related to
the underlying integrity of cardiac vagal control mechanisms. Individuals
who breathe more slowly and more deeply, as well as showing relatively high
levels of IPC, are very likely to exhibit marked resting levels of cardiac
parasympathetic control. Conversely, rapid, shallow breathers, especially
those with low levels of IPC, seem to demonstrate quite modest resting
vagal tone. The interaction between IPC and respiration as illustrated in
Figure 6, suggests that individual differences in IPC play an increasingly
greater role at larger tidal volumes in determining resting vagal tone.
Hence, for any particular RR, differences between high- and low-IPC
individuals in resting vagal tone will become progressively larger, the
greater the tidal volume increases. Furthermore, since RR and tidal volume
are powerfully inversely correlated across individuals (see Table 1), these
findings would then suggest that level of IPC will make little difference
in determining vagal tone among rapid, shallow breathers, whereas sizeable
effects of IPC level would be expected for slow, large-volume breathers.

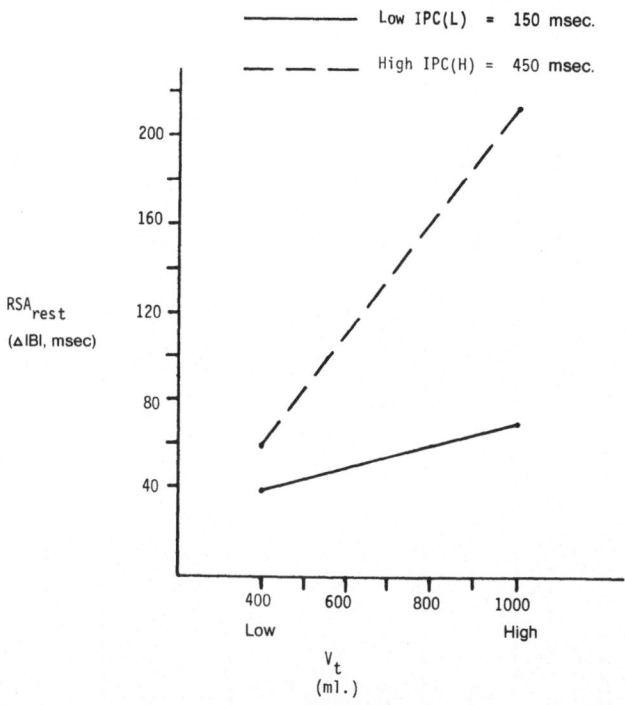

Fig. 6. Interaction between individual differences in parasympathetic
         integrity and respiratory pattern in the determination of RSA
         during rest. Integrity of parasympathetic control (IPC) was an
         index derived from the average RSA magnitude from an individual
         during a three-min period of paced breathing at six cpm and two
         liters tidal volume. Here low IPC = 150 msec (solid line), and
         high IPC = 450 msec (broken line); all RSA values were determined
         with peak-trough differences in heart period. Respiration rate is
         held constant in this figure at 14 cpm. Notice that at a shallow
         tidal volume, IPC contributes relatively little to RSA magnitude,
         whereas at large volumes, it contributes much.

Our investigations of relations between individual differences in cardiac vagal control and respiration appear to complement and extend our other findings concerning intra-individual relationships. Just as we reported that variations in respiratory parameters <u>within the individual</u> seem to influence the efferent expression of inherent rhythmic cardiac vagal activity, individual differences in respiratory pattern seem also to modulate variations in the expression of underlying PI. On the one hand, these data may shed new light upon cardiac vagal control mechanisms by pointing toward the importance of respiratory-cardiac integration for vagal control. On the other hand, since it would appear that vagal control of the heart could be enhanced by behavioral strategies aimed at modification of breathing pattern, these findings may also have relevance for non-intrusive experimental manipulations of vagal tone, both in order to examine potential psychophysiological therapies for cardiovascular disorders associated with deficient vagal outflow (see e.g. Janssen, 1983; Janssen and Beckering, this volume) and in order to explore the significance of interactions between psycho-environmental factors and vagal mechanisms for issues related to cardiovascular competence.

RSA AS INDEX OF VAGAL EFFECTS UPON HEART RATE, NOT CENTRAL PROCESSES

Psychophysiologists utilizing RSA as index of vagal tone, in accord with certain now traditional psychological theories concerning the significance of cardiovascular activity, have suggested that variations in RSA magnitude may be used to reflect general aspects of the status of the central nervous system (Porges, this volume; Porges et al., 1981; Porges, McCabe and Yongue, 1982; Richards, 1985). Thus, differences in RSA between clinical populations and normals within a particular situation (e.g. rest) are hypothesized to reveal differences in, at least, the integrity of central parasympathetic control mechanisms. There are, however, several problems with such a conceptualization.

First of all, RSA magnitude, like cardiac vagal tone, is a situation-specific phenomenon. Both increase under conditions of low activity and physiological quiescence, whereas both decrease quite dramatically when mind or body become active or disturbed (see later). Hence, a clinical population that manifests a higher level of arousal than normal for a resting situation, may have central and peripheral parasympathetic control mechanisms which are just as intact as those of normal individuals; it may only be the inappropriately high general state of physiological activation that masks a perfectly adequate parasympathetic control system. One can only test for and compare the inherent integrity of vagal control across groups when groups are roughly at similar levels of physiological activation. Were it possible to quiet the physiological responses of the clinical group in the direction of normal situation-specific responses, one might just as well expect typical RSA and vagal levels, given the present lack of evidence to the contrary. Conversely, excitation of the normal group under resting conditions might well produce a similar picture of RSA and vagal tone as that seen with the clinical population.

A second problem with the notion that RSA reflects central vagal processes is, perhaps, even more fundamental. Because RSA is a cardiac measure, derived directly from the electrophysiological activity of the heart, it is impossible to deduce from this measure, alone, information about the separate contributions to RSA of the target end-organ itself, the vagal centers in the brain, or the afferent and efferent pathways trafficking neural impulses. This opacity in regard to specific mechanisms is especially evident when RSA magnitude is abnormally low, even when background levels of activation are controlled for: is there something centrally amiss, is the sinus node malfunctioning or are the vagal pathways not communicating their afferent or efferent messages? Information based solely upon end-organ activity precludes the answering of such queries.

A study by Katona, Lipson and Dauchot (1977) concretely illustrates the inadequacy of RSA as index of central vagal activity: using anesthetized dogs, these investigators found that increasing doses of low-dose atropine progressively <u>elevated</u> central vagal efferent activity while at the same time proportionately reducing peripheral cardiac vagal responses (including an RSA-based measure). RSA only reflected peripheral effects, not central ones. That such different peripheral and central effects may also occur in psychophysiological investigations is an obvious possibility that precludes inferences from being made concerning the integrity of central parasympathetic mechanisms, except when the total cardiac vagal control system is functioning well and it is evident that all vagal components must be intact.

RSA, nonetheless, is apparently a very sensitive estimate of the <u>final</u>, summed vagal effects upon heart period. As such, it provides researchers, for the first time, with a tool for observing parasympathetic influences upon cardiac functioning under diverse, naturalistic conditions, and does not require the employment of invasive measurement procedures. On the one hand, this index permits us to begin to illuminate relationships between vagal activity of the heart and other physiological processes in the intact organism, e.g. the manner by which vagal control relates to average heart rate under specific conditions, or the types of respiratory-vagal cardiac interactions previously discussed. On the other hand, such a window to vagal processes enables us to explore cardiac parasympathetic interactions with environmental, psychological and behavioral variations. Our own research using RSA has been oriented to such applications.

In two different studies, we consistently found marked, significant, reductions from resting RSA to occur under mental task conditions. In one study utilizing a memory-comparison reaction-time task with 44 subjects (Grossman and Wientjes, in preparation), RSA during task was, on the average, reduced to 40% of preceding resting, baseline levels (mean RSA during rest = 132 msec during baseline). Furthermore, RSA magnitude significantly varied between the three different task conditions used to manipulate motivation (feedback of performance vs. no feedback vs. extra monetary incentive).

In the second experiment, task-related changes, in which we employed a video game as stressor, were also marked (n = 20; Grossman and Svebak, in preparation). Furthermore, we manipulated the level of psychological stress in the last investigation by introducing the threat of shock for inferior performance during one of the two task conditions. The same video task was used both for threat and no-threat conditions, and the order of presentation of conditions was counterbalanced across subjects. No shocks were actually administered during the threat condition. Results indicated that there was a greater reduction in RSA during the threat conditions than during the no-threat task (mean = 39% and 50% of baseline, resting levels, respectively; p < 0.01). Hence, these data provide substantial evidence that mentally loading tasks reduce parasympathetic control of heart period and that the additional presence of a threatening stimulus (i.e. threat of shock) may further attenuate cardiac vagal tone. Such findings may help to cast light upon cardiac parasympathetic consequences of discrete psychological stressors.

Another relevant question that we explored within this context was, to what degree the task-related tonic heart rate changes were associated with alterations in vagal tone (as indexed by RSA). In the last-mentioned study, we found that changes in HR, from baseline to task, were highly correlated with inverse changes in RSA magnitude across subjects ($r = -0.70$, threat condition; $r = -0.59$, no threat; $p < 0.01$). Similarly, RSA and HR difference scores between the two task conditions were also strongly negatively correlated across subjects ($r = -0.84$). Associations, then, were such that the greater the diminution of RSA, the larger the increase in HR. Furthermore, for both studies mentioned here, across-individual correlations between RSA and HR <u>within mental task conditions</u> were consistently highly negative ($r = -0.63$ to -0.94).

These strong associations, of course, do not necessarily imply that cardiac vagal mechanisms determined the often substantial HR elevations that occurred during tasks (averaging from 4 to 20 bpm depending upon task), although this is, indeed, a possibility. Alternatively, reciprocal sympathetic-parasympathetic interactions may have been responsible for these alterations in HR (i.e. a combination of cardiac sympathetic activation and.vagal withdrawal). In either case, vagal mechanisms do seem to have been directly involved. Future research measuring RSA under more differentiated experimental conditions may point to the responsible causal mechanism.

CONCLUSION

Respiratory sinus arrhythmia is a phenomenon which may provide us with a naturalistic, bird's-eye view of the workings of the cardiac parasympathetic control system. In this Chapter we have attempted to point out some fundamental, and less obvious, issues related to quantification problems and inferential limits inherent to this area of interest. Furthermore, using our own research findings, we have presented evidence of the complex and intimate relationships between RSA and respiratory processes, which seems strongly to suggest important ties between ventilatory and cardiac parasympathetic control mechanisms. Lastly, we have provided experimental data indicating that parasympathetic withdrawal may play a significant role in heart rate responses to psychological stressors.

Our approach to the quantification and application of RSA deviates in several ways from that of other psychophysiological investigators dealing with the phenomenon: (1) we rely upon a simple peak-to-trough estimate of RSA; (2) we stress the significance of respiratory influences upon RSA and the importance of the simultaneous evaluation of RSA and discrete respiratory parameters, and (3) we utilize RSA as an index of the final, summed vagal effects upon heart rate, and not as a reflection of central neural functioning. Our justification for this group of operational premises is strictly based upon inferences drawn from the physiological literature. Consequently, we believe that these guidelines, from a purely empirical perspective, represent the safest boundaries within which to investigate this phenomenon.

REFERENCES

Angelone, A., and Coulter, N.A., 1964, Respiratory sinus arrhythmia: a frequency-dependent phenomenon, <u>J. Appl. Physiol.</u>, 19:479-482.
Ax, A. F., Bamford, J. L., and Fetzner, J. M., 1973, Respiration sinus arrhythmia in psychotic children, <u>Psychophysiology</u>, 10:401-414.
Boer, R. W. de, Karemaker, J., and Strackee, J., 1985, Relationships between short-term blood-pressure fluctuations and heart-rate variability in resting subjects II: a simple model, <u>Med. & Biol. Engineering & Computers</u>, 23:352-358.
Bohrer, R. E., and Porges, S. W., 1982, The application of time-series

statistics to psychological research: an introduction, in: "Psychological Statistics", G. Karen, ed., Hillsdale, N. J.:Erlbaum.

Bristow, J. D., Honour, A. J., Pickering, G. W., Sleight, P., and Smyth, W. S., 1969, Diminished baroreflex sensitivity in high blood pressure, Circulation, 39:48-54.

Clynes, M., 1960, Respiratory sinus arrhythmia: laws derived from computer simulation, J. Appl. Physiol., 15:863-874.

Coker, R., Koziell, A., Olivier, C., and Smith, S. E., 1984, Does the sympathetic nervous system influence sinus arrhythmia in man? Evidence from combined autonomic blockade, J. Physiol, 356:459-564.

Davies, C. T. M., and Neilson, J. M. M.,1967, Sinus arrhythmia in man at rest, J. Appl. Physiol., 22:947-955.

Eckberg, D. L., Kifle, Y. T., and Roberts, V. L., 1980, Phase relationship between human respiration and baroreflex responsiveness, J. Physiol. (London), 304:489-502,

Eckberg, D. L., 1983, Human sinus arrhythmia as an index of vagal cardiac outflow, J. Appl. Physiol., 54:961-966.

Ewing, D. J., Borsey, D. Q., Bellavere, F., and Clarke, B. F., 1981, Cardiac autonomic neuropathy in diabetes: comparison of measures of R-R interval variation, Diabetologica, 32:18-24.

Fouad, F. M., Tarazi, R. C., Ferrario, C. M., Fighaly, S., and Alicandro, C., 1984, Assessment of parasympathetic control of heart rate by a noninvasive method, Am. J. Physiol., 246:H838-H842.

Fox, N. A., and Porges, S. W., 1985, The relation between neonatal heart patterns and developmental outcome, Child Development, 56:28-37.

Gilbey, M. P., Jordan, D., Richter, D. W., and Spijer, K. M., 1984, Synaptic mechanisms involved in the inspiratory modulation of vagal cardio-inhibitory neurones in the cat, J. Physiol., 356:65-78.

Grossman, P., 1983, Respiration, stress and cardiovascular function, Psychophysiology, 20:284-300.

Grossman, P., Wientjes, K., and Defares, P. B., 1984, Individual differences in cardiac parasympathetic control predicted by ventilatory parameters, Psychophysiology, 21:579(A).

Grossman, P. and Wientjes, K., 1985, Respiratory-cardiac coordination as an index of cardiac functioning, in: "Cardiovascular Psychophysiology: Theory and Methods", J.F. Orlebeke, G. Mulder and L.J.P. van Doornen, eds., Plenum, New York, pp. 451-465.

Grossman, P., Wientjes, K. and Defares, P., 1985, Respiratory influences upon individual differences in cardiac parasympathetic control, in: "Stress and the Work Situation", K. Wientjes and P. Grossman, eds., TNO Institute for Perception, Soesterberg, the Netherlands

Haddad, G. G., Jeng, H. J., Lee, S. H., and Lai, T. L., 1984, Rhythmic variations in R-R interval during sleep and wakefulness in puppies and dogs, Am. J. Physiol.,247:H67-H73.

Harper, R. M., Walter, D. O., Leake, B., Hoffman, H. J., Sieck, G. C., Sterman, M. B., Hoppenbrouwers, T., and Hodgman, J., 1978, Development of sinus arrhythmia during sleeping and waking states in normal infants, Sleep, 1:33-48.

Hilsted, J., and Jensen, S. B., 1979, A simple test for autonomic neuropathy in juvenile diabetes, Acta Medica Scand., 205:385-387.

Hinkle, L. E., Carver, S. T., and Plakun, A., 1972, Slow heart rates and increased risk of cardiac death, Arch. Int. Med., 129:732-750.

Hirsch, J. A., and Bishop, B., 1981, Respiratory sinus arrhythmia in humans: how breathing pattern modulates heart rate, Am. J. Physiol., 241:H620-H629.

Janssen, K. H., 1983, Treatment of sinus tachycardia with heart rate feedback: A group outcome study, J. Beh. Med., 6:109-114.

Johnston, L. C., 1980, The abnormal heart rate response to a deep breath in borderline labile hypertension: a sign of autonomic nervous system dysfunction, Am. Heart J., 99:487-493.

Kallenbach, J. M., Webster, T., Dowdeswell, R., Reinach, S. G., Millar, R. N., Scott, and Zwi, S., 1985, Reflex heart rate control in asthma. Evidence of parasympathetic overactivity, Chest, 87:644-648.

Katona, P. G., and Jih, R., 1975, Respiratory sinus arrhythmia: a non-invasive measure of parasympathetic cardiac control, J. Appl. Physiol., 39:801-805.

Lipson, D., and Katona, P. G., 1979, Respiratory sinus arrhythmia: a non-invasive assessment of parasympathetic chronotropic cardiac control in the conscious dog, Federation Proceeding, 38:990 (Abstract).

McCabe, P. M., Yongue, B. G., Ackles, P. K., and Porges, S. W., 1985, Changes in heart period, heart-period variability, and a spectral estimate of respiratory sinus arrhythmia in response to pharmacological manipulations of the baroreflex in cats, Psychophysiology, 22:195-203.

Mulder, G., and Mulder, L. J. M., 1981, Information processing and cardiovascular control, Psychophysiology, 14:392-402.

Mulder, L. J. M., 1985, Cardiovascular measures and models in time and frequency domain, in: "The Psychophysiology of Cardiovascular Control", J. F. Orlebeke, G. Mulder and L. J. P. van Doornen, eds., Plenum, New York.

Orr, W. C., and Naitoh, P., 1976, The coherence spectrum: an extension of correlation analysis with applications to chronobiology, Intern. J. Chronobiol., 3:171-192.

Porges, S. W., Bohrer, R. E., Keren, G., Cheung, M. N., Franks, G. J., and Drasgow, F., 1981, The influence of methylphenidate on spontaneous autonomic activity and behavior in children diagnosed as hyperactive, Psychophysiology, 18:42-48.

Porges, S. W., McCabe, P. M., and Yongue, B. G., Respiratory-heart rate interactions: psychophysiological implications for pathophysiology and behavior, in: "Perspectives in Cardiovascular Psychophysiology", J. J. Cacioppo, ed., R. E. Petty, Guildford:New York.

Raczkowska, M., Eckberg, D. L., and Ebert, T. J., 1983, Muscarinic cholinergic receptors modulate vagal cardiac responses in man, J. Auto. Nervous System, 7:271-278.

Richards, J. E., 1984, The "interrupted stimulus" method for measuring sustained attention in infants from 14 to 26 weeks of age, Psychophysiology, 21:594-595 (A).

Richards, J. E., 1985, Respiratory sinus arrhythmia predicts heart rate and visual responses during visual attention in 14 and 20 week old infants, Psychophysiology, 22:101-109.

Schaefer, K. E., 1958, Respiratory patterns and respiratory response to carbon dioxide, J.Appl.Physiol., 13:1-14.

Schlomka, G., 1937, Untersuchungen über die physiologische Unregelmässigkeit des Herzschlages. III Mitteilung: über die abhängigkeit der respiratorischen Arrhythmie von Schlagfrequenz und vom Lebensalter, Kreislaufforschritte, 29:510-529.

Selman, A., McDonald, A., Kitney, R., and Linkens, D., 1982, The interaction between heart rate and respiration: Part I - experimental studies in man, Automedica, 4:131-139.

Smith, S. A., 1982, Reduced sinus arrhythmia in diabetic autonomic neuropathy: diagnostic value of an age-related normal range, Br. Med. J., 285:1599-1601.

Sundkvist, G., Almer, L. O., and Lilja, B., 1979, Respiratory influence on heart rate in diabetes mellitus, Br. Med. J., 1:924-925.

Wheeler, T., and Watkins, P. J., 1973, Cardiac denervation in diabetes, Br. Med. J., 4:584-586.

White, D. P., Douglas, N. J., Pickett, C. K., Weil, J. V., and Zwillich, C. W., 1983, Sexual influence on the control of breathing, J. Appl. Physiol., 54:874-879.

Wieling, W., Brederode, J. F. M. van, Rijk, L. G. de, and Dunning, A. J., 1982, Reflex control of heart rate in normal subjects in relation to age: a data base for cardiac vagal neuropathy, _Diabetologica_, 22:163-166.

Yuen, C. K., and Fraser, D., 1979, "Digital Spectral Analysis," San Francisco: Pitman.

Zemaityte, D., Varoneckas, G., and Sokolov, E., 1984a, Heart rhythm control during sleep, _Psychophysiology_, 21:279-289.

Zemaityte, D., Varoneckas, G., and Sokolov, E., 1984b, Heart rhythm during sleep in ischemic heart disease, _Psychophysiology_, 21:290-298.

CARDIAC-RESPIRATORY INTEGRATION: IMPLICATIONS FOR THE

ANALYSIS AND INTERPRETATION OF PHASIC CARDIAC RESPONSES

Graham Turpin

Plymouth Polytechnic

INTRODUCTION

Measures of cardiovascular activity have been extensively employed by psychophysiologists to index covert psychological processes. Previous applications of measures such as heart rate have included attempts to quantify such diverse psychological constructs as drive, arousal, activation, anxiety and cognitive effort (Cacioppo and Petty 1982; Obrist, 1981; Orlebeke et al., in press; Siddle and Turpin, 1980). Currently, discrete and subtle phasic heart rate (HR) changes are interpreted as representing different forms of information processing ranging from stimulus registration through to response preparation (Coles et al., in press; Jennings, in press). In contrast, measures of respiration have seldom been adopted as bona fide dependent measures. Instead, they have frequently been relegated to the level of artifact, and obtained only in order to exclude autonomic responses associated with breathing irregularities such as coughing and sighing.

The intention of this chapter is to review the effects of simple sensory stimuli on both respiratory and cardiac responses, and to examine the implications of cardiovascular-respiratory interactions for the analysis and interpretation of phasic cardiac responses. Given the current importance of cardiovascular measures as psychophysiological indices of cognitive activity, it will be argued that a comprehensive understanding of these measures is facilitated if measures of respiratory activity are jointly considered.

In order to illustrate the various levels of interaction between the respiratory and cardiovascular systems, the first section of this chapter will describe basic respiratory-cardiovascular phenomena. The second section will examine the implications of these phenomena for the form of stimulus-elicited phasic cardiac responses. In particular, the influence of concomitant respiratory responses, respiratory sinus arrhythmia, cardiac and respiratory cycle-time, and respiratory-phase modulation on the size and direction of cardiac responses will be explored in some depth. General problems concerning the analysis of phasic cardiac responses will not be covered since these have been resently discussed elsewhere (Siddle and Turpin, 1980; Turpin, 1985).

Stimulus Elicited Cardiac Responses

Various different theoretical frameworks have been proposed in order to encompass the relationship between cardiovascular activity and information processing. Although a comprehensive review of these theories is beyond the scope of the present chapter, some examples will be provided in order to illustrate the application of cardiovascular measures to psychophysiology.

It is claimed that stimuli such as brief tones or white noise pulses elicit several different attentional reflex systems concerned with the current and future processing of environmental information (Graham, 1979; Turpin, 1983). These systems have been characterized in terms of the orienting, defense and startle reflexes and, it is claimed, may be differentiated from one another by their cardiovascular response components and the nature of the eliciting stimulus. Thus, intense auditory stimuli are said to elicit either defensive or startle reflexes which are identified by their accelerative HR response component, whereas low to moderate auditory stimuli elicit orienting responses characterized by HR decelerations. These intensity-dependent transitions in the form of the phasic cardiac response were readily observed in a recent experiment by Turpin and Siddle (1983). Five groups of 15 subjects each received a series of 1000 Hz, 2 sec tones (risetime = 30 msec). The stimulus intensity of each tone series was varied from 105 to 45 dB across the five groups. Several different cardiovascular measures were obtained, and the phasic response to each stimulus was analyzed. The mean HR responses derived from the 5 intensity groups are displayed in Figure 1 and clearly demonstrate the change in direction of the response from cardiac deceleration to acceleration as the intensity of the stimulus is increased. Results such as these are of interest to psychophysiologists since they indicate that different forms of processing might accompany increases in stimulus intensity.

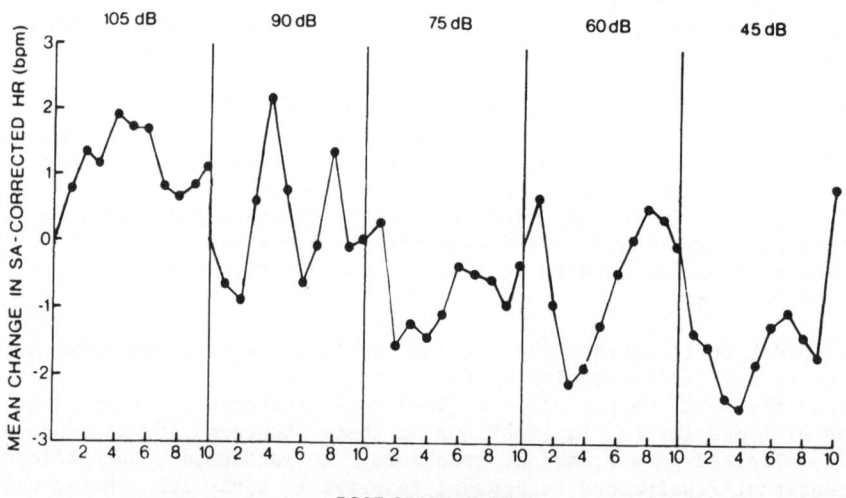

Fig. 1.   Mean HR response averaged across the first three stimulus presentations as a function of intensity and poststimulus beat. Copyright (c) 1983, The Society for Psychophysiological Research. Reprinted with permission of the publishers from "Effects of Stimulus Intensity on Cardiovascular Activity" by G. Turpin and D.A.T. Siddle, Psychophysiology, 20:611-624.

If more complex paradigms are considered, then a variety of orderly cardiac response components may be demonstrated. For example, in a reaction time paradigm consisting of a warning stimulus and imperative stimulus, a tripartite response composed of deceleration, acceleration and deceleration is frequently observed prior to the execution of the motor response. Indeed, a variety of psychological processes which include orienting, uncertainty detection and response preparation have been associated with these cardiac response components (see Bohlin and Kjellberg, 1979). Attempts have also been made to relate the functional significance of these cardiovascular adjustments to proposed psychological processes. An example of this approach concerns the interpretation of the secondary decelerative component in terms of direct sensory facilitation, (Lacey and Lacey, 1978), general body quietening (Obrist, 1981) or increased cardiovascular supply to the musculature (Jennings, 1982). The role of cardiovascular measures as indices of psychological or behavioral processes which are directly concerned with information processing the task performance is implicit in these diverse formulations. The purpose of this chapter, therefore, is to evaluate this role with respect to respiratory-cardiovascular interactions.

Stimulus Elicited Respiratory Responses

Several studies have examined the effects of brief simple stimuli on respiration (see Barry, 1977). Unfortunately, the methods employed to quantify respiratory responses have differed across these studies and preclude any firm conclusions from being reached. For example, changes in respiration have been assessed in terms of both the frequency and amplitude of breathing. They have also been derived either from the breath observed at stimulus onset or from subsequent post-stimulus breathing cycles. Furthermore, a variety of different recording techniques have been employed.

Increases in respiratory amplitude as a function of increased stimulus intensity were said to have been observed in several studies (Davis et al., 1955; McCallum et al., 1969; Smith and Strawbridge, 1969; Steinschneider, 1968). The overall effect of stimulation on either breathing frequency or the duration of various respiratory phases is more difficult to establish. Barry (1977) has claimed that the respiratory component of the orienting reflex (OR) consists of an increase in respiratory cycle length. In reaching this conclusion, he refers to observations made during respiratory response audiology (Bradford, 1975; Poole et al., 1966; Rousey et al., 1964) which demonstrate respiratory slowing at low auditory stimulus intensities (<30 dB). In contrast, however, moderate stimulus intensities (>50 dB) appear to bring about a decrease in respiratory cycle length (Bradford, 1975; Smith and Strawbridge, 1969; Steinschneider, 1968; Turpin and Sartory, 1980). It would seem, therefore, that both respiratory amplitude and frequency are influenced by the intensity of the eliciting stimulus. This conclusion is inconsistent with Barry's claim that the respiratory component of the OR is insensitive to manipulations of stimulus intensity.

A recent study by Harver and Kotses (1983) may help to clarify some of the above issues. They have reported that the exact nature of the respiratory response will depend upon the position of the stimulus in the respiratory cycle. In addition, any stimulus-elicited disturbance in respiration occurs not only during the cycle containing the stimulus onset but also, to varying degrees, in subsequent cycles. Unfortunately, since the stimuli employed in this study were above the intensities (>80 dB) usually employed in studies of the OR, these data are of limited value as regards identifying respiratory components of the OR. However, the study clearly demonstrates the importance of a detailed analysis of the respiratory response, and the presence of respiratory-cycle time effects.

In conclusion, the intensity of simple stimuli would appear to affect the respiratory response in a similar fashion to the cardiac response. It should be noted, however, that in the case of respiration, stimulus intensity effects have not been investigated across a range of intensities comparable to that used in HR research. Similarly, studies which have employed respiration, have tended to adopt a less stringent approach to quantification than research conducted using cardiac measures.

Respiratory Evoked Cardiovascular Changes

The effects of brief intentional changes in the breathing pattern on cardiovascular activity have been examined by several investigators. Westcott and Huttenlocher (1961) demonstrated that sharp inspiratory gasps gave rise to a consistent biphasic pattern of cardiac acceleration followed by deceleration. Stern and Anschel (1968) further manipulated the form of the required respiratory maneuver and studied its effects on HR, skin conductance and digital vascular activity. Subjects were instructed to alter their breathing pattern in a predefined manner for one breath following the presentation of a light signal. In addition to normal breathing, three instructed breathing patterns were examined, consisting of a slightly deeper, slow deep and fast deep inhalations. Skin resistance, respiration, heart rate and digital pulse amplitude responses were measured up to 9 sec following the presentation of the signal stimulus. The average HR response curves produced by the different breathing manipulations are displayed in Figure 2 and clearly demonstrate the effects of manipulating the rate and depth of inspiration. Indeed, the biphasic HR response obtained was almost identical to the findings reported by Westcott and Huttenlocher (1961).

It would appear, therefore, that discrete changes in breathing pattern may produce consistent patterns of cardiovascular activity which are not too dissimilar to those observed in response to auditory stimulation. Since auditory stimuli have themselves been shown to produce changes in the breathing pattern, the possibility arises that cardiovascular responses to such stimuli may only represent concomitant changes to respiration. If this proposition could be substantiated, then the status of cardiac measures as independent indices of central processing might be seriously weakened.

Respiratory Sinus Arrythymia

A second area of cardiovascular-respiratory interaction concerns respiratory sinus arrhythmia (RSA). Many authors have drawn attention to the presence of regular fluctuations in heart rate which appear to be entrained to the respiration frequency (see Porges et al., 1982; Westcott and Huttenlocher, 1961). RSA has generated much research including investigations of the phase relationship between HR and respiration (Angelone and Coulter, 1964; Hirsch and Bishop, 1981; Stoufe, 1971), the biological origins of the rhythm (Clynes, 1960; Davies and Neilson, 1967; Manzotti, 1958; Melcher, 1976; Porges et al., 1982), and its use as a non-invasive measure of parasympathetic tonus (Katona and Jih, 1975, Porges et al., 1982). Since much of this research has been summarized elsewhere in this book, a detailed review of the application of RSA in psychophysiology will not be covered. However, the implications of RSA for the analysis of phasic cardiac responding has received particular attention in psychophysiological research (Siddle and Turpin, 1980) and will be reviewed in the last section of this chapter.

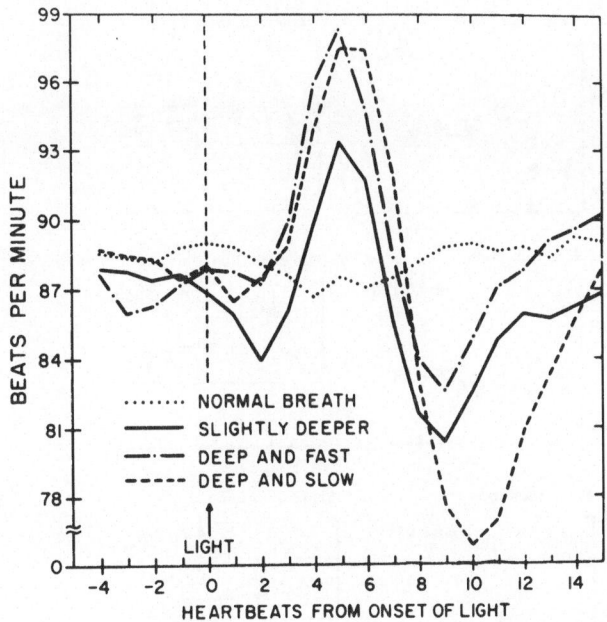

Fig. 2. Mean group heart rate response to four respiratory stimuli.
Copyright (c) 1968, The Society for Psychophysiological Research.
Reprinted with permission of the author from "Deep Inspirations as
Stimuli for Responses of the Autonomic Nervous System" by R.M.
Stern and C. Anschel, Psychophysiology, 5:132-140.

Respiratory Modulation of Cardiac Responses

Phasic cardiac responses would also seem to be directly modulated by
respiratory activity. In particular, it has been hypothesized that the
descending vagal influence on the cardiac motor neurones is either gated or
modulated by respiration (e.g. Lopes and Palmer, 1976; Eckberg et al.,
1980). Cardiac responses such as phasic HR decelerations, which are
presumed to be vagally mediated, would be inhibited during inspiration and
facilitated during expiration.

Evidence for these proposals is derived from two sources. First, a
series of physiological investigations in anesthetized animals has demonstrated that the reflex slowing of the heart, elicited either by baroreceptor or chemoreceptor stimulation, was dependent upon the phase of the
respiratory cycle when the stimulus was delivered. Stimulation during
early or mid-inspiration frequently failed to give rise to reflex cardiac
deceleration, whereas stimuli presented during late inspiration or expiration elicited pronounced decelerations (Iriuchijima and Kumada, 1964;
Katona et al., 1970); Lopes and Palmer, 1976; Davidson et al., 1976).
Similar findings have also been reported in conscious human volunteers
using neck-suction as a baroreceptor stimulus (Eckberg et al., 1980;
Trzebski et al., 1980). Examination of Figure 3, which portrays data from
the Eckberg et al. (1980) study, clearly demonstrates the effects of
respiratory phase on the reflex bradycardia due to neck suction.

Although these physiological data strongly support the notion of
respiratory modulation of vagal effects, there remain some unresolved
issues. Firstly, several studies conducted using direct electrical stimulation either in conscious rabbits (Karemaker, 1980) or humans (Borst and
Karemaker, 1980) have failed to produce reliable respiratory phase effects.

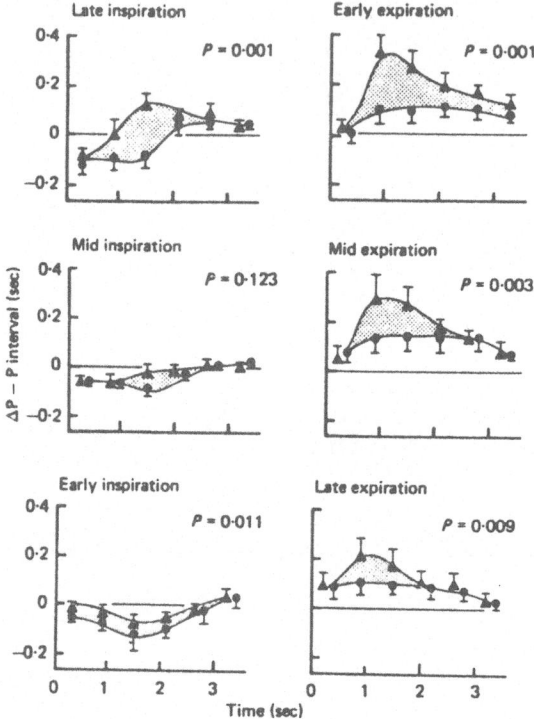

Fig. 3. Average pulse interval changes after each of six tidal volume
threshold crossings, with (triangles) and without (circles) neck
suction. P values were derived from a paired t analysis.
Brackets encompass one S.E. of mean. The stippled areas indicate
the change of pulse interval provoked by baroreceptor stimuli.
Copyright (c) 1980, The Physiology Society. Reprinted with
permission of the author from "Phase Relationship Between Normal
Human Respiration and Baroreflex Responsiveness" by D.L. Eckberg
et al., Journal of Physiology, 304:489-502.

These authors have suggested that the respiratory modulation of cardiac
vagal tone represents an additive effect rather than an absolute respiratory 'gate'. Similarly, Eckberg et al. (1980) present data which demonstrates that the nature of the modulation process is influenced by changes
in respiratory rate. They also conclude that their findings are inconsistent with a simple gating, synchronous with central respiratory neurone
activity.

    A second source of evidence for respiratory modulation of phasic
cardiac activity is derived from several psychophysiological studies.
Gautier (1972) observed respiratory modulation of the decelerative response
to an auditory stimulus which was entirely consistent with reported physiological stimulation studies. Unfortunately, unlike many of the above
studies, he did not allow for the effects of RSA on the quantification of
HR responding which would have been independent of stimulation. A recent
study (Turpin and Sartory, 1980) has re-examined the effects of respiratory
phase on the HR response to auditory stimuli (75 dB 1000 Hz tones) following correction of RSA. The findings from this study are displayed in
Figure 4a and clearly demonstrate phase dependent differences in cardiac
activity. However, greater cardiac deceleration was found for stimuli
presented at mid-inspiration as opposed to the usual finding of vagal
facilitation during the expiratory phase. This shift in phase might be

144

explained by a variety of factors. First, breathing was monitored indirectly using a nasal thermistor as opposed to measurements derived from either a pneumotachograph or phrenic nerve recording. It is possible that different phase relationships between cardiac and respiratory activity may arise due to the time constant of the different recording systems employed. Second, the latencies of the observed cardiac deceleration differed across the various studies. Peak latencies to auditory stimuli varied between 3 and 7 sec (Turpin and Sartory, 1980) whereas latencies of 0.9-1.5 sec were obtained for neck suction (Eckberg et al., 1980). Finally, both individual differences in breathing rate (Eckberg et al., 1980) and mean HR level (Coles et al., 1982) have been said to influence cardiac-respiratory phase relationships. It is possible that these latter factors might explain the sex differences observed in the Turpin and Sartory (1980) study.

A third psychophysiological study by Coles et al. (1982) also provides some support for respiratory modulation of vagal activity. The main purpose of the research was to examine the effect of cardiac cycle time on the primary bradycardia observed in reaction time tasks. However, this study also investigated the influence of respiratory phase on the expression of the cardiac cycle time effect. Their results indicated that the primary bradycardia was attenuated during inspiration but only in subjects with slow HR's. High HR subjects displayed typical RSA but failed to demonstrate any respiratory modulation of cardiac responding.

In summary, there is considerable evidence to support the hypothesis that respiration modulates stimulus-elicited vagal activity. It should also be noted that similar effects have been observed for sympathetically mediated cardiovascular changes (Cohen et al., 1980; Schramm et al., 1980; Seller et al., 1968). However, the exact nature of this interaction remains to be specified (see Koepchen et al., 1981).

Effects of Cardiovascular Responses on Cognitive Activity

Many authors have proposed that stimulus-elicited cardiovascular responses represent functionally significant changes which facilitate information processing in the CNS as opposed to being mere epiphenomena of cognitive processing. Instead of providing a detailed review of these arguments, I propose only to outline some of the working hypotheses which have frequently occurred in the literature. For instance, it has been claimed by several investigators that phasic heart rate responses may actually directly facilitate sensory processing (see Coles et al., in press). The major proponents of this approach are the Laceys who have suggested that afferent input from the baroreceptors modulates brainstem activity and the subsequent early processing of sensory information. Thus any change in baroreceptor activity due to either inherent blood pressure changes (i.e. cardiac cycle time effects) or stimulus-elicited pressor responses, might be expected to modify subsequent sensorimotor processing. For example, reaction time has been said to vary both as a function of the amplitude of the pressure pulse in the cardiac cycle and the size of the anticipatory cardiac deceleration prior to an imperative stimulus (Lacey and Lacey, 1978). Phenomena such as these have received recent critical examination (Carroll and Anastasiades, 1978; Coles et al., in press; Jennings in press). It might be concluded from these reviews that the data support, to varying degrees, a relationship between phasic cardiovascular changes and sensory processing. However, the functional significance of these brief cardiac changes for cognitive processing remains to be demonstrated unequivocably.

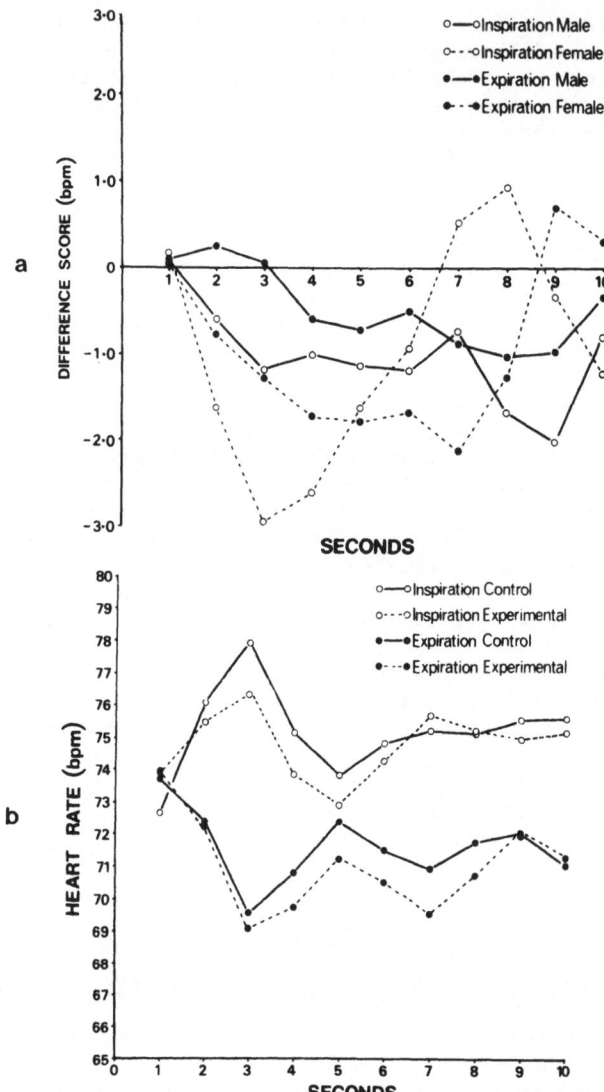

Fig. 4. HR changes as a function of stimulus position in the respiratory cycle. (a) RSA-corrected difference scores following stimulus presentation. (b) HR changes during control and experimental trials. Copyright ©️ 1981, Psychonomic Society. Reprinted with permission of the publishers from "Effects of Stimulus Position in the Respiratory Cycle on the Evoked Cardiac Response" by G. Turpin and G. Sartory, Physiological Psychology, 8:503-508.

Effects of Respiration on Cognitive Activity

Respiration has also been claimed by some investigators (e.g. Flexman et al., 1974; Beh and Nix-James, 1974) to be related or to have a direct influence on cognitive activity. For example, both auditory and visual detection appear to be more efficient when signals are presented in expiration rather than inspiration (Flexman et al., 1974). In contrast, Beh and Nix-James (1974) have reported shorter reaction times for imperative stimuli presented during inspiration as opposed to expiration. Unfortunately, neither of these studies obtained measures of heart rate, so it is impossible to distinguish between respiratory versus cardiac-linked facilitation of processing. There is also some evidence (Jennings and Wood, 1977) to suggest that subjects synchronize their breathing with stimulus presentations in complex cognitive tasks such as reaction time. Indeed, Engel et al. (1972) have suggested that the respiratory phase effects which they observed in a study similar to one conducted by Beh and Nix-James (1974) might have been due to variations in the RT foreperiod. Finally, Diekhoff (1977) has reported that the detection of internal events (i.e. the skin conductance response) is more efficient during inspiration than during expiration. It would appear, therefore, that an association between respiration and cognitive processing may exist but the mechanisms subsuming it remain undefined.

IMPLICATIONS OF RESPIRATORY-CARDIOVASCULAR INTERACTION FOR THE ANALYSIS AND INTERPRETATION OF PHASIC CARDIAC RESPONSES

The previous section has briefly reviewed the various interactions between respiration, cardiovascular activity and information processing. A summary of these effects is provided in Figure 5. The purpose of this section, therefore, is to examine the implications of these effects for the application of cardiac responses as indices of information processing. Issues relating solely to the quantification of cardiac responses will not be considered since they have recently been reviewed elsewhere (Turpin, in press).

The main question with which we are concerned is the construct validity of phasic cardiac changes as indices of information processing. However, as has been discussed in the previous section, the relationship between cardiac change and sensory processing is not a unique, simple function but is moderated by a variety of factors, some of which are illustrated in Figure 5. If we restrict ourselves only to the feed-forward effects of cognitive activity on the HR response, four moderating factors would appear to warrant serious consideration. These are: the effects of concomitant respiratory responding, respiratory phase modulation of cardio-motor efferents, cardiac cycle time effects, and the influence of RSA on the quantification of evoked responses.

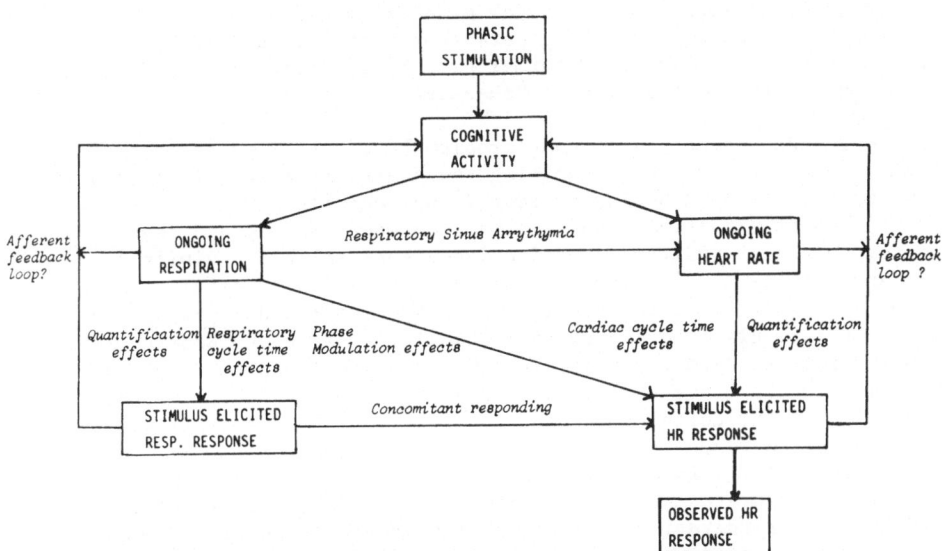

Fig. 5. Summary of the possible effects of respiratory-cardiovascular interactions on stimulus-elicited cardiac responses.

147

Concomitant Respiratory Responding

Simple auditory stimuli give rise to several different forms of respiratory response. Moreover, changes in the breathing pattern also appear to be related to discrete and consistent alterations in cardio-vascular activity. The question of primacy, therefore, must be raised concerning stimulus-elicited changes in heart rate. Are cardiac responses the direct consequence of information processing, a concomitant change to a stimulus-elicited respiratory response or perhaps a combination of both these processes? This question has concerned psychophysiologists ever since interest developed in cardiac responding. For example, the proposition that classically conditioned HR responses were no more than conditioned changes in breathing pattern stimulated much research (Headrick and Graham, 1969; Riege and Peacock, 1968; Smith, 1966; Westcott and Huttenlocher, 1961; Wood and Obrist, 1964).

Generally there have been two approaches to examining the question of respiratory mediation. The first approach has been to control breathing pattern throughout the experimental session, and, typically, this has involved pacing both the frequency and depth of breathing using some external cue such as a light or tone. Classical conditioning studies which have adopted this approach have generally demonstrated differences in the cardiac response between subjects with paced respiration and control subjects who breathed normally (Wood and Obrist, 1964). Although this may implicate respiratory mediation for the overall form of the classically conditioned HR response, it should be stressed that HR response components were also present throughout the controlled breathing conditions. More-over, in a study by Headrick and Graham (1968) differences were only observed with a fast-controlled, as opposed to a normal-controlled, breathing procedure. It would appear that the major components of the classically conditioned HR response are independent of respiratory responding. Furthermore, the adequacy of the controlled breathing approach must also be questioned. A number of problems associated with this procedure have been identified and have probably resulted in its discontinuation as a control technique. For example, subjects frequently experience difficulties in complying exactly with the external breathing cues. This imposes an additional cognitive load which is absent in the uncontrolled breathing groups and may also lead to ambiguities concerning the effectiveness of the breathing manipulation. An additional problem concerns the choice of individually-appropriate breathing parameters for pacing. If the control group does not accurately mimic normal breathing, differences in HR might be expected due to a disruption of homeostatic mechanisms.

More recent approaches to this problem have consisted of measuring both HR and respiration, and examining the degree of association between the two measures. Both Steinschneider (1968) and Klorman et al. (1977) failed to report significant correlations between cardiac and respiratory responses to either auditory or affective-visual stimuli. Similarly, Turpin and Sartory (1980) reported only non-significant correlations between the magnitude of the decelerative HR component and changes in respiration rate elicited by auditory stimuli. Porges and Raskin (1969) have also reported data demonstrating the relative independence of HR and respiration in cognitive tasks. In contrast, Richards (1983) has demonstrated significant correlations between respiration rate/amplitude and cardiac change to visual stimuli in infants. It should also be noted that several authors (e.g. Berg, 1970; Oster et al., 1975) have suggested that some of the cardiovascular response components of the startle reflex might be mediated via respiration. Since cardiac acceleration is frequently identified as a component of startle (Graham, 1979; Turpin, 1983), it might be interesting to speculate that some forms of accelerative HR responses are associated with respiratory activity. This would be consistent with data obtained by Wood and Obrist (1964) and Porges and Raskin (1969) which have demonstrated greater consistency between respiration and cardiac acceleration as opposed to cardiac deceleration. In addition unpublished data from our laboratory have demonstrated significant correlations between the size of cardiac acceleration and increases in respiratory rate. A similar finding between cardiac acceleration and increases in respiration amplitude was also reported by Smith and Strawbridge (1969).

Unfortunately, there have been too few studies which have examined this question to draw any firm conclusions. Clearly, some of the variance associated with cardiac responding originates from concomitant changes in respiration. However, it would appear that respiratory and cardiac responses are not perfectly correlated and that some of the variance of cardiac change is unrelated to changes in respiration.

Respiratory and Cardiac Cycle Time Effects

It is commonly assumed that the evoked cardiac response is unaffected by the position of the stimulus within the experimental paradigm. Thus, stimuli are presented randomly, the only constraints being those imposed by the psychological nature of the experimental paradigm. However, in an earlier section, evidence was presented to suggest that the precise form of vagally mediated cardiac responses was influenced by the relative position of the stimulus with respect to both the cardiac and respiratory cycles. Although these effects may only attenuate or distort the form of the cardiac response, they need to be taken into account if these responses are to be employed as accurate and quantitative measures of cognitive activity. In addition, data of Harver and Kotses (1983) would suggest that the form of the respiratory response may also be determined by respiratory cycle time effects. It would follow, therefore, that cardiac changes concomitant to respiration may also be influenced by stimulus position within the respiratory cycle.

Respiratory Sinus Arrhythmia

Traditionally, cardiac responses have been quantified in terms of HR averaged across a number of trials or subjects. Since there exist large variations in mean HR level, the response is usually expressed as a difference score consisting of the post-stimulus HR response minus a mean pre-stimulus level (Turpin, in 1985). However, this approach assumes that prestimulus HR activity is both stable and non-stationary. The presence of large cyclic variations known as sinus arrythmia (SA), and respiratory sinus arrythmia in particular, poses limitations on such an assumption. This raises several important implications for the use of traditional techniques of HR analysis.

The first is trivial but nevertheless pertinent to many published studies. If a mean is chosen from a number of prestimulus beats or seconds which is smaller than the dominant RSA cycle length, then the position of the stimulus with respect to the RSA cycle will affect the numerical value of the mean obtained. Turpin and Siddle (1978) have illustrated this potential source of error numerically. Clearly the size of the effect will depend upon the amount of RSA present and the length of the prestimulus mean. If subjects display prominent RSA, longer (>4 beats or secs) rather than shorter (<4 beats or secs) prestimulus samples would seem preferable.

It can be argued that RSA poses an even greater problem for the quantification of <u>post-stimulus</u> activity. This issue was first examined in

1941 by Berg and Beebe-Center, who suggested two alternative hypotheses regarding the interaction of RSA and post-stimulus activity. The replacement hypothesis assumes that stimulus-elicited HR change suppresses ongoing RSA. In contrast, the summation hypothesis assumes that post-stimulus activity reflects both the additive effects of cardiomotor efferent activity associated with stimulus presentation and the ongoing variation in vagal efferent activity due to RSA.

These two hypotheses can be tested by examining the effect of stimulus position in the respiratory cycle on the post-stimulus cardiac response. If the replacement hypothesis is correct, stimulus position should have no effect. Alternatively, if the summation hypothesis holds, then the response should vary according to the cyclic HR variation due to RSA present in the post-stimulus period. Indeed, Berg and Beebe-Center (1941) attempted to study the effects of respiratory position of a dramatic startle stimulus on the HR response. They interpreted their data as supporting the replacement hypothesis. However, their findings must be considered inconclusive due to the lack of any statistical analysis and the fact that the response studied was probably atypical since it consisted of a cardiac acceleration which exceeded some 60 bpm. In contrast, two recent studies (Hart, 1975; Turpin and Sartory, 1980) have shown that stimulus position in the respiratory cycle does dramatically determine the form of the HR response. Mean cardiac response curves obtained by Turpin and Sartory (1980) are displayed in Figure 4b and clearly demonstrate differences in the response profile elicited by stimuli delivered either at mid-inspiration or mid-expiration. Further support for the summation hypothesis is derived from a study by Papakostopoulos (1973) which indicated that the extent of cardiac deceleration during a CNV task was dependent upon respiratory phase. Similarly, Williams et al. (1967) showed that the size of the evoked cardiac response was determined by the slope of prestimulus SA activity.

The presence of RSA in the post-stimulus period also has implications for HR analysis when a response has <u>not</u> actually occurred. For example, if RSA cannot be compensated for in some way, it is likely that these variations in HR will be confused with cardiac responses in the absence of stimulus elicited activity. This can be demonstrated using a pseudo-stimulus technique whereby ongoing heart rate is quantified using the same techniques for stimulus-elicited responses. Studies which have included these control periods (Barry, 1978; Eisenberg, 1975; Hart, 1975; Turpin and Siddle, 1978; Turpin and Sartory, 1980) have demonstrated appreciable effects. This confounding of response and non-response due to the presence of RSA has serious implications for HR habituation measurement (Turpin, 1983).

If we accept that RSA can influence both the detection and the form of stimulus-elicited HR responses, it becomes necessary to adopt some form of correction which might remove this confounding influence. Essentially, three methods have been proposed. The first relies on constructing some model of prestimulus SA activity which can then be extrapolated into the post-stimulus period, and removed from the stimulus-elicited cardiac activity (Turpin et al., 1980). The model may either constitute the actual observed pattern of prestimulus RSA (Turpin and Siddle, 1978). A critical account of these techniques has been provided elsewhere (Turpin and Siddle, 1978). Nevertheless, it should be emphasized that several problems arise when these methods are applied to experimental cardiac data. In particular, the modelling of cyclic fluctuations, non-stationarity and the size of the prestimulus sample are issues which require further consideration. The second approach relies on the removal of RSA from ongoing cardiac activity by employing a digital filter (Womack, 1971). Unlike the previous approach, it is specifically directed at RSA and requires quantification of both cardiac and respiratory activity. Unfortunately, this technique has yet to be applied to experimental psychophysiological data. The final attempt at SA-correction relies on subtracting 'cardiac responses' to a pseudostimulus from the post-stimulus cardiac response curve. Essentially this technique involves obtaining cardiac data at positions in the respiratory cycle equivalent to phases when real stimuli had been delivered but without the actual presentation of these stimuli. This technique can either be performed post hoc (Barry, 1978; Coles et al., 1982) or by predetermining stimulus presentation at specific phases in the respiratory cycle (Hart, 1975; Turpin and Sartory, 1980). This approach also attempts to remove only RSA and is thus unable to correct for other sources of cyclic SA activity.

To conclude this section, it appears that SA, and RSA in particular, pose a serious problem to the quantification of phasic cardiac responses. Fortunately, a number of techniques of varying degrees of statistical complexity have been proposed to accommodate this problem. However, Barry (1979a) has recently criticized the rationales underlying these techniques and asserted that they rely on the assumption that the pattern of RSA is unaffected by stimulus presentation. Clearly, the review of stimulus-elicited respiratory responses in a previous section of this chapter makes such an assumption untenable. Indeed, this assumption has never been suggested in the context of SA-correction (Lobstein et al., 1979). Clearly the presence of respiratory responses will lead to respiratory-mediated changes in cardiac activity which could be considered as a change in RSA. The use of a SA-correction procedure would obviously result in changes in cardiac activity which would reflect the change in RSA. The crucial question is whether this change in cardiac activity is considered as a stimulus-elicited cardiac response. Lobstein et al. (1979) have argued that such changes do constitute bona fide responses since they reflect stimulus-bound changes in post-stimulus activity relative to the prestimulus baseline. Alternatively, Barry (1979a,b) has argued that such changes should be considered as artifacts. He suggests that if cardiac activity had been conventionally analyzed using signal averaging, presumably across subjects or trials, this should have resulted in a zero response. However, if the stimulus had been presented at a fixed position in the respiratory cycle, and the individual cardiac response curves averaged, it is difficult to understand why such a response should be lost, as Barry (1979b) has clearly asserted.

A solution to the problem of response definition may be reached if the original purposes underlying this chapter are considered. Assuming that a stimulus has evoked both respiratory and specific cardiac effects, then post-stimulus cardiac activity might reflect respiratory-mediated cardiac responses, a disruption in cyclic background RSA, and a specific cardiac response. If cardiac measures are being employed as an indirect index of some central process, then the variance associated with that process has to be identified and distinguished from other sources of variance such as respiration. We have previously argued that this may be accomplished by examining the shared variance between cardiac, respiratory, somatic and other response modes (Lobstein et al., 1979; Turpin and Siddle, 1978; Turpin, in 1985). Thus, the cardiac response defined by Lobstein et al. (1979) represents an operational definition which is not synonymous with a cardiac response component which might reflect central processing. The issue raised by Barry (1979) does not concern response definition but the mediation of the response. We would argue that the use of techniques such as those advocated by Barry (1978, 1979a, 1983) may actually obscure the distinction between response definition which is atheoretical and response mediation which is theoretical.

CONCLUSION

The aim of this chapter has been to review the interactions between the cardiac and respiratory systems, and their implications for the use of these measures as indices of information processing. It becomes apparent that consideration of an additional system such as respiration more than doubles the complexities that surround HR measurement and its interpretation. If we are seriously concerned with the use of HR as an index of information processing, and also with the mediation of these responses, it is clear that the problem of cardiovascular-respiratory interaction needs to be addressed. This will require that psychophysiologists view measures of respiratory activity as bona fide indices, rather than conceptualizing them as sources of artifact as has previously been the case.

REFERENCES

Angelone, A., and Coulter, N. A., 1964, Respiratory sinus arrhythmia: A frequency dependent phenomenon, J.Appl.Physiol., 19:479-482.

Barry, R. J., 1977, Failure to find evidence of the unitary OR concept with indifferent low-intensity auditory stimuli, Physiol.Psych., 5:89-96.

Barry, R. J., 1978, Disruption of sinus arrhythmia and its relation to the classification of non-habituating OR measures, Physiol.Behav., 21:25-27,

Barry, R. J., 1979a, Correction for sinus arrhythmia in the evoked cardiac response: A timebase problem, Biol.Psych., 9:215-220.

Barry, R. J., 1979b, Fact or artifact? Reply to Lobstein, Turpin and Siddle, Biol.Psych., 9:225-226.

Barry, R. J., 1983, Primary bradycardia and the evoked cardiac response in the OR context, Physiol.Psych., 11:135-140.

Beh, H. C., and Nix-James, D. R., 1974, The relationship between respiration phase and reaction time, Psychophysiology, 11:400-402.

Berg, K. M., 1970, "Heart Rate and Vasomotor Responses as a Function of Stimulus Duration and Intensity," unpublished M.A. thesis, University of Wisconsin.

Berg, R. L., and Beebe-Center, J. G., 1941, Cardiac startle in man, Exp. Psych., 28:262-279.

Bohlin, G., and Kjellberg, A., 1979, Orienting activity in two-stimulus paradigms as reflected in heart rate, in: "The Orienting Reflex of Humans," H.D. Kimmel, E.H. van Olst, and J.F. Orlebeke, eds., Plenum, New York, pp. 169-197.

Borst, C., and Karemaker, J. M., 1980, Respiratory modulation of reflex bradycardia evoked by brief carotid sinus nerve stimulation: additive rather than gating mechanism, in: "Arterial Baroreceptors and Hypertension," P. Sleight, ed., Oxford University Press, Oxford, pp. 276-281.

Bradford, L. J., 1975, Respiration audiometry, in: "Physiological Measures of the Audio-vestibular System," L.J. Bradford, ed., Academic Press, New York, pp. 249-317.

Cacioppo, J. T., and Petty, R. E., 1982, "Perspectives in Cardiovascular Psychophysiology," Guildford Press, New York.

Carroll, D., and Anastasiades, P., 1978, The behavioral significance of heart rate: The Laceys' hypothesis, Biol.Psych., 1:249-275.

Clynes, M., 1960, Respiratory sinus arrhythmia: Laws derived from computer simulation, J.Appl.Physiol., 15:863-874.

Cohen, M. I., Gootman, P. M., and Feldman, J. L., 1980, Inhibition of sympathetic discharge by lung inflation, in: "Arterial Baroreceptors and Hypertension," P. Sleight, ed., Oxford University Press, Oxford, pp. 161-167.

Coles, M. G. H., Jennings, J. R., and Stern, J. A., in press, "Psychophysiological Perspectives: Festschrift for Beatrice and John Lacey," Hutchinson and Ross, Stroudburg, PA.

Coles, M. G. H., Pellegrini, A. M., and Wilson, G. V., 1982, The cardiac cycle time effect: Influence of respiration phase and information processing requirements, Psychophysiology, 19:648-657.

Davidson, N. S., Goldner, S., and McCloskey, D. I., 1976, Respiratory modulation of baroreceptor and chemoreceptor reflexes affecting heart rate and cardiac vagal efferent nerve activity, J.Physiol., 259:523-530.

Davies, C. T. M., and Neilson, J. M. H., 1967, Sinus arrhythmia in man at rest, J.Appl.Physiol., 22:947-955.

Davis, R. C., Buchwald, A. M., and Frankmann, R. W., 1955, Autonomic and muscular responses and their relation to simple stimuli, Psychol. Monogr., 69:1-71.

Diekhoff, G. M., 1977, Effects of phase-of-respiration on GSR detection, Br.J.Psych., 68:499-502.

Eckberg, D. L., Kifle, Y., and Roberts, V. L., 1980, Phase relationship between normal human respiration and baroreflex responsiveness, J.Physiol., 304:489-502.

Eisenberg, R. B., 1975, Cardiotachometry in: "Physiological Measures of the Audio-vestibular System," L.J. Bradford, ed., Academic Press, New York, pp. 319-348.

Engel, B. T., Thorne, P. R., and Quilter, R. E., 1972, On the relationships among sex, age, response mode, cardiac cycle phase, breathing cycle phase, and simple reaction time, J.Gerontol., 27:456-460.

Flexman, J. E., Demaree, R. G., and Simpson, D. D., 1974, Respiratory phase and visual signal detection, Percep.Psychophy., 16:337-339.

Gautier, H., 1972, Respiratory and heart rate responses to auditory stimulations, Physiol.Behav., 8:327-332.

Graham, F. K., 1979, Distinguishing among orienting, defence and startle reflexes, in: "The Orienting Reflex in Humans," H.D. Kimmel, E.H. van Olst, and J.F. Orlebeke, eds., Erlbaum, Hillsdale, New Jersey, pp. 137-168.

Hart, J. D., 1975, Cardiac response to simple stimuli as a function of the respiratory cycle, Psychophysiology, 12:634-636.

Harver, A., and Kotses, H., 1983, The effects of auditory stimuli on breathing period and tidal volume. Paper presented at the Society for Psychophysiological Research, Monterey.

Headrick, M. W., and Graham, F. K., 1969, Multiple-component heart rate responses conditioned under paced respiration, J.Expt.Psych., 79:486-494.

Hirsch, J. A., and Bishop, B., 1981, Respiratory sinus arrhythmia in humans: how breathing pattern modulates heart rate, Amer.J.Physiol., 241:H620-H629.

Iriuchijima, J., and Kumada, M., 1964, Activity of single vagal fibers efferent to the heart, Jap.J.Physiol., 14:479-487.

Jennings, J. R., 1982, Beat-by-beat vascular responses during anticipatory heart rate deceleration, Physiol.Psych., 10:422-430.

Jennings, J. R., in press, Bodily changes during attending, in: "Psychophysiology: Systems, Processes, and Applications," M.G.H. Coles, E. Donchin, and S.W. Porges, eds., Guildford Press, New York.

Jennings, J. R., and Wood, C. C., 1977, Cardiac cycle time effects on performance, phasic cardiac responses, and their interactions in choice reaction time, Psychophysiology, 14:297-307.

Jones, R. H., Cromwell, D. H., Nakagawa, J. K., and Kapuniai, L. E., 1971, An adaptive method for testing for change in digitized cardiotachometer data, IEEE Trans. on Bio-med.Eng., 18:360-365.

Karemaker, J. M., 1980, "Vagal Effects of the Baroreflex on Heart Rate," unpublished PhD thesis, University of Amsterdam.

Katona, P. G., and Jih, F., 1975, Respiratory sinus arrhythmia: Non-

invasive measure of parasympathetic cardiac control, J.Appl.
Physiol., 39:801-805.

Katona, P. G., Poitras, J. W., Barnett, G. O., and Terry, B. S., 1970,
Cardiac vagal efferent activity and heart period in the carotid
sinus reflex, Am.J.Physiol., 218:1030-1037.

Klorman, R., Weissberg, R. P., and Wiesenfeld, A. F., 1977, Individual
differences in fear and autonomic reactions to affective stimulation, Psychophysiology, 14:45-51.

Koepchen, H. P., Klussendorf, D., and Sommer, D., 1981, Neurophysiological
background of central neural cardiovascular-respiratory coordination: Basic remarks and experimental approach, J.Autonom.Nerv.
Syst., 3:335-368.

Lacey, B. C., and Lacey, J. I., 1978, Two-way communication between the
heart and the brain: Significance of time within the cardiac cycle,
Am.Psychol., 33:99-113.

Lobstein, T., 1978, Detection of transient responses in adult heart rate,
Psychophysiology, 15:380-381.

Lobstein, T., Turpin, G., and Siddle, D. A. T., 1979, Comment on Correction
for sinus arrhythmia in the evoked cardiac response: A timebase
problem, Biol.Psychol., 9:221-224.

Lopes, O. U., and Palmer, J. F., 1976, Proposed respiratory 'gating'
mechanism for cardiac slowing, Nature, 264:454-456.

Manzotti, M., 1958, The effect of some respiratory maneuvers on the heart
rate, J.Physiol., 144:541-557.

Melcher, A., 1976, Respiratory sinus arrhythmia in man, Acta Physiol.
Scand., Suppl. 435.

McCallum, M, Burch, N. R., and Roessler, R., 1969, Personality and respiratory responses to sound and light, Psychophysiology, 6:291-300.

Obrist, P. A., 1981, "Cardiovascular Psychophysiology: A Perspective,"
Plenum, New York.

Orlebeke, J. F., Mulder, G., and van Doornen, L. J. P., in press, "Cardiovascular Psychophysiology: Theory and Methods," Plenum, New York.

Oster, P. J., Stern, J. A., and Figar, S., 1975, Cephalic and digital
vasomotor orienting responses: The effect of stimulus intensity and
rise time, Psychophysiology, 12:642-649.

Papakostopoulos, D., 1973, CNV and autonomic function: A review, Electro-
enceph.Clin.Neurophy., Suppl. 33:269-280.

Poole, R., Goetzinger, C. P., and Rousey, C. L., 1966, A study of the
effects of auditory stimuli on respiration, Acta Otolaryngol.,
61:143-152.

Porges, S. W., McCabe, P. M., and Yongue, B. G., 1982, Respiratory-heart
rate interactions: Psychophysiological implications for pathophysiology and behavior, in: "Perspectives in Cardiovascular Psychophysiology," J.T. Cacioppo and R.E. Petty, eds., Guildford Press,
New York, pp. 223-264.

Porges, S. W., and Raskin, D. C., 1969, Respiratory and heart rate
components of attention, J.Exp.Psychol., 81:497-503.

Richards, J. E., 1983, Respiration and respiratory sinus arrhythmia predict
cardiac and visual responses during visual attention in 14 and 20
week old infants. Paper presented at the Society for Research in
Child Development, Detroit.

Riege, W. H., and Peacock, L. J., 1968, Conditioned heart rate deceleration
under different dimensions of respiratory control, Psychophysiology,
5:269-279.

Rousey, C., Snyder, C., and Rousey, C., 1964, Changes in respiration as a
function of auditory stimuli, J.Audit.Res., 4:107-114.

Schramm, L. P., Chornoboy, E. S., and Celler, B. G., 1980, Baroreceptor
modulation of spontaneous and evoked sympathetic activity in rats,
in: "Arterial Baroreceptors and Hypertension," P. Sleight, ed.,
Oxford University Press, Oxford, pp. 135-140.

Seller, H., Langhorst, P., Richter, D., and Koepchen, H. P., 1968, Uber die Abhängigkeit der pressorezeptonschen Hemming des Sympathicus van der Atemphase und ihre Auswirkung in der Vascomotorik, Pflügers Arch. Physiol., 302:300–314.

Siddle, D. A. T., and Turpin, G., 1980, Measurement, quantification and analysis of cardiac activity, in: "Techniques in Psychophysiology," I. Martin and P.H. Venables, eds., Wiley, Chichester, pp. 139–246.

Smith, R. W., 1966, Discriminative heart rate conditioning with sustained inspiration as respiratory control, J.Comp.Physiol.Psych., 61:221–226.

Smith, D. B. D., and Strawbridge, P. J., 1969, The HRR to a brief auditory and visual stimulus, Psychophysiology, 6:317–329.

Sroufe, L. A., 1971, Effects of depth and rate of breathing on heart rate and heart rate variability, Psychophysiology, 8:648–655.

Steinschneider, A., 1968, Sound intensity and respiratory responses in the neonate, Psychosom.Med., 30:534–541.

Stern, R. M., and Anschel, C., 1968, Deep inspirations as stimuli for responses of the autonomic nervous system, Psychophysiology, 5:132–141.

Trezebski, A., Raczowska, M., and Kubin, L., 1980, Influence of respiratory activity and hypocapnia on the carotid baroreceptor reflex in man, in: "Arterial Baroreceptors and Hypertension," P. Sleight, ed., Oxford University Press, Oxford, pp. 282–290.

Turpin, G., 1983, Unconditioned reflexes and the autonomic nervous system, in: "Orienting and Habituation: Perspectives in Human Research," D.A.T. Siddle, ed., Wiley, Chichester, pp. 1–70.

Turpin, G., 1985, Quantification, analysis and interpretation of phasic cardiac responses, in: "Clinical and Experimental Neuropsychophysiology," D. Papakostopoulos, S. Butler, and I. Martin, eds., Croom Helm, London, pp.500–530.

Turpin G., Lobstein, T., and Siddle, D. A. T., 1980, Phasic activity: The influence of prestimulus variability, in: "Techniques in Psychophysiology," I. Martin and P. H. Venables, eds., Wiley, Chichester, pp. 210–217.

Turpin, G., and Sartory, G., 1980, Effects of stimulus position in the respiratory cycle on the evoked cardiac response, Physiol.Psych., 8:503–508.

Turpin, G., and Siddle, D. A. T., 1978, Quantification of the evoked cardiac response: The problem of prestimulus variability, Biol. Psych., 6:127–138.

Turpin, G., and Siddle, D. A. T., 1983, Effects of stimulus intensity on cardiovascular activity, Psychophysiology, 20:611–624.

Westcott, M. R., and Huttenlochner, J., 1968, Cardiac conditioning: The effects and implications of controlled and uncontrolled respiration, J.Expt.Psych., 61:353–359.

Williams, T. A., Schachter, J., and Tobin, M., 1967, Spontaneous variation in heart rates: Relationship to the averaged evoked heart rate response to auditory stimuli in the neonate, Psychophysiology, 4:104–111.

Womack, B. F., 1971, The analysis of respiratory sinus arrhythmia using spectral analysis and digital filtering, IEEE Trans. on Bio-med. Eng., 18:399–409.

Wood, D. M., and Obrist, P. A., 1964, The effects of controlled and uncontrolled respiration on the conditioned heart rate response in human beings, J.Exp.Psychol., 68:221–229.

155

PSYCHOPHYSIOLOGICAL APPROACHES

BEHAVIORAL MODULATION OF CARDIOVASCULAR AND SOMATOMOTOR-CARDIOVASCULAR INTERACTIONS IN THE NON-HUMAN PRIMATE

Bernard T. Engel

Gerontology Research Center (Baltimore), National Institute
on Aging, National Institutes of Health, PHS, US Department
of Health and Human Services, Bethesda, and the Baltimore
City Hospital, Baltimore, MD 21224

INTRODUCTION

It is well-known that one can totally denervate the hearts of mammals, including man, and that these hearts are still capable of maintaining the circulation under a wide variety of conditions such as exercise, hypoxia, hypertension or hypotension. Furthermore, a number of primitive, vertebrate species exist in which there is virtually no innervation to the circulation. Thus, it is clear that myogenic and humoral mechanisms can regulate cardiovascular function relatively well. Since this is so, one needs to ask what role the nervous system performs in the regulation and control of the circulation.

One major role is that neurally-mediated responses of the circulation operate in the service of natural selection. In particular, the wide variety of reflexes which have evolved among the vertebrates enable these animals to operate effectively under a wide range of environmental circumstances. Furthermore, the behavioral implications of these reflexes is great: the reflexes associated with hypoxia and/or hypercapnia enable air breathing animals to survive over a wide range of altitudes; baroreflexes enable animals to perfuse vital organs independent of body posture; reflexes associated with metabolic demands such as dynamic exercise enable terrestial animals to forage or hunt over large territories, and these same reflexes enable other animals to evade many of their natural predators; non-metabolic demands such as the maintenance of homeothermy enable animals to perform continuously in the face of large fluctuations in climate.

While the reflex regulation of the circulation is of unquestionable importance in the facilitation of behavior, it is not sufficient to account for all of the neurally-mediated changes one sees in the circulation in an active animal. Reflexes are inherently reactive; that is, they depend on an eliciting stimulus for their operation. Yet, there are a host of behaviors which are associated with neurally-mediated circulatory adjustments which occur under conditions where one could not ascribe the circulatory responses to eliciting stimuli. These behaviors are proactive and are emitted to obtain environmental consequences or to avoid adverse environmental events. The concomitant circulatory response normally occur either before the behavior has been emitted, or before reflex-eliciting stimuli could have occurred in sufficient degree to account for the cardiovascular responses one observes. A noteworthy example of such responses are the cardiovascular adjustments to exercise which can be seen to occur either before any somatomotor responses are emitted (Petro, Hollander and Bouman, 1970; Borst, Hollander and Bouman, 1972; Freyschuss, 1970), or in the absence of any movement of the joint (Goodwin, McCloskey and Mitchell, 1972). Furthermore, there is evidence that these responses to exercise can be organized in the brain and emitted as patterns of somatomotor, pulmonary and cardiovascular behaviors without the need for any eliciting stimuli (Eldridge, Millhorn and Waldrop, 1981; Hobbs, 1982). My colleagues and I have been concerned with the questions of behavioral-cardiovascular inter- actions for many years. In 1970 we (Engel and Gottlieb) described a non- human primate model of learned heart rate control. In a number of sub- sequent experiments we have used this animal model to examine some of the physiological or behavioral mechanisms which mediate the interactions between experience and circulatory activity or reactivity. In this chapter I will review results from a number of studies we have done which show that many of the responses of the circulation which have been assumed to be reflexes are in fact conditional responses which occur only in specific contexts such as those in which the animal has been trained to emit certain cardiovascular response.

STABILITY OF CARDIOVASCULAR RESPONSE PATTERNS

A demonstration of instability of cardiovascular responses during similar circumstances would be a strong test of the reflex model of neural control of the circulation since one would expect reflexes to be relatively stable as long as they were measured under comparable conditions. We have examined this question in a number of studies.

In one such study we monitored heart period and blood pressure con- tinously over 18 hour periods for several weeks in each of six animals. The protocol was very simple: we implanted an arterial cannula in an external iliac artery and maintained the cannula patent by continuous infusion of heparinized saline (e.g., see Engel and Gottlieb, 1970). Throughout the observation period the animal was maintained in a primate chair which was enclosed in a primate booth. Observations began only after the animal had recovered fully from its surgery. All observations followed the same protocol. At 1700 hours the booth door was closed and the animal sat, undisturbed with free access to water but no food. At 1800 hours our computer automatically turned the recording system on and began measuring heart period and blood pressure on a beat to beat basis. Every 128 second these data were analyzed and the means and standard deviations were stored on magnetic tape for subsequent analysis. This process continued for 18 hours (until noon the following day). At 2000 hours the light in the booth was automatically turned off and remained off until 0800 hours the next day. Finally, at 1200 hours the computer completed its data analysis at which time we opened the booth door and cleaned and fed the animal. At 1700 hours this procedure was repeated. Animals were observed this way for 5 days/week over periods of 4 to 5 weeks.

We correlated heart period with blood pressure during each of three time periods: 1800 to 2000 hours when the booth light was on but there were no people in the laboratory; 2000 to 0800 hours when the booth light was off and the laboratory was relatively quiet; 0800 to 1200 hours when the booth light was on and people were in the laboratory carrying out various experiments. The individual correlations for each time period within the 18 hour "day" were converted to z-scores and averaged across days.

Since the animals merely sat, undisturbed in their booths, and since this situation did not change from one day to the next, one would predict

160

from a pure reflex control model of the circulation that the correlations between heart period and blood pressure would be stable and independent of time period. In fact, this was not so. As can be seen in Table 1, the correlation between heart period and systolic blood pressure was consistently low in the light off period relative to either of the light on periods (diastolic pressure shows a similar pattern). Clearly, even under the benign conditions described above, the integration among specific components of the circulation is not invariant as one might expect from a purely reflexive system, but is instead quite variable and conditional.

A second study in which we explored the reflex control of the circulation involved the elicitation of the baroreflex. The baroreflex is probably the most important, neurally-mediated mechanism through which acute responses of blood pressure are buffered. This dynamic reflex has several important physical properties. One of these is called the gain or sensitivity and can be measured by the beat to beat rate of change of heart period as a function of the change in blood pressure. Because this reflex is mediated from receptors located in diverse sites in the arterial tree, one might expect its gain to be very stable over a wide variety of experimental conditions. However, a number of studies have shown that this is not so. Bristow, Brown, Cunningham et al. (1971) have shown that the reflex gain is attenuated in man during bicycle exercise; Brooks, Fox, Lopez et al. (1978) have shown a similar effect during mental arithmetic; Goldstein, Harris and Brady (1977) have reported that baboons which are maintaining their mean blood pressures elevated during experiments in which they have been operantly trained to raise blood pressure, also have attenuated baroreflexes; finally, we (Engel and Joseph, 1982) have shown that monkeys which are trained to slow or speed their hearts also attenuate the gain of their baroreflexes.

We have described our procedure for training monkeys to slow or speed their hearts in detail in a number of papers, several of which are cited in the bibliography of this chapter. Therefore, I will describe our technique only briefly here. There is a panel of three lights arranged in a horizontal array on the door of the monkey's booth. When the door is shut, this panel is directly in front of the animal. One of the end lights is red, and when it is turned on it signals the animal that it should slow its heart. The other end light is green and it is the signal to the monkey to speed its heart. The red or green lights function as cues to the animal to perform; only one can be on at any time, and it remains lit throughout an entire session. In some experiments the session is 1024 seconds in duration, in others it lasts 2048 seconds. The center light is white or

Table 1. Correlations between heart period and systolic blood pressure during 18 hour monitoring periods. Period I is based on 55 pairs of observations, period II on 339 observations and period III on 116 pairs of values.

| Number of | | Monitoring periods | | |
Animals	Sessions	I 1800 - 2000	II 2000 - 0800	III 0800 - 1200
1	23	−0.08	−0.07	−0.87
2	22	−0.58	0.01	−0.76
3	18	−0.72	−0.24	−0.79
4	24	−0.51	−0.07	−0.63
5	13	−0.72	−0.05	−0.79
6	17	−0.60	−0.17	−0.81

yellow and functions as an indicator of performance to the monkey. When it is on, the animal is performing successfully; when it is off the animal is not meeting its criterion and is vulnerable to receive an electric shock to its tail. The shock (10 ma., 0.45 sec.) can occur at any time after the light goes off. Moreover, if the animal fails to perform correctly after having received a shock, the center light will remain off and the animal will receive subsequent shocks at the rate of one every eighth second - it should be noted here that a well-trained animal normally receives very few shocks and almost never fails to avoid subsequent shocks.

The criterion heart rate which determines whether the center light remains on or goes off is determined during a baseline period which immediately precedes the onset of the session. During the baseline period no lights are ever lit, and the animal is never shocked. The criteria are set so that the animal must slow or speed its heart rate relative to baseline heart rate.

Once an animal had learned to speed and slow its heart, baroreflex testing was carried out. Animals were given either a bolus, IV injection of phenylephrine which causes a vasoconstriction, a rapid rise in blood pressure and a reflex slowing of heart rate, or a bolus, IV injection of nitroglycerin which causes a vasodilation, a rapid drop in blood pressure and a reflex speeding of heart rate. Our hypothesis was that the baroreflex, elicited by phenylephrine while the monkey was maintaining a relative tachycardia, would be attenuated relative to a control test during which the animal was sitting quietly without any requirement for heart rate control. Similarly, we hypothesized that an animal would show an attenuated baroreflex to nitroglycerin during sessions when it was maintaining a relative bradycardia.

As the data in Table 2 clearly show, both hypotheses were confirmed. Each of the three monkeys tested attenuated the gain of its baroreflex during periods when it was controlling its heart rate. Since the baroreflexes are elicited by changes in blood pressure, and since the animal had no way to know when its barorelexes would be elicited, it seems likely that the inhibition of the reflex reflected a tonic, neurally-mediated state associated with learned heart rate control.

We also studied the consistency of the relationship between heart rate and blood pressure in two other studies. In one study we looked at the beat-to-beat changes in heart rate and mean arterial pressure during the 30

Table 2. Baroreflex sensitivities (beats/min./mm Hg.) during control and operant cardiac conditioning sessions. All differences between conditioning and control values are significant.

A. Nitroglycerin Animal	Control	Slow
1	1.81	1.15
2	2.56	0.23
3	1.13	0.68

B. Phenylephrine Animal	Control	Speed
1	1.69	0.91
2	2.64	0.21
3	4.18	1.93

seconds prior to the moment when an animal received a tail shock for not performing correctly, and the 30 seconds following the shock (Engel, 1974). The results were very striking (Figure 1). Despite large changes in heart rate, blood pressure remained very stable throughout the entire 60 seconds period thus illustrating once again that the close associationship between heart rate and blood pressure that one often sees is not inherent to the circulation but is a function of the conditions under which those responses are measured.

The last study I will describe in which we studied the relationship between heart rate and blood pressure was one in which we created a co-variation between these two responses experimentally, and then modified the relationship through subsequent training (Ainslie and Engel, 1974). In this study we classically conditioned monkeys to associate a click which sounded for 128 seconds with an unavoidable tail shock. The conditioned responses in this situation include a tachycardia and a pressor response which can be measured during the 128 seconds while the click is sounding but before the shock is delivered – in this experiment we always compared the "warning" click to a neutral click of a different frequency which is easily discriminated, and which is never paired with tail shock. After the animals were responding reliably to the clicks, we trained two of them to slow their hearts and two of them to speed heart rate using the operant conditioning procedure I described above. Then we combined the two procedures by superimposing the click stimuli on the operant conditioning in the same experiment. We found that under these conditions the classically conditioned heart rate response was reversed by the operant procedure among

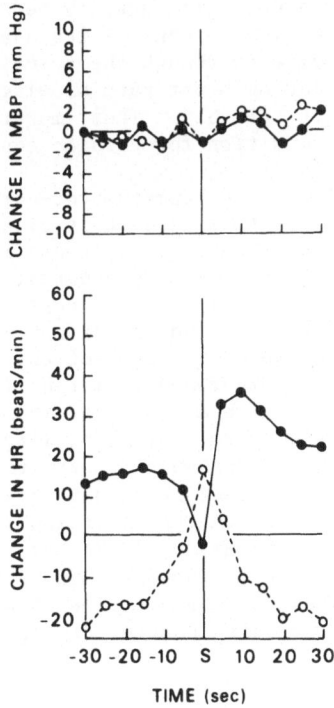

Fig. 1   Heart rate and mean blood pressure changes from baseline during the 30 sec. prior to and following shock(s) in slowing and speeding sessions. Data are averages for three highly trained animals. Note the large changes in heart rate which are not accompanied by correlated changes in blood pressure. (Open and closed dots).

those animals which were required to slow heart rate, but it remained a
tachycardia among those animals that had been trained to speed their
hearts. Furthermore, when the animals which were originally trained to
speed their hearts were retrained to slow heart rate, they too emitted a
bradycardia to the warning clicks relative to the neutral clicks even
though the warning clicks were always followed by inescapable shocks.

What was especially interesting in the context of the present discussion is that the classically conditioned pressor response which was not
affected by the operant cardiac training also was not affected during the
combined procedures, i.e., it remained a pressor response. Thus, this
study showed that the covariation of heart rate and blood pressure which
was elicited during a classical conditioning procedure could be reversed by
changing the contingencies between the classically conditioned response and
the putatively noxious stimulus, the tail shock.

CARDIOVASCULAR-SOMATOMOTOR INTEGRATION

We have observed a reliable relationship between cardiovascular
responses and somatomotor responses in our operant conditioning experiments. Specifically, animals which are slowing their hearts show a
reliable tendency to decrease their motor behavior, and when they are
speeding their hearts they show a tendency to increase motor activity
(Engel, Gottlieb and Hayhurst, 1976). In order to learn whether this motor
behavior was necessary or merely sufficient to increase heart rate, we
tested an animal in our cardiac conditioning procedure while it was under
the influence of a potent, cataleptic agent, phencyclidine (Engel, 1979).
The question was: "would this drug, which greatly reduces the monkey's
movements, also abolish its ability to control its heart rate". Table 3
presents the results. Clearly, even though the animal no longer showed
differential motor responses during heart rate slowing or speeding, it
still sped and slowed its heart reliably. Thus, motor activity is a sufficient, but not a necessary condition for cardiac control.

Certainly, the classical model of somatomotor-cardiovascular integration is physical exercise. In this case it is clear that the metabolic
demands associated with exercise require an increase in blood flow to
working muscles, and it is well-known that the normal physiological mechanism for increasing systemic blood flow is to increase cardiac output by
increasing heart rate. However, it is not clear how much of an increase in
cardiac output is essential to the performance of the exercise, and how
much is associated either with an increase in metabolic demand by "inappropriate" working muscles, or with an increase in non-metabolic demands
such as those normally associated with thermal cooling. In any case, it
was of interest to see whether the monkey can learn to attenuate the tachycardia of exercise. I should point out here that experiments in our
laboratory (Perski and Engel, 1980) and in other laboratories (Clemens and
Shattock, 1979; Goldstein, Ross and Brady, 1977) have shown that human
subjects can learn to attenuate their increases in heart rate while exercising. However, it is difficult to characterize physiological mechanisms
in man, and an animal model of cardiac control during exercise would be
very helpful.

Thus, in an experiment which is part of an on-going program of
research in our laboratory, we set out to learn whether we could teach a
monkey to attenuate its heart rate while it was exercising. We first
taught the animal to slow its heart rate using the procedure I have already
outlined. Then, we taught the animal to lift a weight repeatedly. Figure
2 illustrates the system we used. The weight that the monkey was trained
to lift was 8.2 kg - the animal weighed 8.0 kg - and the distance it had to

Table 3. Effects of phencyclidine (1.0 mg/kg, IM) on heart rate and motor reactivity during control and operant conditioning sessions.

A. Baseline Levels

	Activity (Movements/10 sec.)		Heart Rate (Beats/min.)	
	Control	Phencyclidine	Control	Phencyclidine
Slowing	8.1 *	3.6	176.6	162.4
Speeding	6.7 *	4.3	173.6	169.5

B. Change from Baseline during conditioning

	Activity		Heart Rate	
Slowing	-3.1 *	-0.2	-11.8 *	-5.4
Speeding	1.1*	-0.6	6.2*	5.6*

* $P < 0.05$

raise the weight was 4.5 cm. By using appropriately placed photocells it was possible to force the animal to lower the weight each time in order to meet our experimental conditions. If the monkey did not lift the weight within 2 seconds after the previous lift, a clicker would begin sounding, and after 4 seconds it would receive a tail shock. Furthermore, if the monkey failed to lift the weight within another 4 seconds, the clicker would continue to sound and it would receive another tail shock. It should be noted here that this monkey was so proficient that it almost never received a shock for failing to lift the weight in any of the experiments I will summarize below. Furthermore, it never received consecutive tail shocks.

After the monkey learned to exercise reliably, it was trained to attenuate its heart rate and to exercise during the same session. The results given below are based on 74 sessions, each 1024 seconds in duration. During half of these the monkey exercised only, and during the other 37 sessions it exercised while at the same time it was required to slow heart rate. In order to obviate any systematic errors attributable to changes in work performance, the sessions were counterbalanced within each day (4 sessions/day, 2 exercise only and 2 combined) as well as across days.

In addition to heart rate and blood pressure we also measured O_2 and CO_2 in the expired air. In this paper I will report only the O_2 results. All response were measured on a beat-to-beat basis. However, the results given below have been summarized and will be based on averages taken every 64 seconds throughout the session.

Figure 3 shows the changes in heart rate from baseline during consecutive sets of sessions. As can be seen from this Figure, the increase in heart rate during exercise-only sessions was relatively consistent across sessions whereas the heart rate response during the combined sessions fell monotonically from the first to the last block of sessions just as one would expect if this was a learned skill. Figure 3 also shows that while the heart changes differed systematically across the two conditions, systolic pressure did not. It is noteworthy that the correlations between number of weights lifted/session and session number was 0.04 for the exercise-only sessions, and -0.02 for the combined sessions. These insignificant correlations indicate that the monkey did not change its weight lifting behavior systematically in the course of study.

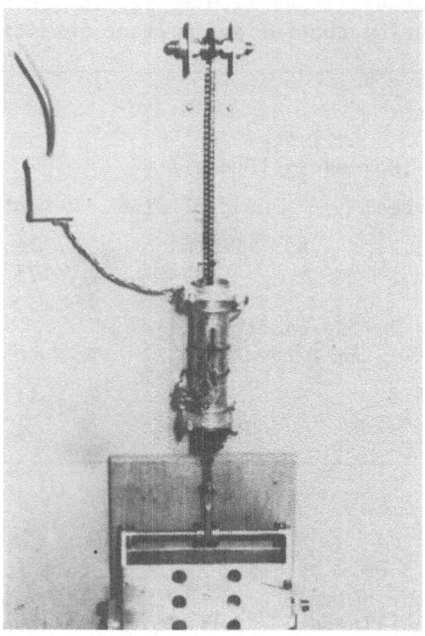

Fig. 2. Weights lifted by the monkey during exercise sessions. The
weights are attached to a lever inside the booth (not shown) by
which the animal raises and lowers them. Photocells positioned
near the weights detect their movement.

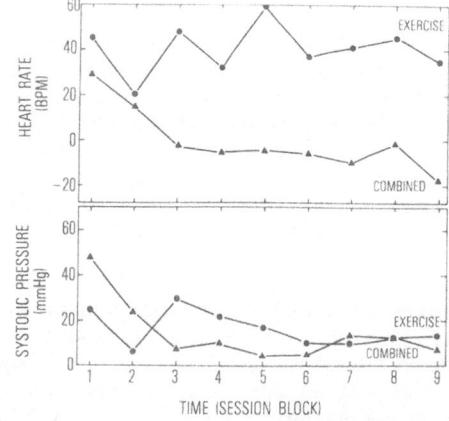

Fig. 3. Average changes in heart rate and systolic blood pressure across
exercise only and combined exercise and heart rate slowing
sessions. The first point is based on the first 5 sessions and
each subsequent point is based on consecutive, 4 session blocks.
Note that as training progresses, heart rate falls in the combined
sessions but remains unchanged in the exercise only sessions.
Note also that systolic blood pressure changes are similar in the
two exercise conditions.

Figure 4 shows the relationship between cardioavascular performance
and % O_2 in the expired air relative to room air. The point on each curve
shows the mean levels for the particular response, and the slope of each

line shows the least squares fit through the respective 37 pairs of values. Since we did not measure ventilation, we cannot measure O_2 consumption. However, the slope of cardiovascular performance as a function of O_2 extraction would be the same irrespective of ventilation. The data in Figure 4 show clearly that the monkey was able to attenuate its heart rate from baseline - baseline heart rates during exercise-only and during the combined sessions, 181.4 beats/min. and 188.3 beats/min., respectively, were not significantly different. The average increase in heart rate was 40.4 beats/min. for exercise only, and -0.7 beats/min. for the combined sessions. Average % O_2 extraction was similar in the exercise-only (2.2%) and combined (2.1%) sessions. Systolic pressure changes also were similar between the exercise only (16.3 mm Hg) and combined (14.5 mm Hg) sessions. The rate pressure products, indices of myocardial work, reflected the heart rate differences (exercise-only = 9.65 x 10^3, combined = 2.72 x 10^3).

The cardiovascular results show clearly that the animal's cardiovascular system was working far more efficiently during the combined sessions than it was during the exercise-only sessions, and the results showed further, as did most of the results cited above in previous experiments, that the relationship between heart rate and blood pressure is not invariant as a pure reflex model of the circulation would imply, but is instead highly dependent on the conditions operating at the time the measurements are made.

PLASTICITY OF CENTRAL NERVOUS CONTROL OF THE CIRCULATION

Experimental studies on the relationship between central neural activity and cardiovascular responses have grown in number substantially in the past decade (e.g., Randall, 1977; Galosy, Clarke, Vasko et al., 1980; Schneiderman, 1983). The findings from this research has forced a number of revisions of older concepts about the interaction between the nervous system and the cardiovascular system. Among these changing concepts two are especially relevant to the present discussion: first, it has become clear that the notion of a cardiovascular center in the brain is no longer tenable; instead it now is clear that centrally mediated control functions are widely distributed throughout the brain and spinal cord. And second, it is clear that associated with this diversity of control, there exists hierarchical regulation such that some control systems can be modulated by other systems.

We are exploring the extent to which behaviorally mediated processes can modulate the neural control of the cardiovascular system. I described one such experiment above when I noted that it is possible for the monkey to modulate the sensitivity of its baroreflexes when it is operantly slowing or speeding its heart. In the experiment that I will describe now, we observed that the monkey can even override the effects of direct stimulation of its brain when it is controlling its heart rate (Joseph and Engel, 1981).

As in some of the previous studies I described above, we began this experiment by first teaching animals to slow and to speed their hearts. After the animals had become proficient in controlling their heart rates, we carried out electrophysiological studies of their brains. Specifically, we identified telencephalic and diencephalic sites which when stimulated electrically resulted in reliable increases in heart rate and mean blood pressure. After establishing that these sites would respond reliably when stimulated, we carried out a series of experiments in which we systematically examined the abilities of the animals to control their heart rates while receiving electrical stimulation of the brain. We discovered that there were sites which when stimulated resulted in consistent increases in

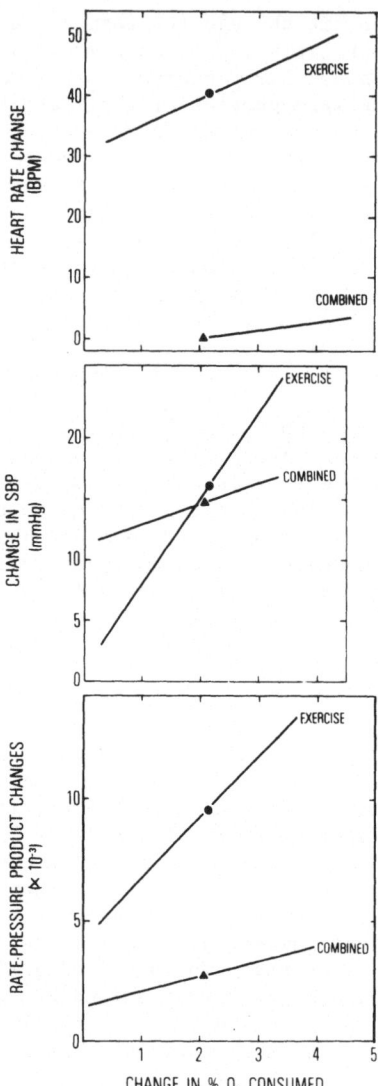

Fig. 4. Heart rate, systolic pressure and rate-pressure product responses during exercise only and combined sessions. The abcissa is the change in O_2 (relative to baseline) in expired air relative to room air. The slope of each cardiovascular response during the combined sessions is significantly less than during the exercise only session. Since each line is derived from 37 sessions, the findings reflect cardiovascular performance across a wide range of work.

heart rate and blood pressure irrespective of the operant conditions extant. However, there also were some sites where the effects of brain stimulation could be overcome during operant performance, i.e., the animals were able to continue to slow their hearts even though the imperative brain stimulation was going on at the same time. Figure 5 shows the behavior of an animal to a single bout of brain stimulation during control, speeding or slowing sessions. It illustrates the findings that: 1) all animals could slow their hearts even while being stimulated in the posterior hypothalamus; 2) stimulation in the same site during control or heart rate speeding sessions resulted in increases in heart rate; and 3) even though

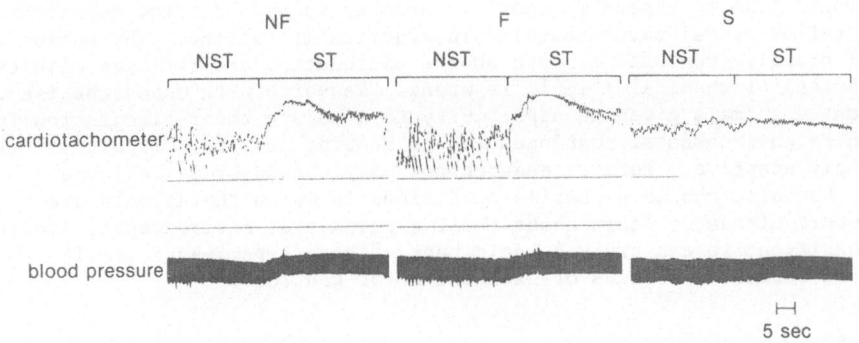

Fig. 5. Beat to beat heart rate and blood pressure responses during
control, speeding and slowing sessions. Note the large rise in
heart rate during electrical stimulation of the brain (ST) during
speeding or control sessions, and the absence of any change in
heart rate response during the slowing sessions. Note further
that even in the absence of heart rate responses, one can see
blood pressure responses during the slowing sessions. Recordings
of periods when there is no brain stimulation (NST) also are
included to show the magnitude of the brain stimulation effect.

heart rate increases were inhibited during brain stimulation, blood
pressure responses still were present. Thus, the findings from this experiment vividly underscore a central thesis of this paper: although many
cardiovascular responses are elicited through reflex pathways, not all
cardiovascular responses are invariably bound to stimuli, nor are the
relationships among component responses invariably linked: the responses
can be conditional, and the correlations among responses also can be conditional.

CONCLUSION

Throughout most of the history of physiology, inferences about the
relationship between the nervous system and the circulation have been based
on experiments doen with anesthetized animals under conditions where the
nervous system has not been allowed to function adaptively. Presently, one
can see a strong emphasis on studies with animals which are awake and are
allowed to behave (e.g., Smith, Galosy and Weiss, 1982; Engel and
Schneiderman, 1984). Thes experiments are showing that many of the reflex
relationships seen in the anesthetized animal are overridden in the
behaving animal. Furthermore, these studies are finding that when the
animal is allowed to interact with its environment and to profit from its
experiences, the cardiovascular effects one observes are different from
those that might have been predicted from studies with the anesthetized
preparation. In 1977 Wurster, writing on the spinal sympathetic control of
the heart, wrote that:

"The monolithic view of mass sympathetic discharge has fallen. The
understanding of the differential nature of sympathetic outflow to
different structures under various conditions will continue to evolve
... Much of the past and present sympathetic neurophysiology has been
studied under anesthetized and paralyzed conditions. The role of
various 'sympathetic' pathways in skeletal motor control or ascending
afferent transmission is unclear. Almost all concepts of sympathetic
control require testing in the unanesthetized, instrumented animal.
These experiments may follow the course of studies of skeletal motor
control".

I would like to expand Wurster's statement to say that the monolithic view of reflex neural-cardiovascular interaction is falling. The notion that all neurally-mediated effects on the circulation are reflexes elicited by mechanical or chemical stimuli is wrong. Research with unanesthetized, instrumented animals given an opportunity to modulate their circulation in relation to environmental contingencies is showing that the circulation is exceedingly adaptive. Future research not only should study behaving animals, but also should emphasize conditions in which the animals are given opportunities to learn about their experimental environments. Under these conditions it can truly be said that, "these experiments (will) follow the course of studies of skeletal motor control".

REFERENCES

Ainslie, G. W., and Engel, B. T., 1974, Alteration of classically conditioned heart rate by operant reinforcement in monkeys, J. Com. Physiol. Psychol., 87:373.

Borst, C., Hollander, A. P., and Bouman, L. N., 1972, Cardiac acceleration elicited by voluntary muscle contractions of minimal duration, J. Appl. Physiol., 32:70.

Bristow, J. D., Brown, E. B. Jr., Cunningham, D. J. C., Howson, M. G., Petersen, E. S., Pickering, T. G., and Sleight, P., 1971, Effect of bicycling on the baroreflex regulation of pulse interval, Circ. Res., 28:582.

Brooks, D., Fox, P., Lopez, R., and Sleight, P., 1978, The effect of mental arithmetic on blood pressure variability and baroreflex sensitivity in man, Proc. Physiol. Soc., 280:75P.

Clemens, W. J., and Shattock, R. J., 1979, Voluntary heart rate control during static muscular effort, Psychophysiology, 16:327.

Eldridge, F. L., Millhorn, D. E., and Waldrop, T. G., 1981, Exercise hyperpnea and locomotion: parallel activation from the hypothalamus, Science, 211:844.

Engel, B. T., 1974, Electroencephalographic and blood pressure correlates of operantly conditioned heart rate in the restrained monkey, Pavlov J. Biol. Sci., 9:222.

Engel, B. T., 1980 Somatic mediation of heart rate: a physiological analysis, in: "Biofeedback and Self-Regulation", N. Birbaumer and H. D. Kimmel, eds., Lawrence Erlbaum Ass., Hillsdale, NJ.

Engel, B. T., and Gottlieb, S. H., 1970, Differential operant conditioning of heart rate in the restrained monkey, J. Comp. Physiol. Psychol., 73:217.

Engel, B. T., Gottlieb, S. H., and Hayhurst, V., 1976, Tonic and phasic relationships between heart rate and somato-motor activity in monkeys, Psychophysiology, 13:288.

Engel, B. T., and Joseph, J., 1982, Attenuation of baroreflexes during operant cardiac conditioning, Psychophysiology, 19:609.

Engel, B. T., and Schneiderman, N., 1984, Operant conditioning and the modulation of cardiovascular function, Annu. Rev. Physiol., 46:199.

Freyschuss, U., 1970, Elicitation of heart rate and blood pressure increase on muscle contraction, J. Appl. Physiol., 28:758.

Galosy, R. A., Clarke, L. K., Vasko, M. R., and Crawfor, I. L., 1980, Neurophysiology and neuropharmacology of cardiovascular regulation and stress, Neurosci. Biobehav. Rev., 5:137.

Goldstein, D. S., Harris, and Brady, J. V., 1977, Baroreflex sensitivity during operant blood pressure conditioning, Biofeedback & Self-Regulation, 2:127.

Goldstein, D. S., Ross, R. S., and Brady, J. V., 1977, Biofeedback heart rate training during exercise, Biofeedback & Self-Regulation, 2:107.

Goodwin, W. M., McCloskey, D. I., and Mitchell, J. H., 1972, Cardiovascular and respiratory responses to changes in central command during isometric exercise at constant muscle tension, J. Physiol., 226:173.

Hobbs, S. F., 1982, Central command during exercise: parallel activation of the cardiovascular and motor systems by descending command signals, in: "Circulation, Neurobiology and Behavior", O. A. Smith, R. A. Galosy and S. M. Weiss, eds., Elsevier, New York.

Joseph, J. A., and Engel, B. T., 1981, Instrumental control of cardio-acceleration induced by central electrical stimulation, Science, 214:341.

Perski, A., and Engel, B. T., 1980, The role of behavioral conditioning in the cardiovascular adjustments to exercise, Biofeedback & Self-Regulation, 5:91.

Petro, J. K., Hollander, A. P., and Bouman, L. N., 1970, Instantaneous cardiac acceleration in man induced by a voluntary muscle contraction, J. Appl. Physiol., 29:794.

Randall, W. C., ed., 1977, "Neural Regulation of the Heart", Oxford University Press, New York.

Schneiderman, N., 1983, Behavior, autonomic function and animal models of cardiovascular pathology, in: "Biobehavioral Bases of Coronary Heart Disease", T. M. Dembroski, and T. H. Schmidt.

Smith, O. A., Galosy, R. A., and Weiss, S. M., eds., 1982, "Circulation, Neurobiology and Behavior", Elsevier, New York.

Wurster, R. D., 1977, Spinal sympathetic control of the heart, in: "Neural Regulation of the Heart", W. C. Randall, ed., Oxford University Press, New York.

FACTORS INFLUENCING THE COVARIATION OF HEART RATE

AND OXYGEN CONSUMPTION

Jasper Brener

University of Hull
England

Numerous experimental phenomena indicate that activity in the highest levels of the nervous system is associated with predictable changes in cardiac performance. This may be due to the effects of the implicated neural processes on striate muscular (and respiratory) activity which in turn produces neural, chemical and mechanical stimuli that elicit variations in cardiac activity through known reflex pathways. Since striate muscular activity is a major source of variation in energy expenditure, it is to be expected that alterations in cardiac performance that are produced through this route will covary strongly with variations in metabolic rate. However, experimental evidence indicates that the higher nervous system may also produce systematic alterations in cardiac performance through pathways that do not involve the striate muscles. Thus, predictable cardiac responses may be produced in curarized subjects by stimulation of the motor brain, by instructions and by conditioning procedures. Changes in cardiac performance that are produced independently of striate muscular performance would be expected to occur relatively independently of variations in metabolic rate. The research reported is based on the premise that cardiac activities which covary with metabolic rate are produced via feedback from striate muscular activity whereas cardiac variations that occur independently of metabolic ions are produced by higher nervous system processes acting directly on pontine-medullary circuits involved in the extrinsic control of the heart. This work developed from an attempt to understand the mechanisms involved in learned HR control.

LEARNED HEART RATE CONTROL

It is readily demonstrable that with minimal training (perhaps none), naive individuals are able to comply with instructions to increase and decrease their HRs. Since compliance with instructions has emerged as a standard operational means for classifying responses as "voluntary" or not, these demonstrations qualify certain HR variations for inclusion in this category. It seems improbable that the neural processes involved in such instances of voluntary control are the same as or even similar to those involved in the voluntary control of the striate muscles. However, this hypothesis is difficult to test because our knowledge of the processes underlying voluntary striate muscular control are far from complete.

173

Work on learned control of the viscera has been valuable in drawing attention on the need for a more precise specification of the processes of "voluntary behavior" (Brener, 1981). However, until such a specification has been provided, the question of whether voluntary control of the heart, exists in the same sense as voluntary control of the striate muscles is at least unanswerable and perhaps, meaningless. On the other hand, it may be possible to account for the phenomena of learned HR control in terms of well-established pathways by which the nervous system influences the heart and indeed a considerable amount of data relevant to such an account has been reported.

Much experimental data suggest that in the freely-moving subject, learned HR control is one manifestation of a generalized behavioral adjustment that also involves prominent striate muscular and respiratory components. For example, Brener, Phillips and Connally (1977) conditioned tonic heart rate changes in freely-moving animals using a shock-avoidance procedure. It was found that the very substantial conditioned increases (+ 20%) and decreases (- 20%) in HR levels were accompanied by equally significant alterations in energy expenditure as measured by oxygen consumption (VO_2). The groups also exhibited profound differences in their rates of ambulation although variations in this response were not required for shock avoidance.

If the nervous system were capable of being programmed to control HR independently of striate muscular and respiratory activities, these group differences in ambulation rate and VO_2 would not have been expected. Certainly, the VO_2 differences observed are far greater than would have been produced by cardio-specific adjustments. This apparent inefficiency of learned HR control suggests that the nervous system may interpret external demands for alterations in HR as demands for alterations in general activity. Given the importance of feedback from striate muscular and respiratory activity in cardiovascular regulation, individuals may comply with requirements to alter their HRs by appropriate alterations of striate muscle or respiratory activity. Although this strategy may have a relatively high metabolic cost, its information-processing demands are minimal.

The central idea of this hypothesis was examined in an experiment by Brener, Phillips and Connally (1980) which compared the HR, metabolic and ambulation adjustments induced by operant reinforcement contingencies that required either increases in HR or in ambulation rate in order to avoid electric shock. Animals that learned to avoid the shock under the HR contingencies exhibited behavioral adaptations that were indistinguishable from those exhibited by animals that learned shock avoidance under the running contingencies. In both cases, successful avoidance was characterized by an ergotropic response incorporating elevations in HR, energy expenditure and ambulation rates. These and similar results do not suggest the operation of any special mechanisms of cardiac learning. Neither do they imply that the nervous system is capable of independent cardiac control.

Investigators who have sought to question the view that learned cardiac control is a reflexive consequence of striate muscular activity have presented evidence that environmental contingencies may modify HR independently of striate muscular activity. For example, over a relatively short period of time much data were published indicating that even when the striate muscles are paralyzed and respiration is artificially controlled, HR is amenable to operant conditioning (Miller, 1969). Insofar as the curarization procedures were effective in eliminating striate muscular and respiratory variations, these experiments appeared to negate the hypothesis that learned cardiac control was an artefact of learned alterations in respiratory or striate muscular activity. Although it is well known that the curare studies have proven difficult to replicate (Brener, Eissenberg and Middaugh, 1974; Miller and Dworkin, 1974), it should be noted that these difficulties apply mainly to replication of the very large effects reported in the initial studies. Since the difficulties in replication were first reported, smaller but statistically-reliable effects have been reported independently by several investigators (Cabanac and Serres, 1976; Middaugh, Eissenberg and Brener, 1975; Thornton and Van Toller, 1973; Gliner, Horvath and Wolfe, 1975).

In principle, evidence of cardiac conditioning in curarized organisms rules out the possibility that the observed alterations in cardiac activity are reflexively mediated by feedback (neural, chemical or mechanical) from the striate muscles. However, since curare acts primarily at the motor end plates and does not interfere with the generation or transmission of efference towards the striate muscles, the experiments cannot be said to provide conclusive evidence that cardiac activity is conditionable independently of striate muscular processes in general. This is because the curarization procedure does not take account of more central pathways linking striate muscular and cardiac control.

Several transfer studies have yielded data that are consistent with the view that HR variations learned under curare are due to the influence of motor outflow processes on cardiac control (Black, 1967; Note 1). For example, DiCara and Miller (1969) conditioned one group of curarized rats to increase their HRs when presented with a conditioned stimulus and another group of curarized rats to decrease their HRs when the conditioned stimulus occurred. Two weeks later, and in a freely-moving state, subjects were again presented with the conditioned stimuli but not the reinforcing (shock) stimuli. It was found that subjects which had been trained to increase their HRs exhibited significantly higher respiration and general activity rates than subjects that had been trained to decrease their HRs. Since during the curare conditioning sessions, subjects had been paralyzed and had been maintained under the same parameters of artificial respiration, there was no chance for the reinforcement contingencies to have programmed the control of these responses directly. This implies that the conditioning procedure was responsible for modifying activity in brain circuits that are involved in the coordinated regulation of striate muscular, respiratory and cardiovascular performance.

Another experiment which favors this conclusion was reported by Goesling and Brener (1972) who employed a shock-avoidance procedure to condition high tonic levels of general activity in one group of rats (the Active Group) and low tonic levels of general activity in another group (the Immobile Group). Once these behavior patterns had been established, subjects in both groups were curarized and submitted to further conditioning sessions. Half the subjects in the Active and Immobile groups were permitted to avoid shocks by increasing their HRs and the other half by decreasing their HRs. It was found that the precurare training of the subjects, and not the reinforcement contingencies applied during the curare sessions, was the principle determinant of the HR changes exhibited under curare. Regardless of whether they were reinforced for increasing or decreasing their HRs, during the curare session subjects that had been trained to increase their activity levels in the undrugged state (Active Group) exhibited HR increases whereas subjects that had been trained to decrease their activity (Immobile Group) exhibited HR decreases.

These data indicate that, at best, curarization controls for the possible influences on HR of feedback from the striate muscles. Because of central coupling between the neural processes responsible for cardiac, striate muscular and respiratory control, HR variations observed under curare cannot be said to have occurred independently of striate muscular control processes.

An alternative approach to the question broached by the curare studies has been to examine the capacity of intact individuals to modify their noraml HR responses to exercise challenges involving controlled levels of striate muscular activity. The relevant studies have shown that individuals may learn to decrease their normal HR responses to dynamic exercise demands (Goldstein, Ross and Brady, 1977; Perski and Engel, 1980) and to increase and decrease their normal HR responses to static exercise demands (Clemens and Shattock, 1979). The method employed in these studies was first of all to record the subject's HR response to fixed muscular work loads (Exercise Condition). Then, with exteroceptive feedback of HR available, subjects were instructed to alter their HRs whilst engaging in the exercise (Control Condition). In all cases it was found that subjects were able to alter their unconditioned HR responses to exercise in the direction(s) demanded by instructions. Since compliance with instructions necessarily implies learning, these results appear to support the hypothesis that the nervous system may be programmed to alter HR independently of striate muscular activity. However, this conclusion is based on the questionable assumption that constant rates of striate muscular activity will be associated with constant rates of external work.

Trotter (1956), amongst others, has pointed out that the relationship between external work and energy expenditure may be influenced by such factors as the muscles employed to execute the work and the efficiency with which the selected muscles are regulated. Thus, increases in motor skill tend to be associated with reductions in the unit metabolic costs of external work (Brener, 1984; Sparrow, 1983). This increase in behavioral efficiency may be attributed to the elimination of motor activities that are superfluous to meeting the task demands. For example, as a motor skill improves, the background level of isometric muscular contraction may decline and so too may the involvement of energy-consuming fast-twitch muscle fibers. Subtle changes of this sort, which might otherwise escape detection, would be reflected by reductions in the rate of energy expenditure. Since energy expenditure was not recorded in any of the studies cited above, the possibility remains open that when subjects were successful in altering their HRs whilst maintaining fixed levels of external work, their overall rates of striate muscular and respiratory activity were changing together with their HRs. If this were true, the data could not be said to offer new evidence of cardio-specific control but it would be consistent with the proposition that HR variations are driven by feedback produced by the striate muscles.

Moses, Clemens and Brener (1984; Note 2) have recently explored this possibility by examining HR control while subjects were engaging in static muscular contractions of the forearm equal to 10%, 30% and 50% of the maximum voluntary contractions. Relevant results for their 30% contractions are displayed in Figure 1 where it will be seen that although subjects were able to increase and decrease their HRs relative to exercise-only levels, these alterations were accompanied by correlated variations in VO_2. Thus again the data fail to provide evidence that learning processes may modify the cardiac response to metabolic demand.

Although these studies indicate that HR learning is strongly linked to striate muscular processes, they do not elucidate the nature of linkage. In freely-moving subjects, the consequences of striate muscular adjustments could provide the eliciting stimuli for HR variation. But so too could centrally-initiated neural activity which is directed at the striate muscles and which, for example, is held responsible for conditioned HR changes in curarized subjects.

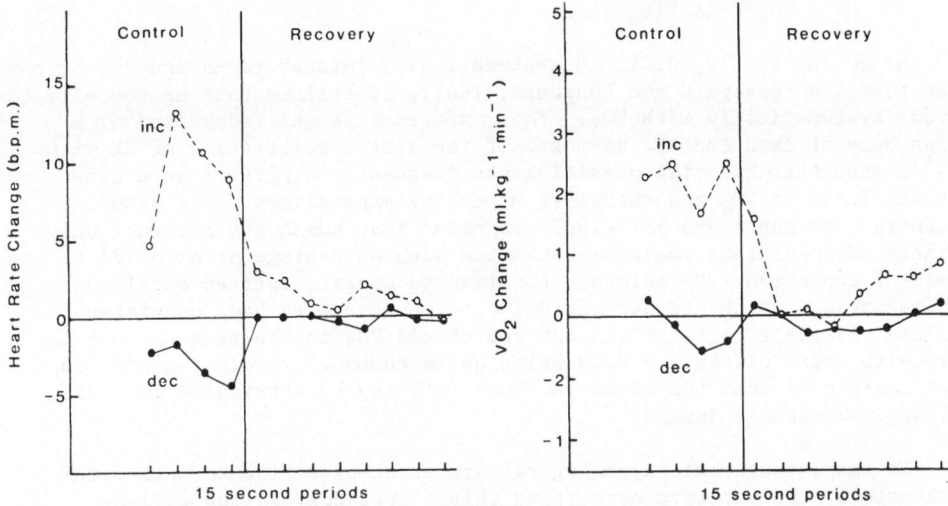

Fig. 1.   "Voluntary" changes in heart rate during exercise and accompanying
          changes in oxygen consumption. [The data illustrated were
          obtained by substracting heart rate and oxygen consumption means
          recorded during exercise-only conditions from equivalent means
          recorded while subjects were exercising and attempting to either
          increase (inc) or decrease (dec) their heart rates with the aid of
          biofeedback.]

ENERGY EXPENDITURE, STRIATE MUSCULAR ACTIVITY AND HEART RATE

     Variations in activity, whether attributed to psychological factors or
not, imply variations in energy expenditure. Since O_2 is required by the
tissues to sustain the processes of energy metabolism, the rate at which
the cardiovascular system perfuses the tissues is closely related to the
organism's overall rate of activity. The relationship between variations
in O_2 consumption (VO_2) and cardiac performance is described by the
equation,

$$VO_2 = CO \cdot (A-V)O_2 \text{ diff} \tag{1}$$

where CO is the Cardiac Output and $(A-V)O_2$ diff. is the difference in O_2
concentration between the arterial (aortic) and mixed venous (pulmonary
artery) blood.

     In the transition from rest to maximal exercise, VO_2 may increase by a
factor of 20 whereas cardiac output (CO), the product of HR and stroke
volume (SV), only increases by a factor of approximately six. The balance
of the tissues' O_2 needs is met by alterations in the rate at which they
extract O_2 from the blood. Under conditions of maximal exercise the
$(A-V)O_2$ diff. is approximately four times that observed under conditions of
rest.

     Over the maximum range of VO_2 variation, changes in CO are accounted
for by a two-fold increase in SV and a three-fold increase in HR. However,
much of the SV variations tends to occur at the lower extremes of the VO_2
range. In the region of light to heavy steady-state activity, SV remains
more-or-less constant and most of the increase in CO is borne by HR. Thus
for the normal range of activity, SV may be treated as a constant (k) and
solving equation (1) for HR we get:

$$HR = VO_2/k \cdot (A-V)O_2 \text{ diff} \tag{2}$$

Since the $(A-V)O_2$ diff. is systematically related to HR and VO_2 by the same function (Bevegard and Shepherd, 1967), it follows that HR too will covary systematically with VO_2. This inference is well supported by a large body of data and the strength of the linear covariation of HR with VO_2 is such that exercise physiologists frequently employ HR as a convenient index of VO_2 and therefore of energy expenditure. For example, Malhotra, Sen Gupta and Rai (1963) reported that human HRs recorded under a variety of conditions could be estimated with an average error of 7% on the basis of concurrent VO_2 values. Experiments on rats carried out in our laboratory and which are described in the next section have consistently yielded bivariate correlations between HR and VO_2 in the range of 0.6 to 0.95 with coefficients = > 0.80 being quite common. In other words, in many cases more than 60% of HR variance (r^2) may be attributed to variations in metabolic demand.

To the extent that psychological processes give rise to metabolic alterations, the pathways supporting this strong correlation will be involved in producing HR variations. Striate muscular activity through which organisms do commerce with their environments is systematically associated with most, if not all, psychological processes. Since variations in the activity of this effector system are the most important source of variations in energy expenditure, it is unsurprising that evolution has favored the development of a strong linkage between striate muscular and cardiac control. The striate muscles which comprise 50% of the total body mass absorb approximately 20% of the total VO_2 at rest but approximately 90% of the total VO_2 under conditions of heavy exercise in which the VO_2 may be 20 times greater than at rest. This enormous increase in O_2 utilization by the striate muscles is associated with a parallel increase in the proportion of the total CO received by them (17% at rest versus 80% in heavy exercise).

When the striate muscles become active they cause increases in cardiac activity through a variety of pathways. Short latency cardiac accelerations have been attributed to the activation of Types III and IV afferents in the contracting muscle (Mitchell, Kauffman and Iwamoto, 1983). These afferents, some of which respond to metabolic factors, may influence cardiac activity through segmental, intersegmental and suprasegmental pathways. Heart rate changes within one beat of muscular activation have been attributed to a vagally-mediated muscle-heart reflex (Gelsema, 1983). The "long-loop" suprasegmental reflex pathway produces sympathetically-induced vasomotor responses which act in concert with the blood-pumping action of the muscles to increase venous return to the heart. This elevates right atrial pressures which, in turn, elicit changes in left ventricular function giving rise to increases in stroke volume. Profound elevations of right atrial pressure activate the Bainbridge reflex which causes sympathetically-mediated HR increases. However, more subtle changes in arterial blood pressure acting through the baroceptors of the carotid bodies and aortic arch produce short-latency reflexive alterations in HR.

Within 3 to 15 seconds of the onset of muscular activity, depletion in local O_2 produces autoregulatory vasodilation which further augments venous return. Changes in blood gas composition produced by muscular energy expenditure also act on the chemoreceptors of the brain, the aortic arch and the carotid bodies to bring about reflex augmentations in respiration and HR. Increased inspiratory activity alters the tissue-heart pressure gradient to increase venous return and also elevates HR by augmenting cardiac vagal inhibition. These influences of respiration on cardiac performance provide further linkages between the level of cardiac output and the prevailing metabolic demand. In all of these cases, cardiac acceleration is a response to prior striate muscular activity. Therefore it is to be expected that HR variations that are mediated by these "feedback" pathways will be highly correlated with variations in VO_2.

As indicated earlier, much HR variation attributed to psychological processes can be explained in terms of these mechanisms. However, cardiac performance may also vary independently of metabolic demand. In this case the normally strong covariation of HR with VO_2 is degraded and HR values deviate from predictions that are based on concurrent VO_2 rates. These metabolically-independent variations in cardiac activity are of special significance in that they reflect a mismatch of blood supply (or the potential for blood delivery) and demand. When sustained, such states of disequilibrium are non-adaptive and, in some cases, they may be pathogenic. For example, sustained metabolically-excessive elevations in cardiac output have been implicated in the etiology of cardiovascular disease including hypertension and coronary heart disease (Obrist, 1981; Steptoe, 1981).

If the rate of tissue perfusion is either too high or too low, the plasma pH will be changed thereby impairing the functional efficiency of the tissues. Although the cardiovascular system is endowed with numerous mechanisms to prevent such a state from enduring, it would appear that certain environmental demands induce nervous system states which can override these regulatory processes. For example, tissue overperfusion, characterized by abnormally low $(A-V)O_2$ diffs., suggesting tissue alkalosis and attributable to psychological factors, is illustrated in the experimental findings of Langer, Obrist and McCubbin (1979). These investigators demonstrated that when dogs engage in striate muscular work to avoid electric shock they exhibit lower $(A-V)O_2$ diffs. at each level of CO than they do when they engage in exercise that is not motivated by shock-avoidance. The early work of Grollman (1929) also illustrates this process. He found that medical students exhibited significant increases in cardiac output with accompanying decreases in $(A-V)O_2$ diff. when they were accused by their professor of laxity in their physiology course. A more recent demonstration of the effect is provided by Gliner, Horvath and Biddy (1979) in an examination of hemodynamic alterations associated with public speaking.

The functional value of tissue overperfusion in human psychological stress is unclear. Perhaps it is an evolutionary vestige of a mechanism for priming the tissues in anticipation of metabolically-demanding defense or other maintenance activities. Such a process could facilitate short-latency, high energy activities and enable more sustained performance by retarding the moment at which the involved tissues reach a state of energy depletion (Folkow and Neil, 1971). However, the cardiovascular control system will not tolerate long periods of overperfusion and excessive blood flow will be reduced by autoregulatory and chemoceptively-elicited vasoconstriction (Forsyth, 1971). This elevates the Total Peripheral Resistance (TPR) reducing the CO but, at the same time, increasing the systemic blood pressure and thereby the cardiovascular workload. Thus, cardiovascular adjustments that in the short term, may assist in promoting rapid, high-energy activity could, if sustained, decrease cardiovascular efficiency and create conditions for the development of cardiovascular disease.

Several sources of evidence support Krogh and Lindhard's (1913) view, more recently articulated by Brod, Fencl, Hejl and Jerka (1959) and then Obrist (1981), that cardiac responses which antedate metabolic demand are triggered by the neural circuits responsible for control of the striate muscles. For example, following his review of central control of cardiovascular functions, Smith (1974) concluded that stimulation of virtually all brain structures that elicit striate muscular activity also produces predictable variations in cardiovascular performance. This is apparent even when the striate muscular targets of brain stimulation have been immobilized (Eldridge, Millhorn and Waldrop, 1981). Freyschuss (1970) has demonstrated that cardiac and blood pressure responses to voluntary isometric contractions of the forearm in man are not eliminated by neuro-muscular paralysis of the target effectors. Another example of cardiac control by "Central Command" or feedforward control is reported by Goodwin, Mitchell and McCloskey (1972) who employed mechanical vibration of the implicated muscles to manipulate the perceived effort associated with the performance of standard levels of muscular work. They found that cardio-vascular responses were related more closely to the levels of "Central Effort" required to contract the muscles than they were to the metabolic costs of the activity.

Although such cardiac responses cannot be attributed to feedback produced by the consequences of striate muscular activity, their exper-imental demonstration has frequently involved striate muscular demand. For example Rushmer, Smith and Lasher (1960) observed that exercise-trained dogs exhibited increases in cardiac output when the experimenter laid his hand on the treadmill switch. The strong central linkage between cardiac and striate muscular control is illustrated by many reports that antici-pation of exercise produces substantial HR increases (e.g. Kozar, 1964). Lang (1979) has reported data which indicate that merely thinking about activity is sufficient to produce significant augmentations in HR. Because such cardiac responses anticipate rather than follow striate muscular activity, they will occur relatively independently of variations in VO_2. Assuming the relative constancy of stroke volume, they will be reflected by HRs that are elevated above metabolic requirements. Such dissociations of HR and VO_2 have been observed under conditions requiring high levels of motor readiness (Blix, Stromme and Ursin, 1974; Turner, Carroll and Courtney, 1983).

The research to be described here is concerned with distinguishing HR variations that are due to metabolic demand from those that occur independ-ently of metabolic variation and are attributable to "Central Command". The experiments reported represent some initial attempts to identify envir-onmental demand conditions that give rise to cardiac variations produced by these two routes.

EXPERIMENTAL FACTORS INFLUENCING THE HR/VO_2 RELATIONSHIP

An example of the influence of psychological or environmental demand factors on the relationship between HR and VO_2 is provided in Figure 2. These curves illustrate the mean levels of HR recorded at different VO_2s over 10 successive days of operant conditioning of ambulation in two groups of six rats each. Subjects in the Food Group were reinforced with food pellets on a 90-second Variable-Interval schedule for running a criterion distance. The same ambulation criterion was imposed by a Variable-Interval 90-second shock-avoidance schedule to sustain running in the Shock Group. These schedules of reinforcement led to similar rates of work as reflected by rates of ambulation and the ranges of VO_2 recorded from the two groups. It will also be seen that the changes in HR per unit change in VO_2 are similar for the Food and Shock conditions.

However, the Shock Group have significantly higher mean HRs than the Food Group over the full VO_2 range. This tonic HR difference is super-imposed on similar HR/VO_2 gradients and generates essentially parallel curves for the two groups. In this case it seems reasonable to attribute the tonic HR difference between groups to the different demands imposed respectively by the Food and Shock reinforcement schedules. Because these

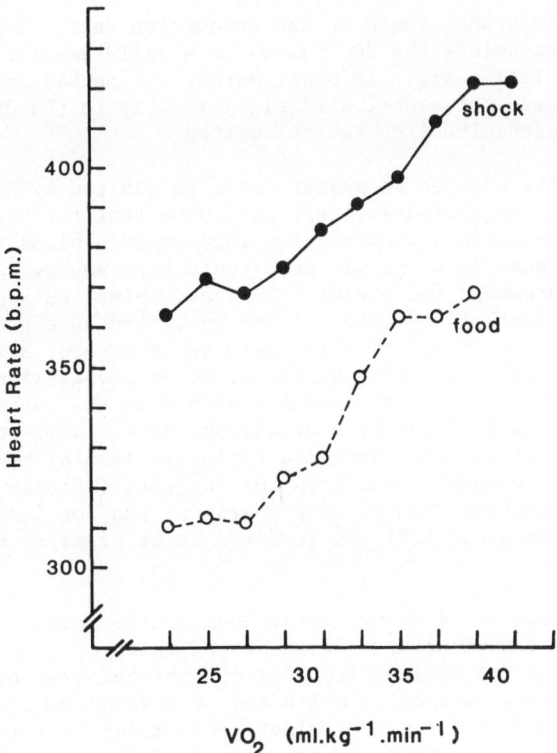

Fig. 2. Heart rate means at different levels of oxygen consumption
recorded from animals running to get <u>food</u> or to avoid <u>shock</u>.

tonic HR differences are unrelated to metabolic demand, they may be attributed to the operation of feedforward or Central Command pathways. In
terms of the relationship between VO_2 and HR described by Equation 2 in the
previous section, the data imply that the Shock condition led to smaller
$(A-V)O_2$ diffs. than did the Food condition. However, the case is not
conclusive since the comparison does not control for the possibility that
subjects in the Shock Group had intrinsically higher HRs than subjects in
the Food Group. This consideration led to the adoption of the following
method for assessing the metabolic appropriateness of HR levels:

(a) Concurrent recordings are made of HR and VO_2 under reference (minimal
     stress) conditions.
(b) A linear regression line is fitted to the data: an equation of the
     form $HR_e = m(VO_2) + k$ for this regression line describes the reference
     HR/VO_2 relationship.
(c) Concurrent recordings are then made of HR and VO_2 under test (stress)
     conditions.
(d) For each data point (i) the regression equation derived in steps (a)
     and (b) is used to estimate a HR value (HR_{ei}) for each VO_2 value
     (VO_2i) recorded under (c). These values are notated HR_{ei} (<u>e</u>stimate
     for measure <u>i</u>).
(e) The HR_e associated with each recorded VO_2 value is then subtracted
     from the actual HR value recorded concurrently with that VO_2 value
     yielding a HR_{di} value for each couplet of HR_i and VO_2i measures
     recorded under the test conditions, i.e. $HR_{di} = HR_i - HR_{ei}$.

Inferences regarding the metabolic appropriateness of HRs recorded
under the test condition are drawn from the mean values of its associated
HR_d values. If the mean HR_d differs significantly from zero, it is
inferred that nonmetabolic sources of influence are at work. It will be

recognized that this inference rests on the assumption that the regression equation employed to calculate the HR_d values is a valid description of the "non-stress" HR/VO_2 relationship. In other words, the method assumes that nonmetabolic factors have not contributed significantly to the HR variations on which the regression line was calculated.

The capacity of the muscles to sustain work is limited by blood perfusion rates, and as suggested earlier, it may be that the biological value of feedforward mechanisms in producing increases in blood flow (or in potential blood flow rate) is to permit more rapid high-energy responses and to increase the threshold for muscular fatigue. Since this process anticipates increased metabolic demand, it may be viewed as a pre-execution or preparatory motor adaptation. On this basis we (Sherwood, Brener and Moncur, 1983) hypothesized that tonic states of motor preparation would be associated with metabolically-unwarranted elevations in HR. States of motor preparation were manipulated by controlling the temporal predictability of Imperative Stimuli that demanded explosive running responses for the avoidance of electric shock. One group of subjects (HP) was submitted to a procedure which required them to be prepared to run for 5 seconds in every minute. The other group (LP) was required to be prepared for 30 seconds in every minute.

Both groups were submitted to two seven-hour sessions each of which started with a four-hour habituation period during which no experimental stimuli were presented. The habituation periods were followed immediately by three-hour conditioning periods in which the avoidance contingencies were applied. For all subjects a Discriminative Stimulus (SD) was presented for fixed periods of thirty seconds on the average of once per minute (mean ISI = 30 seconds; range = 10 - 50 seconds). During the presence of the SD but not in its absence, subjects in both groups were presented with three-second Imperative Stimuli (ISs). Each IS was followed by a one-second electric shock unless the subject ran a criterion distance during the presence of the IS. Although subjects in the two groups received an equal number of ISs on each session, these stimuli were presented in such a way as to produce a higher state of motor preparation in one group of subjects than in the other.

In particular, in the High Predictability (HP) condition one IS was always presented in each SD and it always occurred five seconds following the onset of the SD. On the other hand in the Low Predictability (LP) condition, subject to the constraint that no more than two ISs occurred in each DS, they were programmed to occur with equal probabilities (p = 0.033) in each second of the SD. The rationale of this arrangement was that in the HP condition, preparation for running was functional only during the 5 seconds immediately following the onset of the SD. However in the LP condition where between zero and two ISs could occur at unpredictable times during the course of each SD, preparation for running continued to be functional throughout the SD.

In order to avoid electric shock, subjects had to run 12 centimeters against a wheel rotation torque of 100 grams within the three-second period of the Imperative Stimulus. This was a taxing motor demand that had been selected on the basis of previous experimentation. Ambulation involves a substantial muscle mass in the rat and we wished to minimize ambulation differences between groups. This is because our previous observations were consistent with reports that at given levels of VO_2, HR is influenced by the size of the muscle mass involved in performing the work. Small muscle masses tend to give rise to higher HRs than large muscle masses (Lewis et al., 1983; Stenberg, Astrand, Ekblom, Royce and Saltin, 1967). Thus we have observed that at given levels of VO_2, HR tends to be inversely related to rate of ambulation.

Regression lines were computed for each subject on the basis of the 240 one-minute means for HR and VO_2 recorded during the Habituation period of Session 1. The regression equations describing these lines were then employed to compute HR deviation (HR_d) scores for each 30-minute period of each session by the method that has been described. Figure 3 presents the mean HR_d data for Sessions 1 and 2 for the HP and LP groups. It will be seen here that both groups exhibited increasingly negative HR deviations during the first habituation period. However, at the onset of conditioning, the HR deviations displayed a strong positive tendency that was more marked in the LP than the HP group. On Session 2, a similar pattern of scores is evident although the distinction between the groups is even more marked. Subjects in the LP group exhibited more positive HR deviations during the habituation period and this was maintained during conditioning.

The results of this experiment are consistent with the hypothesis that preparation for motor activity is associated with metabolically-excessive elevations in HR. If the assumption of relatively constant stroke volumes is maintained, the results imply that as subjects habituated to the experimental chamber, tissue perfusion decreased. Then when the avoidance contingencies were applied, tissue perfusion increased and it increased significantly more under the LP condition where a relatively high state of motor readiness was required than it did under the HP condition. Of course, if stroke volume decreased and compensated for the increases in HR, cardiac output and hence tissue perfusion rates may have been maintained at levels appropriate to the metabolic load. In this case, variations in the HR/VO_2 relationship signified by the HR deviation scores may be interpreted as changes in the permissive pumping level of the heart (Guyton, 1977), viz. changes in the heart's potential for blood delivery rather than changes in actual perfusion rates.

However, the observation of substantial negative HR deviation scores during the latter parts of the habituation phases suggests that the regression model employed to assess the deviations did not provide an accurate picture of the normal "non-stress" relationship between HR and

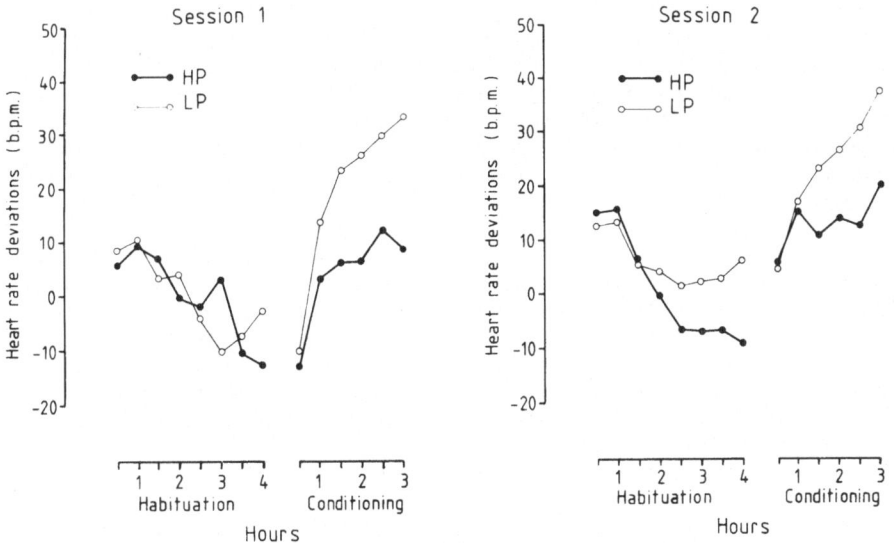

Fig. 3.   Heart rate deviations during habituation and shock-avoidance conditioning on two sessions in two groups of rats. [HP animals were required to be ready to run for 5 seconds in every 60 whereas LP animals were required to be ready for 30 seconds in every 60.]

VO_2. This is plausible since the data employed to compute the model included the initial part of the habituation period during which the subjects may have been highly aroused due to transport to the experimental room and introduction to the apparatus.

This possibility was reinforced by the results of a recent attempt to determine whether methods for inducing heightened states of motor preparation that do not involve electric shock would also give rise to metabolically-excessive elevations in HR (Brener and Myers, 1984; Note 3). In this case motor preparation was manipulated by restricting unconditioned species-characteristic motor responses. It is well established that within certain limits, rats exhibit a strong monotonic relationship between running rates and food-deprivation levels (Richter, 1927). We reasoned that if this instinctive hunger-induced tendency to ambulate was prevented, levels of motor preparation would increase. Similar methods were employed for computing HR deviations, but in this experiment subjects were run for two three-hour habituation sessions to provide 360 one-minute HR and VO_2 measures for the computation of the regression lines. The habituation sessions were followed by six 100-minute experimental sessions during which food was delivered independently of behavior. Using regression lines fitted to the habituation data, heart rate deviation scores (HR_d) were calculated on the basis of 20-minute HR and VO_2 means recorded during the experimental sessions (5 HR_d estimates per session).

Two groups of six rats each were studied under conditions of 23 hours food deprivation, in a running wheel environment where they were presented with food pellets independently of their behavior on a variable-time schedule with a mean of 90 seconds. During food-delivery sessions but not during habituation, the running wheel was locked for Experimental subjects (Wheel-Locked Food Group, WLF). However, it was always free to rotate for Control subjects (Wheel-Free Food Group, WFF). Since Experimental (WLF) subjects were prevented by the locked wheel from engaging in hunger-induced ambulation, we anticipated that they would be more motorically prepared and hence would exhibit greater positive HR deviations than Control (WFF) subjects. A further comparison group was provided by six subjects which were submitted to two three-hour habituation sessions followed by six 100-minute sessions in which inescapable electric shocks were presented on a 90-second variable-time schedule (Wheel-Free Shock Group, WFS). These subjects were run in non-deprived states with the wheel free to rotate. It was anticipated that the WFS subjects would exhibit positive HR deviations during the initial post-habituation sessions but that these deviations would decline as a function of sessions since, unlike the previous shock experiment, no motor requirement was implied by the contingencies and hence motor preparation was not functional.

The results of this study are illustrated in Figure 4 where it will be seen that although the HR deviations recorded from the WLF Group were significantly less negative than those recorded from the WFF Group, both groups exhibited HRs that were substantially lower than predictions based upon the habituation regression lines. No significant differences in HR_d scores were found between the WFS and WLF groups, both of which exhibited positive HR deviations on the first experimental session followed by successively more negative HR deviations until the final session. In terms of the theoretical proposals outlined earlier, the similarity of the HR_d scores in these two groups suggests the procedures to which they were submitted served to maintain a stronger contribution from feedforward processes to HR control (motor preparation?) than did the WFF condition. However, the observation of negative HR deviations in all three group and particularly in the WFF group, suggests that regression lines based on two three-hour habituation sessions does not provide an adequate model of the "non-stress" relationship between HR and VO_2. Since estimates of HR based on these lines were higher than those recorded during the experimental sessions, it is suggested that during the the habituation sessions, subjects exhibited supranormal HRs or were motorically prepared. Then as they adapted to the experimental environment, motor preparation waned and HR tended to fall relative to metabolic rate.

In order to explore this process more fully, multiple regression analysis using VO_2 and Experimental Session as predictors of HR was undertaken on the 600 one-minute group means of HR and OC recorded during the six experimental sessions. Each of the 100 one-minute HR and VO_2 group means for each session was obtained by averaging the measures recorded from the six subjects in that group for that minute. The results of this analysis are provided in Table 1. Whereas a simple regression model with only VO_2 as a predictor of HR provided the best regression equation for the Shock and Experimental Food groups, the best regression equation for the Control Food animals incorporated VO_2 and Days as predictors. In the

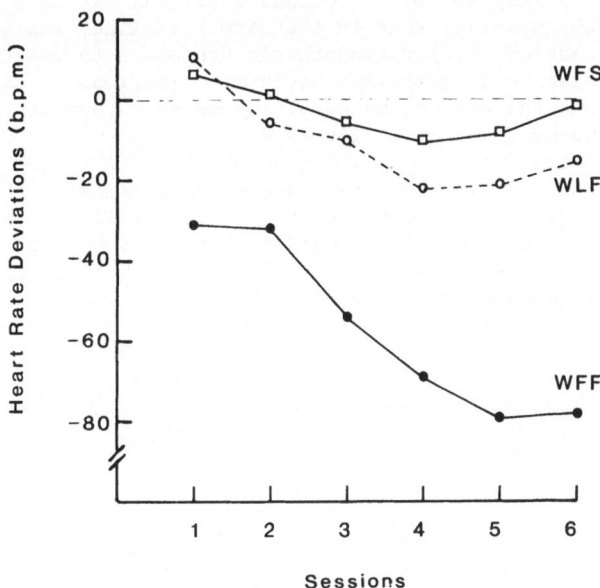

Fig. 4. Heart rate deviations as a function of daily sessions in three groups of rats. [See text for explanation.]

Table 1. Best Regression Equations for Predicting HR with VO_2 and Session Number (S) as Possible Predictors. By multiple regression methods, best regression equations were selected using 600 concurrently recorded one-minute means (100 per session for six sessions) of HR and VO_2. The mean for each minute was obtained by averaging measures recorded for that minute from the six subjects comprising each group. (VO_2 measured in $ml.kg^{-1}.min^{-1}$; Six consecutive experimental sessions numbered 1-6.)

Conditions:	Best Regression Equation:
Wheel-Locked Food:	$HR(+18.465) = 5.361(VO_2) + 218.739$
Wheel-Free Shock:	$HR(+12.486) = 5.301(VO_2) + 233.292$
Wheel-Free Food:	$HR(+12.326) = 5.117(VO_2) - 10.731(S) + 242.762$

latter case, the curves for each session were parallel but the Y-intercept of the regression line decreased by approximately 10 bpm on each successive session. As suggested below, this days effect may be attributed to an adaptation-related shift in the balance of sympathetic and parasympathetic tones responsible for maintaining HR level.

Sympathetic and parasympathetic blockade influence the HR/VO$_2$ relationship in the manner depicted in Figure 5. These data represent the means of 4 subjects from the Brener, Phillips and Connally (1980) experiment that were injected with blocking doses of beta-adrenergic (propranolol), parasympathetic (methyl atropine) or combined (propranolol + methyl atropine) antagonists whilst they were engaged in shock-avoidance behavior. The results are typical and we have observed similar effects in many subsequent experiments. The effects illustrated in this Figure also conform closely to those reported by Ekblom, Goldbarg, Kilbom and Astrand (1972) for humans. In particular, when VO$_2$ is low sympathetic blockade has relatively little effect on mean HR whereas parasympathetic blockade has a large effect. As VO$_2$ increases the effect of sympathetic blockade increases and that of parasympathetic blockade declines. It is a reasonable inference from these curves that in the normal (saline) state, as VO$_2$ increases, the contributions of the sympathetic processes to the control of the heart increase relative to parasympathetic contributions. This model suggests that the potential effects on HR of increases in sympathetic activity are likely to be greatest at low VO$_2$s.

It is hypothesized that introduction to the experimental situation elevates sympathetic activity. Effects on the heart are likely to be caused by the action of the sympathetic cardiac nerves as well as by circulating catecholamines. These factors serve to elevate HR above the levels appropriate to the concurrent rate of energy expenditure and their oper-

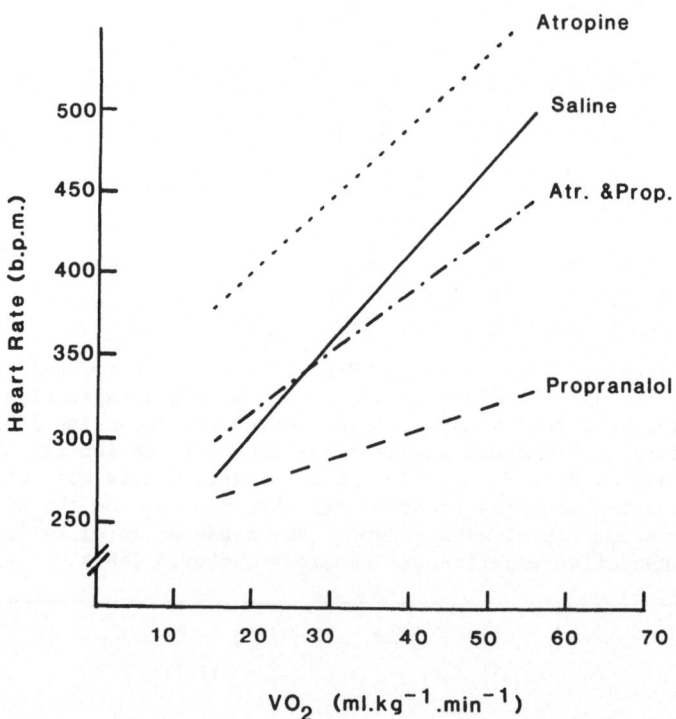

Fig. 5. Heart rate as a function of oxygen consumption during autonomic blockade.

ation reflects a motor preparatory process. To the extent that the contingencies operating in the experimental environment permit a behavioral adaptation on the basis of the subject's preformulated, naturally-occurring motor responses, this tonic preparatory process will wane. As it does so, the HR/VO_2 curve will move closer to that observed when the beta-adrenergic receptors are blocked (Figure 5). However, if the contingencies prevent the occurrence of these naturally-occurring responses (WLF group) or if naturally-occurring responses do not permit a satisfactory adaptation (WFS group), the tonic sympathetic influences wane less rapidly and HR is maintained at high levels relative to VO_2. This also occurs if the experimental contingencies explicitly demand sustained states of motor preparation as in the LP condition of the Sherwood, Brener and Moncur (1983) study. Another observation that is consistent with this general hypothesis comes from a recent experiment by Brener, Phillips and Sherwood (1983). Here it was found that subjects which were required to run for food maintained higher HRs relative to VO_2 than did subjects which were given food independently of their behavior. This difference emerged as the experiment progressed although the two groups showed no differences in ambulation rates or VO_2.

It is therefore suggested that environmental conditions that require a new motor adaptation may sustain high levels of activity in the feedforward pathways responsible for controlling the heart and thereby induce metabolically-excessive elevations in HR. The data presented are consistent with Obrist's (1981) proposal that such elevations are mediated by sympathetic influences on the heart. These hypotheses may be tested by examining the effects of sympathetic and parasympathetic agonists and antagonists on the HR/VO_2 relationship under conditions that vary in their demands for motor preparation. Data on plasma catecholamine levels under different demand conditions would also be helpful (McCubbin, Richardson, Langer, Kizer and Obrist, 1983). However, it is very difficult to provide definitive evidence that preparation for striate muscle activity is at the source of disturbances in the HR/VO_2 relationship. Perhaps relevant data may be acquired from concurrent recordings of activity in brain structures associated with motor programming. Alternatively it may be possible to monitor reflexological methods (Bonnet, Requin and Semjen, 1980; Brunia, 1983).

REFERENCES

Bevegard, B. S., and Shepherd, J. T., 1967, Regulation of the circulation during exercise in man, Physiol. Rev., 47:178-213.
Blix, A. S., Stromme, S. B., and Ursin, H., 1974, Additional heart rate - an indicator of psychological activation, Aerospace Med., 11:1219-1222.
Bonnet, M., Requin, J., and Semjen, A., 1981, Human reflexology and motor preparation, Exer. & Sport Sci. Rev., 9:119-157.
Brener, J., 1981, Control of internal activities, British Medical Bull., 37:169-174.
Brener, J., 1984 (in press), Operant Reinforcement, feedback and the efficiency of learned motor control, in: "Psychophysiology: Systems, Processes and Applications, Vol II", M. Coles, E. Donchin and S. Porges, eds., Guildford Press, New York.
Brener, J., Eissenberg, E., and Middaugh, S., 1974, Respiratory and somato-motor factors assocaited with operant conditioning of cardiovascular responses in curarized rats, in: "Cardiovascular Psychophysiology", P. A. Obrist, A. H. Black, J. Brener and L. V. DiCara, eds., 251-275, Aldine Press, Chicago.
Brener, J., Phillips, K., and Connally, S. R., 1977, Oxygen consumption and

ambulation during operant conditioning of heart rate increases and
decreases in rats, Psychophysiology, 14:483-491.

Brener, J., Phillips, K., and Connally, S., 1980, Energy expenditure, heart
rate and ambulation during shock-avoidance conditioning of heart
rate increases and ambulation in freely-moving rats, Psychol-
physiology, 17:64-74.

Brener, J., Phillips, K., Sherwood, A., 1983, Energy expenditure during
response-dependent and response-independent food delivery in rats,
Psychophysiology, 20:384-392.

Brod, J., Fencl, V., Hejl, Z. E., and Jirka, J., 1959, Circulatory changes
underlying blood pressure elevation during acute emotional stress
(mental arithmetic) in normotensive and hypertensive subjects, Clin.
Sci., 18:269-.

Brunia, C. H. M., 1983, Motor preparation: Changes in amplitude of Achilles
Tendon reflexes during a fixed foreperiod of one second, Psychophysiology, 20:658-664.

Cabanac, M., and Serres, P., 1976, Peripheral heart as a reward for heart
rate response in the curarized rat, J. Comp. & Physiol. Psychol.,
90:435-441.

Clemens, W. J., and Shattock, R. J., 1979, Voluntary heart rate control
during static muscular effort, Psychophysiology, 16:327-332.

DiCara, L. V., and Miller, N. E., 1969, Transfer of instrumentally learned
heart-rate changes from curarized to noncurarized state: Implications for a mediation hypothesis, J. Comp. & Physiol. Psychol.,
68:159-162.

Eldridge, F. L., Millhorn, D. E., and Waldrop, T. G., 1981, Exercise
hyperpnea and locomotion: Parallel activation from hypothalamus,
Science, 211:844-846.

Folkow, B., and Neil, E., 1971, Circulation, Oxford University Press, New
York.

Forsyth, R. P., 1971, Regional blood flow changes during 72 hour avoidance
schedules in monkeys, Science, 173:546-548.

Freyschuss, U., 1970, Cardiovascular adjustment to somatomotor activation,
Acta Physiol. Scand., Suppl. 342:1-63.

Gelsema, A. J., De Groot, G., and Bouman, L. N., 1983, Instantaneous
cardiac acceleration in the cat elicited by peripheral nerve stimulation, J. Appl. Physiol., 55(3):703-710.

Gliner, J. A., Bedi, J. F., and Horvath, S. M., 1979, Somatic and non-
somatic influences on the heart: hemodynamic changes, Psychophysiology, 16:358-362.

Gliner, J. A., Horvath, S. M., and Wolfe, R. R., 1975, Operant conditioning
of heart rate in curarized rats - hemodynamic changes, Am. J.
Physiol., 228:870-874.

Goesling, W. J., and Brener, J., 1972, Effects of activity and immobility
conditioning upon subsequent heart-rate conditioning in curarized
rats, J. Comp. & Physiol. Psychol., 81:311-317.

Goldstein, D. S., Ross, R. S., and Brady, W. W., 1977, Biofeedback heart
rate training during exercise, Biofeedback & Self-Regulation, 2:107-
126.

Goodwin, G. M., McCloskey, D. I., and Mitchell, J. H., 1972, Cardiovascular
and respiratory responses to changes in central command during
isometric exercise at cosntant muscle tension, J. Physiol., 226:173-
190.

Grollman, A., 1929, Physiological variations in the cardiac output of man,
Am. J. Physiol., 89:584-588.

Guyton, A. C., 1977, "Textbook of Medical Physiology", W. B. Saunders
Company, Philadelphia.

Kozar, A. J., 1964, Anticipatory heart rate in rope climbing, Ergonomics,
7:311-315.

Krogh, A., and Lindhard, J., 1913, The regulation of respiration and circu-

lation during the initial stages of muscular work, J. Physiol.
(London), 47:112-136.

Lang, P. J., 1979, A bio-informational theory of emotional imagery, Psychophysiology, 16:512.

Langer, A. W., Obrist, P. A., and McCubbin, J. A., 1979, Hemodynamic and
metabolic adjustments during exercise and shock avoidance in dogs,
Am. J. Physiol: Heart & Circ. Physiol., 5:H225-H230.

Malhotra, M. S., Sen. Gupta, J., and Rai, R. M., 1963, Pulse count as a
measure of energy expenditure, J. Appl. Physiol., 18:994-996.

McCubbin, J. A., Richardson, J. E., Langer, A. W., Kizer, J. S., and
Obrist, P. A., 1983, Sympathetic neuronal function and left ventricular performance during behavioral stress in humans: The
relationship between plasma catecholmaines and systolic time
intervals, Psychophysiology, 20:102-110.

Middaugh, S., Eissenberg, E., and Brener, J., 1975, The effect of artificial ventilation on cardiovascular status and on heart rate conditioning in the curarized rat, Psychophysiology, 12:520-526.

Miller, N. E., 1969, Instrumental learning of heart rate changes in
curarized rats: Shaping and specificity to discriminative stimulus,
Science, 163:434-445.

Miller, N. E., and Dworkin, B. R., 1974, Visceral learning: Recent difficulties with curarized rats and significant problems for human
research, in: "Cardiovascular Psychophysiology", P. A. Obrist, A. H.
Black, J. Brener and L. V. DiCara, eds., 312-331, Aldine Press,
Chicago.

Mitchell, J. H., Kaufman, M. P., and Iwamoto, G., 1983, The exercise
pressor reflex: Its cardiovascualr effects, afferent mechanisms, and
central pathways, Ann. Rev. Physiol., 45:229-242.

Obrist, P. A., 1981, "Cardiovascular Psychophysiology: A Perspective",
Plenum Press, New York.

Perski, A., and Engel, B. T., 1980, The role of behavioral conditioning in
the cardiovascular adjustments to exercise, Biofeedback & Self-
Regulation, 5:91-104.

Richter, C. P., 1927, Animal behavior and internal drives, Quarterly Rev.
Biol., 2:307-343.

Rushmer, R. F., Smith, O. A., and Lasher, E. P., 1960, Neural mechanisms of
cardiac control during exertion, Phsyiol. Rev., 40 Suppl. 4:27-34.

Sherwood, A., Brener, J., and Moncur, D., 1983, Information and states of
motor readiness: Their effects on the covariation of heart rate and
energy expenditure, Psychophysiology, 20:513-529.

Smith, O. A., 1974, Reflex and Central Mechanisms involved in the corol of
the heart and circulation, Ann. Rev. Physiol., 36:93-123.

Stenberg, J., Astrand, P., Ekblom, B., Royce, J., and Saltin, B., 1967,
Hemodynamic response to work with different muscle groups, sitting
and supine, J. Appl. Physiol., 22:61-70.

Steptoe, A., 1981, "Psychological Factors in Cardiovascular Disorders",
Academic Press, London.

Sparrow, W. A., 1983, The efficiency of skilled performance, J. Motor
Behavior, 15:237-261.

Thornton, E. W., and Van Toller, C., 1973(a), Effect of immunosympathectomy
on operant heart rate conditioning in the curarized rat, Physiol. &
Behavior, 10:983-988.

Thornton, E. W., and Van Toller, C., 1973(b), Operant conditioning of heart
rate changes in the functionally decorticate curarized rat, Physiol.
& Behavior, 10.

Trotter, J. R., 1956, The physical properties of bar-pressing behavior and
the problem of reactive inhibition, Quarterly J. Exp. Psychol.,
8:97-106.

Turner, J. R., Carroll, D., and Courtney, H., 1983, Cardiac and metabolic
responses to "Space Invaders": An instance of metabolically-
exaggerated cardiac adjustment?, Psychophysiology, 20.

REFERENCE

1. Black, A. H., October 1967, Operant conditioning of heart rate udner
    curare, (Technical Report 12), Hamilton, Ontario, Canda; McMaster
    University, Department of Psychology.
2. Moses, J., Clemens, W. J., and Brener, J., in preparation, 1984, Energy
    expenditure varies during voluntary heart rate control while engag-
    ing in static exercise.
3. Brener, J., and Myers, C., in preparation, 1984, Changes in the
    relationship between heart rate and oxygen consumption during food
    and shock delivery.

THE INTEGRATION AND DIFFERENTIATION OF CARDIOVASCULAR

AND METABOLIC RESPONSES TO STRESS

Alan W. Langer*, Catherine M. Stoney*, Paul A. Obrist**
and James R. Sutterer*

*Behavioral Physiology Laboratory, Department of Psychology
Syracuse University, Syracuse, New York 13210
**Department of Psychiatry, School of Medicine
University of North Carolina, Chapel Hill
North Carolina 27514

INTRODUCTION

The problem of clarifying how cardiac and metabolic (somatic) processes interact over a wide range of behavioral conditions which have been
variously characterized as stressful has been of long standing interest to
both physiologists and psychophysiologists alike. Not only are the
relationships among these events rather complex from a physiological point
of view, but also from a behavioral standpoint. For example, the term
stress refers to a rather heterogeneous set of events such as heat stress,
cold stress, exhaustion, infection, trauma, anxiety, nervous tension,
strain, and even physical exertion and exercise. Furthermore, even when
the analysis is limited to only one type of stress, such as psychological
stress, the welter of results that emerge are somewhat difficult to summarize. This difficulty can, in part, be ascribed to the facts that many of
the studies reported frequently operationalize stress using different
experimental paradigms and involve experiments conducted on various
species. Moreover, even where the focus is limited to outcomes with human
volunteers, the populations from which samples have been selected often
vary along many important dimensions. Notwithstanding these difficulties,
the scope of the present chapter will be delimited to one which focuses on
the cardiac-metabolic (somatic) interactions which take place during
physical (exercise) and psychological stress. The rationale for this
approach is twofold. First, it is clear from an evolutionary perspective
that the capacity to engage in intensive and extensive dynamic exercise
provides the organism with a greater opportunity to survive. This is
complimented by an ever increasing body of evidence which suggests that the
physiological consequences of exercise may be directly salutory and beneficial in terms of diminishing the risk of future cardiovascular morbidity
and mortality (Bjorntorp, 1982; Paffenbarger and Hale, 1975; Paolone,
Lewis, Lanigan and Goldstein, 1976; Patterson, Shephard, Cunningham, Jones
and Andrews, 1979). Secondly, in contrast to exercise, it has become
something of a "zeitgeist" that so-called psychological or behavioral
stress may often play a crucial role in the etiology of various cardiovascular pathophysiologies (i.e. cardiovascular-based psychosomatic formulations). Therefore, these two classes of stress have been more or less
distinguished along a dimension of physiological adaptation-maladaptation,

with exercise stress localized on the adaptation side of the continuum and psychological stress on the maladaptation side. In light of these circumstances, it would be rather important to determine whether or not the cardiovascular and metabolic responses elicited by these two types of stressors can be differentiated.

CARDIAC-METABOLIC INTEGRATION DURING STRESS

The integration of cardiac responses (i.e. cardiac output and heart rate) on the one hand and metabolic function (i.e. pulmonary ventilation and gas exchange) on the other represents one of the most fundamental concepts in exercise physiology because physical exercise is one of the most demanding conditions imposed on the cardiovascular and pulmonary systems. Thus, during dynamic exercise under aerobic conditions, the increased demands for energy expenditure (oxygen consumption ($\dot{V}O_2$)) is directly mediatated through alterations in pulmonary ventilation ($\dot{V}_E$) and blood flow (cardiac output). As a result cardiac output varies as a direct function of the workload imposed and hence $\dot{V}O_2$ (Bevegard, and Shepherd, 1967; Ekelund and Holmgren, 1967; Smith, Guyton, Manning, and White, 1976), an effect that is primarily due to a widening of the arteriovenous oxygen $(a-v)O_2$ difference (blood oxygen extraction) and an exercise induced tachycardia (Bruce and McDonough, 1975; Rushmere, 1959; Wang, Marshall, and Shepherd, 1960). Indeed, the failure to elicit adequate increases in pulmonary ventilation and/or cardiac output during exercise challenge has become a clinical marker for the diagnosis and treatment of cardiac and pulmonary dysfunction (Auchincloss, Gilbert, Potts, Watts, Kuppinger, Dickstein, Gorelick, and Peppi, 1982; Hickam and Cargill, 1948; McDonough, Danielson, Wills, and Vine, 1974).

In contrast, the cardiovascular and metabolic responses to behavioral stress are less well understood even though this type of stress continues to be implicated in the etiology of various cardiovascular disorders including hypertension (Harrell, 1980; Langer, Obrist, and McCubbin, 1979), coronary artery disease (Herd, 1983; Jenkins, 1976; Schneiderman, 1983), sudden cardiac death (Corley, Mauck, and Shiel, 1975; Engel, 1978; Richter, 1957) and related increased susceptibility to life threatening cardiac arrhythmias (Lawler, Botticelli, and Lown, 1976; Lown, Verrier and Corbalan, 1973). The bulk of the evidence for these claims is derived almost entirely from demonstrations of stress-induced pathology in infrahuman species, whereas the confirmation of any link between psychological events and cardiovascular disease in man remains either correlational or anecdotal and hence merely speculative. Despite these shortcomings, a sizable literature has evolved which details a broad range of cardiovascular and metabolic responses to various behavioral stressors in man. These include alterations in systolic and diastolic arterial blood pressure (Ax, 1953; Jost, Ruilman, Hillman, and Gulo, 1952; Obrist, Gaebelein, Teller, Langer, Grignolo, Light, and McCubbin, 1978), cardiac output (Brod, Fencl, Hejl, and Jirka, 1959; Gliner, Bedi, and Horvath, 1979; Grollman, 1929), systolic time intervals (McCubbin, Richardson, Langer, Kizer, and Obrist, 1983), respiratory rate and end-tidal carbon dioxide (Suess, Alexander, Smith, Sweeney, and Marion, 1980) and most typically heart rate (HR) (Berg and Beebe-Center, 1941; Petry and Desiderato, 1978). Collectively, these responses have not been shown to be essential components of a common physiological response pattern and are frequently noted when the data are partitioned with respect to individual differences (Lacy, 1967; Manuck and Schaeffer, 1978; Obrist, 1981). Whether these individual differences predict greater or lesser future susceptibility to cardiovascular pathology, though frequently suggested (Falkner, Onesti, Angelakos, Fernandes and Langman, 1979; Hastrup, Light, and Obrist, 1982; Manuck and Proietti, 1982), has yet to be adequately demonstrated.

Historically, the concept that cardiac and metabolic processes are integrated during emotional stress dates back to Cannon's pioneering work on the emergency theory of emotions (1916) which proposed that similar physiological reactions accompanied pain, fear, anger, and rage. In particular, Cannon noted that these emotional stressors augmented the rate and forcefulness of cardiac contractions, elevated arterial blood pressure, and increased pulmonary ventilation, all of which was seen as a preparatory response to fight or flight. Given this frame of reference, the physiological adjustments to emotional stress could be viewed as adaptive since engaging in either fight or flight engenders both survival potential and involves the organism in intense physical activity. The notion that such preparatory responses could be potentially debilitating and maladaptive was later proposed by Cannon (1942) to result when "the bodily forces are fully mobilized for action, and if this state of extreme perturbation continues in uncontrolled possession of the organism for any considerable period, without the occurrence of activity, dire results may ensue". According to this scheme, the physiological changes elicited by emotional stress are potentially deleterious when they are protracted in the absence of actual fight or flight and corresponding modifications in physical activity. Selye (1956) enlarged upon the concept of nonspecificity by arguing that both eustress and distress produced a generalized alarm reaction which involved the same physiological consequences. Interestingly, empirical support for specificity in cardiac and respiratory function to diverse emotional states was first described by Wundt (see Ruckmick, 1936) who noted differential patterns of HR, pulse strength, respiratory rate and strength to states of pleasantness and unpleasantness. Evidence for patterning in a wide range of autonomic and somatic measures was later reported to accompany experimentally induced states of fear and anger (Ax, 1953). Despite the fascinating nature of this work, the search for the presence or absence of differential physiological reactions to different emotions has typically emphasized the direction rather than the magnitude of change in physiological reactivity. Consequently, these efforts have not substantially clarified the precise interrelationship between cardiac and somatic adjustments to emotional stress.

A more direct and comprehensive assessment of the degree of integration among cardiac and somatic processes to behavioral stress was later extensively explored in a series of studies by Obrist and associates. This work generally found a consistent concomitance among HR and somatic activity in both man and animal during several experimental procedures including simple reaction time and classical aversive conditioning. Moreover, this coupling among HR and somatic activity was found to be consistent with respect to the direction of change, viz., HR and somatomotor activity either both increasing or decreasing, as well as the magnitude of the effects obtained. For example, the authors noted in human subjects (Obrist, 1968; Obrist, Webb, Sutterer, and Howard, 1970; Webb and Obrist, 1970) a marked concomitance between phasic cardiac deceleration and cessation of ongoing somatic activity (respiratory frequency and amplitude, eye movements and blinks, and electromyographic bursts in and around the mouth and chin) during a simple reaction time task and in anticipation of an aversive UCS (shock) on non-reinforced test trials during aversive classical conditioning. On the other hand, phasic increases in HR and somatomotor activity were observed during the first part of a preparatory interval of an RT task (Obrist et al., 1969) and immediately following CS onset during classical aversive conditioning (Wood and Obrist, 1964). Subsequently, this pattern of cardiac-metabolic integration in humans was replicated by other investigators using a variety of somatic and respiratory measures during both classical aversive conditioning (Cohen and Johnson, 1971) and reaction time tasks (Holloway and Parsons, 1972; Jennings, Averill, Opton, and Lazarus, 1971). Also, these effects have been documented in infrahuman species subjected to classical aversive

conditioning procedures (Black and DeToledo, 1972; Hein, 1969) and naturalistic stressors (Adams, Baccelli, Mancia, and Zanchetti, 1969; Hofer,
1971). On balance these results suggested a significant degree of integration between HR and various somatic indices to these types of behavioral
challenges, consistent with the predictable relationship among HR and
metabolism during dynamic aerobic exercise.

CARDIAC-METABOLIC DIFFERENTIATION DURING STRESS

However, not all behavioral stress interventions have been found to
produce alterations in HR that covary with somatomotor activity. For
instance, Obrist, Lawler, Howard, Smithson, Martin, and Manning (1974)
reported that a signalled shock avoidance reaction time task elicited
phasic elevations in HR at a point in time when shock was expected but not
delivered, with little or no change in gross somatic activity. The authors
proposed that this type of behavioral stress differed from those eliciting
an integrated pattern of cardiac-somatic responding (i.e. classical
aversive conditioning) because it provided subjects with an opportunity to
cope (exercise control over the delivery of nociceptive stimulation) which
putatively is perceived as more stressful. Similar findings have been
reported by others who have examined tonic alterations in several parameters of somatic functioning during exposure to various types of behavioral stress. However, in one study capitalizing on threat of shock as a
stressor, Petry and Desiderato (1978) noted that subjects who were anticipating shock delivery after a six minute interval and who were provided
with a clock to indicate the time remaining before shock, showed elevations
in both HR and anxiety at the end of the anticipation interval, with little
or no correspondence in forearm EMG activity. These results suggest that
the degree of perceived stress (anxiety) need not always be related to the
opportunity to control aversive outcomes; however, it is important to note
that aversive stimulation was never actually delivered to subjects in this
study. Using $\dot{V}O_2$ as a direct index of metabolic activity, Blix, Stromme,
and Ursin (1974) reported that the HR of pilots during flight operations
such as take off and landing was greater than that predicated based on the
linear relationship between HR and $\dot{V}O_2$ during exercise. The average HR
during these maneuvers, which can be perceived as stressful and dangerous,
was 102 bpm which was associated with a level of $\dot{V}O_2$ that was significantly
below that which occurs when HR is elevated to similar levels during
aerobic exercise. The authors referred to this as an "additional" HR
response. Similarly, Gliner, Bunnell, and Horvath (1982) found negative
correlations characterizing the relationship between cardiac output and the
$(a-v)O_2$ difference for subjects purportedly experiencing anxiety prior to
giving a speech.

In an attempt to further explore this problem we (Langer et al., 1979)
compared the cardiovascular and metabolic adjustments of chronically
instrumented dogs exposed to both treadmill exercise (at 1 (slow), 3
(medium), and 5 (fast) mph) and signalled shock avoidance training. This
study permitted continuous recording of cardiac output, stroke volume, HR,
systolic and diastolic arterial blood pressures, total peripheral resistance (TPR) and discrete determinations of the $(a-v)O_2$ difference. In order
to compare the cardiac-metabolic relationships during exercise and behavioral stress, separate linear regression equations were calculated for the
relationship between cardiac output or HR and the $(a-v)O_2$ difference. An
example of the results depicting the relationship between cardiac output
and the $(a-v)O_2$ difference in one animal is provided in Figure 1. The
individual data points represent the actual observations which were made
during signalled shock avoidance training. These values have been superimposed over the line of best fit and the corresponding 95% prediction
interval calculated on the basis of the exercise data. Notice that from a

total of 21 observations during shock avoidance, more than 50% fall below
the lowest prediction band where the expected frequency is only 2.5%. This
effect is also revealed when the data are averaged by conditions. Referring to Table 1 it can be seen that for the same animal the cardiac output
at 3 mph (3.7 liters/minute) is quite comparable to the level elicited
during avoidance conditioning (3.5 liters/minute). In contradistinction,
the $(a-v)O_2$ difference during exercise rises to a level of 7.1 volumes %
whereas during avoidance the $(a-v)O_2$ difference (5.4 volumes %) exhibits no
significant departure from resting levels (5.2 volumes %). This differentiation between cardiac output and the $(a-v)O_2$ difference during behavioral
relative to exercise stress was found to be reliable for four of the six
animals tested. Moreover, when the same analysis was conducted on the
relationship between HR and the $(a-v)O_2$ difference five of six animals
exhibited a similar pattern, viz., comparable elevations in HR during
exercise and avoidance were associated with a lower $(a-v)O_2$ difference
during avoidance. In addition, we found larger pressor responses in these
animals during the behavioral stressor (Figure 2) which was partially due
to a significantly larger fall in TPR during exercise.

While the exercise data are in agreement with previous studies
delineating the cardiovascular and metabolic correlates of the exercising
dog (Bailie, Robinson, Rostorfer, and Newton, 1961; Barger, Richards,
Metcalfe, and Gunther, 1956; Fixler, Atkins, Mitchell, and Horwitz, 1976),
behavioral stress elicited a differentiated pattern among cardiac and
metabolic processes relative to exercise. We have described this cardiac
output response as an example of overperfusion of the systemic circulation
because the cardiac output is relatively excessive in relation to blood
oxygen extraction $((a-v)O_2$ difference) and hence metabolic demand. This
finding was somewhat unexpected in light of the fact that local blood flow
in many if not most tissues of the body is primarily modulated according to
the existing metabolic activity level of the tissues, despite changes in
other factors that might affect the capacity of the blood to deliver oxygen
and nutrients and to remove CO_2 and other waste byproducts from the
tissues. This process, referred to as local autoregulation, can be seen in
most vascular beds including skeletal (Jones and Berne, 1964), cardiac
(Berne, 1964), cerebral (Rapela and Green, 1964), hepatic (Torrance, 1959),
renal (Thurau, 1964), and intestinal (Johnson, 1964) beds. Furthermore,
this phenomenon also characterizes the regulation of blood flow throughout
the entire systemic circulation, a process known as whole body autoregulation (Folkow, 1952; Granger and Guyton, 1969). Therefore, behavioral
stress can elicit overperfusion which by definition represents a failure to
regulate systemic blood flow in accordance with actual metabolic demand.

AUTONOMIC MEDIATION OF CARDIAC-METABOLIC INTERACTIONS

A related problem is to determine the role of the autonomic nervous
system in modifying the cardiovascular response to these stressors because

Table 1. Relationship between Cardiac Output and the $(a-v)O_2$ Difference
during Rest, Exercise, and Shock Avoidance in One Dog.

			Rest		Exercise (3 mph)		Avoidance	
cardiac output (liters/min)	Mean ±	S.E.	2.0	.24	3.7	.16	3.5	.09
$(a-v)O_2$ (vol. %)	Mean ±	S.E.	5.2	.24	7.1	.30	5.4	.22

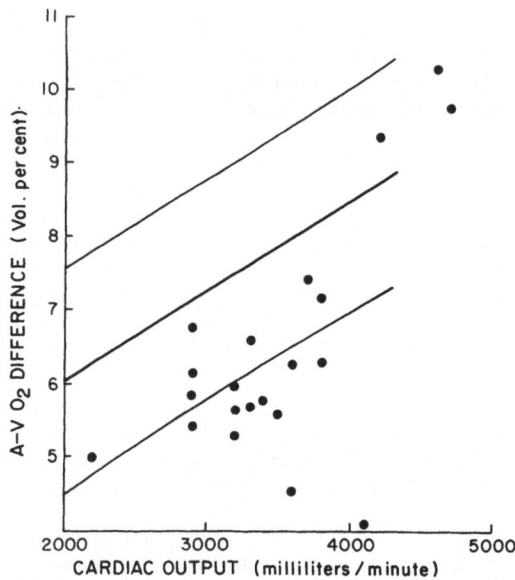

Fig. 1. Line of best fit and 95% prediction interval representing
relationship between cardiac output and $(a-v)O_2$ difference
determined on the basis of exercise stress for one dog. Data
points represent actual observations during shock avoidance.
Copyright 1979, The American Physiological Society. Reprinted
with permission.

many of the changes in human cardiac performance observed during both
exercise and behavioral stress resemble those that result from stimulation
of the sympathetic nervous system. For example, with reference to exercise, considerable evidence shows that the beta-adrenoceptor blocking agent
propranolol hydrochloride significantly attenuates both cardiac output and
HR during constant load exercise (Brown, Wasserman and Whipp, 1976;
Twentyman, Disley, Gribbin, Alberti and Tattersfield, 1981; Williams,
Singh, Ambler and Dorrington, 1976). Although propranolol prolongs the
time constants for changes in HR and $\dot{V}O_2$ during exercise (Petersen, Whipp,
Davis, Huntsman, Brown and Wasserman, 1983), its does not reduce either
cardiac output or HR to resting levels. Rather, it produces a compensatory
widening of the $(a-v)O_2$ difference, thereby maintaining $\dot{V}O_2$ at preblockade
levels (Ekblom, Goldbarg, Kilbom and Astrand, 1972; Furberg and
Schmalensee, 1968; Petersen et al., 1983). In contrast, beta-blockade has
been shown to attenuate both phasic (Obrist et al., 1974) and tonic (Obrist
et al., 1978) HR acceleration during shock avoidance reaction time stress,
suggesting that cardiac output may have been reduced to pre-stress levels.
Furthermore, the phasic HR pattern noted by Obrist et al. (1974) failed to
include significant differences in gross somatomotor activity between the
beta-blocked and saline control groups, despite clear-cut differences in
HR. Along similar lines, Imhof, Blatter, Fuccella and Turri (1969) compared the effects of exercise and emotional stress on the HR of ski jumpers
and found that the beta-adrenergic blocking agent oxprenolol entirely
blunted the emotional tachycardia, but only partially diminished the exercise tachycardia. Ostensibly, unlike exercise, during behaviorally stressful conditions which produce a differentiation in HR and somatic activity,
the positive cardiac chronotropic response is almost entirely due to
enhanced beta-adrenergic stimulation. On the other hand, behavioral
stressors which engender integrated cardiac-somatic patterning such as
simple reaction time and classical aversive conditioning are associated
with HR effects that are primarily mediated by changes in vagal tone
(Obrist, 1981).

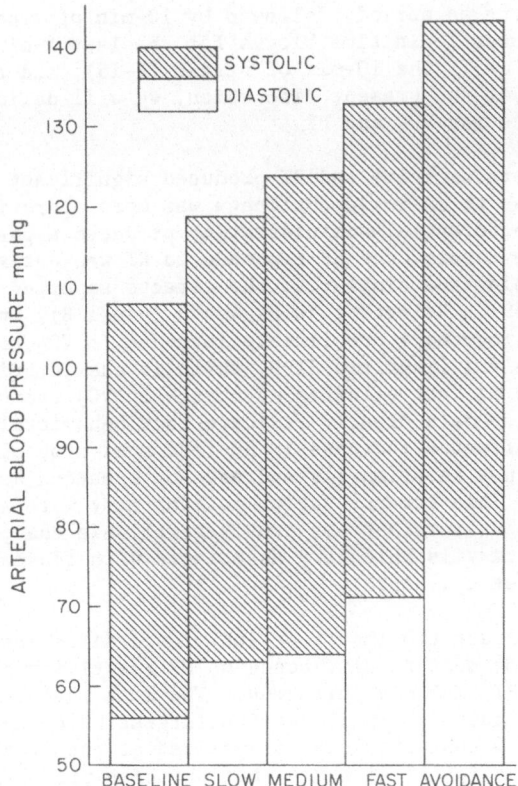

Fig. 2. Average systolic and diastolic blood pressure responses of 6 dogs during rest, 3 grades of treadmill exercise, and shock avoidance stress. Copyright 1979, The American Physiological Society. Reprinted with permission.

RECENT EVIDENCE ON CARDIAC-METABOLIC INTERACTIONS DURING STRESS

Since we have previously reported (Lnager et al., 1979) that behavioral stress, when compared to exercise stress elicited a relative systemic overperfusion, viz., an elevation in cardiac output and HR in excess of metabolic demand in dogs, we have recently (Langer, McCubbin, Stoney, Hutcheson, Charlton and Obrist, 1985b) evaluated whether the tachycardia which accompanies behavioral stress in humans represents a normal cardiac adjustment to an increased demand for oxygen, similar to the exercise response. A second objective of this study was to identify the precise role that beta-adrenergic mechanisms play in mediating this type of cardiac adjustment. Finally, this study assessed whether individual differences in HR reactivity during behavioral stress are also manifested during exercise. Thirty-four healthy males were randomly assigned to two experimental treatment groups with 14 subjects (beta-blocked group (BBG)) receiving 4 mg propranolol hydrochloride (iv) 15 minutes before stress testing while the remaining 20 subjects (intact group (IG)) were stress tested without any pharmacological pretreatment. Oxygen consumption ($\dot{V}O_2$), carbon dioxide production ($\dot{V}CO_2$), minute ventilation ($\dot{V}_E$), the partial pressures of end-tidal oxygen ($P_{ET}O_2$) and carbon dioxide ($P_{ET}CO_2$) were continuously monitored in real time on a breath-to-breath basis by means of an automated minicomputerized system (Langer, Hutcheson, Charlton, McCubbin, Obrist, and Stoney, 1985a). On two separate sessions all subjects were exposed to upright bicycle exercise at 300 kpm·min^{-1} and an unsignalled shock avoidance reaction time (RT) task. Both tasks incorporated a 10-min rest or baseline, a 10-min stress period, followed by 10-min of recovery. These data were averaged over 1-min time blocks for the last 5-min of rest (designated minutes 1-5), the 10-min of stress (6-15), and the 10-min of recovery (16-25). For the present discussion, we will delimit our presentation to the results for VO_2 and HR.

As expected, both exercise and RT produced significant increases in HR although the response to exercise challenge was more appreciable (Figure 3, panel A). Whereas propranolol administration produced a partial diminution of the exercise tachycardia, the HR response to RT was entirely abolished by beta-adrenergic blockade similar to the effects reported for oxprenolol by Imhof et al. (1969). Referring to Figure 3 (panel B), it can be readily seen that exercise produced a predictable increase in VO_2 to a steady-state level of approximately 1 liter/min STPD, which is characteristic for this work load, while the RT task elicited no change in VO_2 from resting levels. We conclude that these data clearly indicate that behavioral stress induced a metabolically unwarranted increase in HR (and most probably cardiac output), an effect that is primarily mediated by enhanced beta-adrenergic drive on the heart. This interpretation is consonant with a recent report demonstrating that behavioral stress provokes reliable changes in both HR and systolic time intervals which are associated with plasma catecholamine responses (McCubbin et al., 1983).

In order to evaluate the impact of individual differences in stress reactivity, a post-hoc median split based on HR reactivity of the intact subjects during the RT task was performed. The most reactive group (MRG) refers to the 10 subjects who exhibited the largest HR change from rest while the remaining 10 subjects were categorized as the least reactive group (LRG). Figure 4 (panel A) shows that exercise produced a comparable augmentation in HR for both groups. However, during RT stress the MRG realized a significantly larger HR response. This pattern was not evident with respect to VO_2 as both groups had similar and predictable elevations in VO_2 which reached a steady state during exercise, with no reliable change from rest noted for either group during RT (Figure 4, panel B). These observations are in agreement with those recently described by Turner, Carol, and Courtney (1983) who noted that high HR reactors and low HR reactors did not differentiate in terms of their VO_2 levels during a "space invaders" task. Within the context of our study, the fact that the MRG and the LRG differentiate on the basis of HR but not metabolism (VO_2) suggests that the metabolically excessive HR response to behavioral stress is exacerbated in reactive subjects. Finally, these data also reveal that the differential HR responsivity to the RT task was not a feature of the exercise response, where the MRG and LRG showed similar adjustments in HR. Apparently, these individual differences in HR stress reactivity engender an element of stressor specificity similar to the situational stereotypy described by Lacey (1967).

DISCUSSION AND IMPLICATIONS

At the beginning of the chapter, we outlined a position that has incorporated exercise stress within a biologically adaptive conceptual framework, including experimental evidence that suggests that this type of stress offers the organism potentially greater immunity from the development of cardiovascular disease. This view was contrasted with the notion that psychological stress may foster maladaptive consequences vis a vis its putative role in the etiology of various cardiovascular diseases. To date, one of the major obstacles confronting the viability of this distinction has been the fact that many of the cardiovascular effects which occasion both exercise and psychological stress are rather similar. For example, both conditions have been found to augment arterial blood pressure, HR and

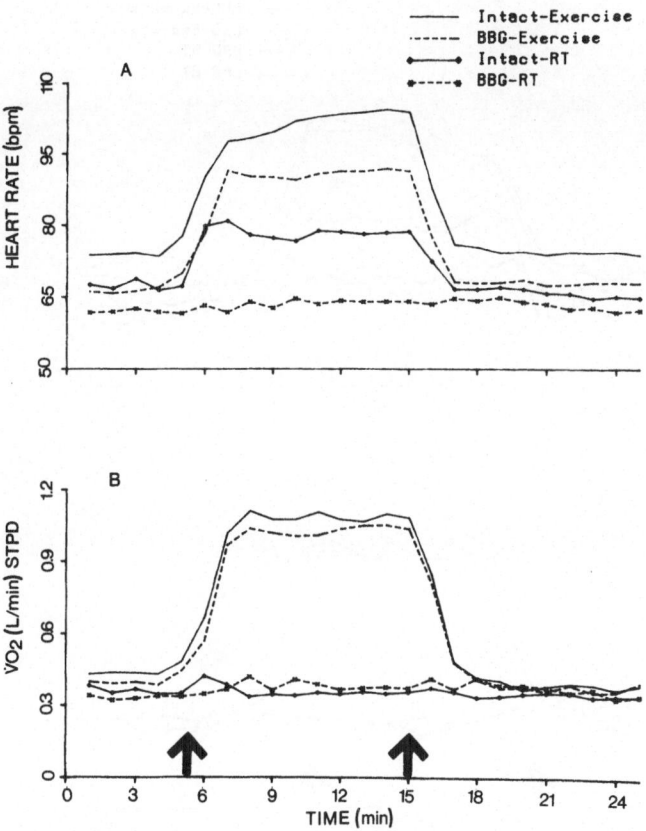

Fig. 3.   Average min-by-min HR (panel A) and $\dot{V}O_2$ (panel B) during 5-min of
rest, 10-min of exercise or RT, and 10-min of recovery with and
without beta-adrenergic blockade.

cardiac output.   Consequently, if both types of stressors produce similar
cardiovascular and metabolic adjustments, it becomes increasingly difficult
to impute pathogenic significance to behavioral stress.   In light of this
problem, the results of both our animal and human studies provides reasonable support to argue that the cardiac and metabolic responses to these
stressors are not similar.   Thus, we have clearly elaborated a dissociation
among cardiac and metabolic processes, relative to exercise, during
psychological stress.   The animal work has definitively established that
behavioral stress induces episodes of systemic overperfusion, a circulatory
state that was accompanied by appreciable pressor responses.   In human
subjects, we have found that the HR response to behavioral stress is
exaggerated with respect to actual metabolic demand ($\dot{V}O_2$), an effect that
was potentiated in reactive subjects.   Therefore, these stressors do produce discriminable cardiac-metabolic response patterning which would seem
necessary for the establishment of any cardiovascular-based psychosomatic
hypothesis.

     A more specific implication of these results is that they generally
conform to the autoregulatory theory of essential hypertension (Coleman,
Granger and Guyton, 1971; Ledingham and Cohen, 1963; Smith and Hutchins,
1979) which posits that episodes of overperfusion of the systemic circulation precipitates local vascular autoregulatory vasoconstriction that
effectively reduces cardiac output to normal levels, but at the expense of
an elevated arterial pressure.   Several lines of evidence support such a
proposed mechanism.   For instance, Coleman, Bower, Langford and Guyton

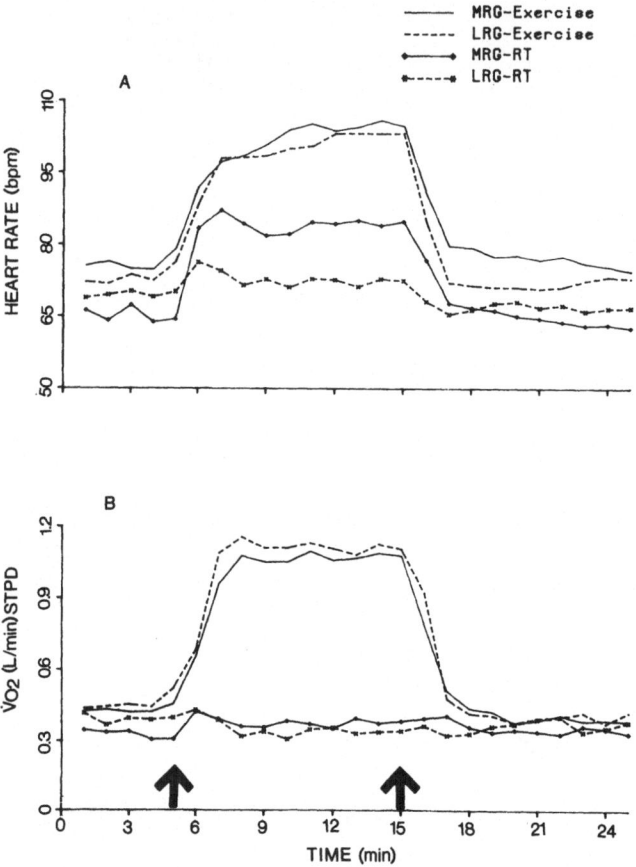

Fig. 4.   Average min-by-min HR (panel A) and VO$_2$ (panel B) during 5-min of
rest, 10-min of exercise or RT, and 10-min of recovery for the MRG
and LRG.

(1970) reported that fluid volume loading of anephric patients sustained by
artificial dialysis resulted in an elevated arterial pressure which was
initially mediated by a large increase in cardiac output. Subsequently,
overhydration evoked a fall in cardiac output that was accompanied by an
appreciable rise in peripheral resistance which served to sustain blood
pressure at abnormal levels. More recently, Smith and Hutchins (1979)
found that young spontaneously hypertensive rats (SHR) exhibited a hyperkinetic circulatory state (high cardiac index), which preceded increases in
TPR that resulted in a normal cardiac output while elevating mean arterial
pressure. Also, an elevated cardiac output has been found to be characteristic of both mild (Sannerstedt, 1969) and borderline (Julius and Conway,
1968) hypertension, conditions which frequently develop into a sustained
hypertension later in life (Julius and Shork, 1971). However, Julius and
Conway (1968) did not find that the elevated cardiac output in labile
hypertensives was necessarily coincident with normal levels of metabolism.

Nonetheless, this elevation in cardiac output can be substantially
reduced by beta-adrenergic blockade (Julius, Pascual, Sannerstedt, and
Mitchell, 1971), which has led various investigators to conclude that this
phenomenon is primarily mediated by either enhanced activity or outflow of
the cardiac sympathetic innervations and/or hyperresponsivity of the
cardiac beta-adrenergic receptors (Frohlich, Tarazi and Dustan, 1969;
Julius, Esler and Randall, 1975). Our human data are in accord with these
findings in terms of the fact that the tachycardia provoked by behavioral

stress was entirely blunted by beta-adrenoceptor blockade. Of related
interest is the finding that overperfusion has been elaborated in cases of
idiopathic hyperkinetic circulation, a clinical syndrome which is frequently accompanied by a labile blood pressure. Thus, Gorlin, Brachfeld,
Turner, Messer and Salazar (1959) reported a high cardiac output state in
these patients which was associated with a low (a-v)O_2 difference.
Curiously, when these patients were subjected to exercise, cardiac output
realized little or no change in spite of a significant increase in $\dot{V}O_2$
which was mediated entirely on the basis of a widening of the (a-v)O_2
difference. The relevance of our findings to this clinical literature is
that it shows that behavioral stress can induce circulatory changes that
are similar to those which are implicated in the etiology of essential
hypertension. The fact that the effects we observed in both the animal and
human studies were of a relatively brief duration does not rule out the
possibility that protracted behavioral stress could produce a sustained
hyperkinetic circulatory state which in turn could trigger compensatory
increases in arteriolar resistance and hence arterial blood pressure. This
is not to say that other intervening influences may not exert a profound
impact on the course of development of essential hypertension. Guyton
(1981) has emphasized that the elevation in cardiac output, which may
elicit autoregulatory processes is primarily mediated by an expanded intravascular volume due to an impairment of renal function. In this connection, Light, Koepke, Obrist, and Willis (1983) reported that experimental
stress attenuated urinary sodium and fluid excretion, which was directly
related to the magnitude of the HR increase to the stressor. This may
indicate a common sympathetic influence of cardiac and renal functioning
during behavioral stress. In addition, Folkow and collaborators (Folkow,
Grimby and Thulesius, 1958; Folkow, Hallback, Lundgren, Sivertsson, and
Weiss, 1973) have proposed that structural changes in the vascular wall of
the major resistance vessels (hypertrophic rebuild) occur in response to
alterations in transmural pressure, a phenomenon which could result from an
elevated cardiac output due to increased sympathetic tonus on the heart
and/or expanded intravascular volume. Obviously, the confirmation of these
potentially interrelated etiological pathways awaits direct assessment of
cardiac output, renal, metabolic and hemodynamic functions in a carefully
controlled longitudinal paradigm.

Finally, several converging lines of evidence suggest that increased
sympathetic nervous system activation in response to emotional stress may
serve an important role in the initiation and progression of coronary
artery disease (Herd, 1983; Schneiderman, 1983). According to
Schneiderman, the sequelae includes both an increase in blood pressure and
the release of catecholamines, which may compromise the endothelial lining
of arterial vessels. However, a second etiological route involves the
effect of catecholamine release on the mobilization of lipid stores.
Usually, the mobilized lipids are converted to free fatty acids as an
energy substrate during muscular activity. During fight or flight
reactions that do not result in physical activity, excess free fatty acids
are converted by the liver to triglycerides, a portion of which are then
converted to very low-density and low-density lipoproteins, the latter of
which have been implicated in pathogenesis of coronary artery disease.
Despite the fact that all the elements of this model have not been directly
evaluated, it is rather interesting that the lipid contribution to coronary
artery disease may reflect a situation where free fatty acids are mobilized
in excess of metabolic demand. Like systemic overperfusion, this would
represent yet another example of how a differentiated pattern of cardiovascular and metabolic processes during behavioral stress, unlike exercise,
could set the stage for the development of cardiovascular pathology.
Therefore, the relative degree of integration/differentiation of cardiovascular and metabolic processes may offer an important link in the understanding of the etiology of cardiovascular-based psychosomatic disorders.

REFERENCES

Adams, D. B., Baccelli, G., Mancia, G., and Zanchetti, A., 1969, Cardio-vascular changes during naturally elicited fighting behavior in the cat, Am. J. Physiol., 216:1226-1235.

Auchincloss, J. H., Gilbert, R., Potts, J. L., Watts, J. P., Kuppinger, M., Dickstein, R. A., Gorelick, D. E., and Peppi, D., 1982, J. Card. Rehab., 2:280-286.

Ax, A. F., 1953, The physiological differentiation between fear and anger in humans, Psychosomatic Med., 15:433-442.

Bailie, M. D., Robinson, S., Rostorfer, H. H., and Newton, J. L., 1961, Effects of exercise on heart output of the dog, J. Appl. Physiol., 16:107-111.

Barger, A. C., Richards, V., Metcalfe, J., and Gunther, B., 1956, Regulation of the circulation during exercise. Cardiac output (direct Fick) and metabolic adjustments in the normal dog, Am. J. Physiol., 184:613-623.

Berg, R. L., and Beebe-Center, J.G., 1941, Cardiac startle in man, J. Exp. Psychol., 28-29:262-279.

Berne, R. M., 1964, Regulation of coronary blood flow, Physiol. Rev., 44:1-29.

Bevegard, B. S., and Shepherd, J. T., 1967, Regulation of the circulation during exercise in man, Physiol. Rev., 47:178-213.

Bjorntorp, P., 1982, Hypertension and exercise, Hypertension, 4(Suppl. III):56-59.

Black, A. H., and DeToledo, L., 1972, The relationship among classically conditioned responses: Heart rate and skeletal behavior, in: "Classical Conditioning II: Current Theory and Research", A. H. Black and W. F. Prokasy, eds., Appleton-Century-Crofts, New York.

Blix, A. S., Stromme, S. B., and Ursin, H., 1974, Additional heart rate: An indicator of psychological activation, Aerospace Med., 45:1219-1222.

Brod, J., Fencl, V., Hejl, Z., and Jirka, J., 1959, Circulatory changes underlying blood pressure elevation during acute emotional stress (mental arithmetic) in normotensive and hypertensive subjects, Clin. Sci., 18:269-279.

Brown, H. V., Wasserman, K., and Whipp, B. J., 1976, Effect of beta-adrenergic blockade during exercise on ventilation and gas exchange, J. Appl. Physiol., 41:886-892.

Bruce, R. A., and McDonough, J. R., 1975, Cardiac output at rest and during exercise, Cardiovas. Clin., 6:353-369.

Cannon, W. B., 1916, "Bodily Changes in Pain, Hunger, Fear and Rage", D. Appleton and Company, New York.

Cannon, W. B., 1942, Voodoo death, Am. Anthropol., 44:169-181.

Cohen, M. J., and Johnson, H. J., 1971, Relationship between heart rate and muscular activity within a classical conditioning paradigm, J. Exp. Psychol., 90:222-226.

Coleman, T. G., Bower, J. D., Langford, H. G., and Guyton, A. C., 1970, Regulation of arterial pressure in the anephric state, Circulation, 42:509-514.

Coleman, T. G., Granger, H. J., and Guyton, A. C., 1971, Whole-body circulatory autoregulation and hypertension, Circ. Res., 28-29 (Suppl. 2):76-81.

Corley, K. C., Mauck, H. P., and Shiel, F. O'M., 1975, Cardiac responses associated with "yoked-chair" shock avoidance in squirrel monkeys, Psychophysiology, 12:439-444.

Ekblom, B., Goldbarg, A. N., Kilbom, A., and Astrand, P. O., 1972, Effects of atropine and propranolol on the oxygen transport system during exercise in man, Scand. J. Clin. Lab. Investigation, 30:35-42.

Ekelund, L. G., and Holmgren, A., 1967, Central hemodynamics during exercise, Circ. Res., 10 (Suppl. I):133-143.

Engel, G. L., 1978, Psychological stress, vasodepressor (vasovagal) syncope and sudden death, Ann. Int. Med., 89:403-412.

Falkner, B., Onesti, G., Angelakos, E. T., Fernandes, M., and Langman, C., 1979, Cardiovascular responses to mental stress in normal adolescents with hypertensive parents, Hypertension, 1:23-30.

Fixler, D. E., Atkins, J. M., Mitchell, J. H., and Horwitz, L. D., 1976, Blood flow to respiratory, cardiac, and limb muscles in dogs during graded exercise, Am. J. Physiol., 231:1515-1519.

Folkow, B., 1952, Study of the factors influencing the tone of denervated blood vessels perfused at various pressures, Acta Physiol. Scand., 27:99-117.

Folkow, B., Grimby, G., and Thulesius, O., 1958, Adaptive structural changes of the vascular walls in hypertension and their relation to the control of the peripheral resistance, Acta Physiol. Scand., 44:255-272.

Folkow, B., Hallback, M., Lundgren, R., Sivertsson, R., and Weiss, L., 1973, Importance of adaptive changes in vascular design for establishment of primary hypertension studies in man and SHR, Circ. Res., 32-33 (Suppl. 1):2-13.

Frohlich, E. D., Tarazi, R. C., and Dustan, H. P., 1969, Hyperdynamic beta-adrenergic circulatory state: Increased beta-receptor responsiveness, Arch. Int. Med., 123:1-7.

Furberg, C., and Schmalensee, G. V., 1968, Beta-adrenergic blockade and central circulation during exercise in sitting position in healthy subjects, Acta Physiol. Scand., 73:435-446.

Gliner, J. A., Bedi, J. F., and Horvath, S. M., 1979, Somatic and non-somatic influences on the heart: Hemodynamic changes, Psychophysiology, 16:358-362.

Gliner, J. A., Bunnell, D. E., and Horvath, S. M., 1982, Hemodynamic and metabolic changes prior to speech performance, Physiol. Psychology, 10:108-113.

Gorlin, R., Brachfeld, N., Turner, J. D., Messer, J. V., and Salazar, E., 1959, The idiopathic high cardiac output state, J. Clin. Investigation, 38:2144-2153.

Granger, H. J., and Guyton, A. C., 1969, Autoregulation of the total systemic circulation following destruction of the central nervous system in the dog, Circ. Res., 25:379-388.

Grollman, A., 1929, Physiological variations in the cardiac output of man. The effect of psychic disturbance on the cardiac output, pulse, blood pressure and O_2 consumption of man, Am. J. Physiol., 89:584-588.

Guyton, A. C., 1981, The relationship of cardiac output and arterial pressure control, Circulation, 64:1079-1088.

Harrell, J. P., 1980, Psychological factors and hypertension: A status report, Psychol. Bull., 87:482-501.

Hastrup, J. L., Light, K. C., and Obrist, P. A., 1982, Parental hypertension and cardiovascular response to stress in healthy young adults, Psychophysiology, 19:615-622.

Hein, P. L., 1969, Heart rate conditioning in the cat and its relationship to other physiological responses, Psychophysiology, 5:455-464.

Herd, J. A., 1983, Physiological basis for behavioral influences in arteriosclerosis, in: "Biobehavioral Bases of Coronary Heart Disease", T. M. Dembroski, T. H. Schmidt and G. Blumchen, eds., Karger, Basel.

Hickman, J. B., and Cargill, W. H., 1948, Effect of exercise on cardiac out-put and pulmonary arterial pressure in normal persons and in patients with cardiovascular disease and pulmonary emphysema, J. Clin. Investigation, 27:10-23.

Hofer, M. A., 1970, Cardiac and respiratory function during sudden prolonged immobility in wild rodents, Psychosomatic Med., 32:633-647.

Holloway, F. A., and Parsons, O. A., 1972, Physiological concomitants of reaction time performance, Psychophysiology, 9:189-198.

Imhof, P. R., Blatter, K., Fuccella, L. M., and Turri, M., 1969, Beta-blockade and emotional tachycardia, radiotelemetric investigations in ski jumpers, J. Appl. Physiol., 27:366-369.

Jenkins, C. D., 1976, Recent evidence supporting psychologic and social risk factors for coronary disease, Part I, New Eng. J. Med., 294:987-994.

Jennings, J. R., Averill, J. R., Opton, E. M., and Lazarus, R. S., 1971, Some parameters of heart rate change: Perceptual versus motor task requirements, noxiousness, and uncertainty, Psychophysiology, 7:194-212.

Johnson, P. C., 1964, Origin, localization and homeostatic significance of autoregulation in the intestine, Circ. Res., 14-15 (Suppl. 1):225-232.

Jones, R. D., and Berne, R. M., 1964, Local regulation of blood flow in skeletal muscle, Circ. Res., 14-15 (Suppl. 1):30-38.

Jost, H., Ruilmann, C. J., Hill, T. S., and Gulo, M. J., 1952, Studies in hypertension II. Central and autonomic nervous system reactions of hypertensive individuals to simple physical and psychologic stress situations, J. Nervous & Mental Disease, 115:152-162.

Julius, S., and Conway, J., 1968, Hemodynamic studies in patients with borderline blood pressure elevation, Circulation, 38:282-288.

Julius, S., Esler, M.D., and Randall, O. S., 1975, Role of the autonomic nervous system in mild human hypertension, Clin. Sci. & Molecular Med., 48:2435-2525.

Julius, S., Pascual, A. V., Sannerstedt, R., and Mitchell, C., 1971, Relationship between cardiac output and peripheral resistance in borderline hypertension, Circulation, 43:382-390.

Julius, S., and Shork, M. A., 1971, Borderline hypertension - A critical review, J. Chronic Diseases, 23:723-754.

Lacey, J. I., 1967, Somatic response patterning and stress: Some revisions of activation theory, in: "Psychological Stress: Issues in Research", M. H. Appley and L. Trumbell, eds., Appleton-Century-Crofts, New York.

Langer, A. W., Hutcheson, J. S., Charlton, J. D., McCubbin, J. A., Obrist, P. A., and Stoney, C. M., 1985a, On-line minicomputerized measurement of cardiopulmonary function on a breath-by-breath basis, Psychophysiology, 22:50-58.

Langer, A. W., McCubbin, J. A., Stoney, C. M., Hutcheson, J. S., Charlton, J. D., and Obrist, P. A., 1985b, Cardiopulmonary adjustments during exercise and an aversive reaction time task: Effects of beta-adrenoceptor blockade, Psychophysiology, 22:59-68.

Langer, A. W., Obrist, P. A., and McCubbin, J. A., 1979, Hemodynamic and metabolic adjustments during exercise and shock avoidance in dogs, Am. J. Physiol., 236:H225-H230.

Lawler, J. E., Botticelli, L. J., and Lown, B., 1976, Changes in cardiac refractory period during signalled shock avoidance in dogs, Psychophysiology, 13:373-377.

Ledingham, J. M., and Cohen, R. D., 1963, Role of the heart in the pathogenesis of renal hypertension, Lancet, 2:979-981.

Light, K. C., Koepke, J. P., Obrist, P. A., and Willis, P. W., 1983, Psychological stress induces sodium and fluid retention in men at high risk for hypertension, Science, 220:429-431.

Lown, B., Verrier, R., and Corbalan, R., 1973, Psychologic stress and threshold for repetitive ventricular response, Science, 182:834-836.

McCubbin, J. A., Richardson, J. E., Langer, A. W., Kizer, J. S., and Obrist, P. A., 1983, Sympathetic neuronal function and left ventricular performance during behavioral stress in humans: The relationship between plasma catecholamines and systolic time intervals, Psychophysiology, 20:102-110.

McDonough, J. R., Danielson, R. A., Wills, R., and Vine, D. L., 1974, Maxima cardiac output during exercise in patients with coronary artery disease, The Am. J. Cardiology, 33:23-29.

Manuck, S. B., and Proietti, J. M., 1982, Parental hypertension and cardio-vascular response to cognitive and isometric challenge, Psycho-physiology, 19:481-489.

Manuck, S. B., and Schaefer, D. C., 1978, Stability of individual differ-ences in cardiovascular reactivity, Physiology & Behavior, 21:675-678.

Obrist, P. A., 1968, Heart rate and somatic-motor coupling during classical aversive conditioning in humans, J. Exp. Psychol., 77:180-193.

Obrist, P. A., 1981, "Cardiovascular Psychophysiology: A Perspective", Plenum, New York.

Obrist, P. A., Gaebelein, C. J., Teller, E. S., Langer, A. W., Grignolo, A., Light, K. C., and McCubbin, J. A., 1978, The relationship among heart rate, carotid dP/dt, and blood pressure in humans as a func-tion of the type of stress, Psychophysiology, 15:102-115.

Obrist, P. A., Lawler, J. E., Howard, J. L., Smithson, K. W., Martin, P. L., and Manning, J., 1974, Sympathetic influences on cardiac rate and contractility during acute stress in humans, Psychophysiology, 11:405-427.

Obrist, P. A., Webb, R. A., and Sutterer, J. R., 1969, Heart rate and somatic changes during aversive conditioning and a simple reaction time task, Psychophysiology, 5:696-723.

Obrist, P. A., Webb, R. A., Sutterer, J. R., and Howards, J. L., 1970, Cardiac deceleration and reaction time: An evaluation of two hypotheses, Psychophysiology, 6:695-706.

Paffenbarger, R. S., and Hale, W. E., 1975, Work activity and coronary heart mortality, The New Eng. J. Med., 292:545-550.

Paolone, A. M., Lewis, R. R., Lanigan, W. T., and Goldstein, M. J., 1976, Results of two years of exercise training in middle-aged men, Physician & Sports Med., 4:72-77.

Patterson, D. J., Shephard, R. J., Cunningham, D., Jones, N. L., and Andrew, G., 1979, Effects of physical training on cardiovascular functioning following myocardial infarction, J. Appl. Phsyiol., Resp., Environ. & Exer. Physiol., 47:482-489.

Petersen, E. S., Whipp, B. J., Davis, J. A., Huntsman, D. J., Brown, H. V., and Wasserman, K., 1983, Effects of beta-adrenergic blockade on ventilation and gas exchange during exercise in humans, J. Appl. Physiol., Resp., Environ. & Exer. Physiol., 54:1306-1313.

Petry, H. M., and Desiderato, O., 1978, Changes in heart rate, muscle activity, and anxiety level following shock threat, Psycho-physiology, 15:398-402.

Rapela, C. E., and Green, H. D., 1964, Autoregulation of canine cerebral blood flow, Circ. Res., 15 (Suppl. 1):1205-1211.

Richter, C. P., 1957, On the phenomenon of sudden death in animals and man, Psychosomatic Med., 19:191-198.

Ruckmick, C. A., 1936, "The Psychology of Feeling and Emotions", McGraw-Hill, New York.

Rushmer, R. F., 1959, Constancy of stroke volume in ventricular response to exertion, Am. J. Physiol., 196:745-750.

Sannerstedt, R., 1969, Hemodynamic findings at rest and during exercise in mild arterial hypertension, Am. J. Med. Sci., 258:70-79.

Schneiderman, N., 1983, Behavior, autonomic function and animal models of cardiovascular pathology, in: "Biobehavioral Bases of Coronary Heart Disease", T. M. Dembroski, T. H. Schmidt and G. Blumchen, eds., Karger, Basel.

Selye, H., 1956, "The Stress of Life", McGraw-Hill, New York.

Smith, T. L., and Hutchins, P. M., 1979, Central hemodynamics in the devel-opmental stage of spontaneous hypertension in the unanesthetized rat, Hypertension, 1:508-517.

Smith, E. E., Guyton, A. C., Manning, R. D., and White, R. J., 1976, Integrated mechanisms of cardiovascular response and control during exercise in the normal human, Progress in Cardiovascular Disease, 18:421-443.

Suess, W. M., Alexander, A. B., Smith, D. D., Sweeney, H. W., and Marion, R. J., 1980, The effects of psychological stress on respiration: A preliminary study of anxiety and hyperventilation, Psychophysiology, 17:535-540.

Thurau, W. C., 1964, Autoregulation of renal blood flow and glomerular filtration rate, including data on tubular and peritubular capillary pressure and vessel wall tension, Circ. Res., 14-15 (Suppl. 1):132-141.

Torrance, H. B., 1958, Control of the hepatic arterial circulation, J. Royal College Surgeons of Edinburgh, 4:147.

Turner, J. R., Carroll, D., and Courtney, H., 1983, Cardiac and metabolic responses to "space invaders": An instance of metabolically-exaggerated cardiac adjustment?, Psychophysiology, 20:544-549.

Twentyman, O. P., Disley, A., Gribbin, H. R., Alberti, K. G. M. M., and Tattersfield, A. E., 1981, Effect of beta-adrenergic blockade on respiratory and metabolic responses to exercise, J. Appl. Physiol., Resp., Environ. & Exer. Physio., 51:788-793.

Wang, Y., Marshall, R. J., and Shepherd, J. T., 1960, The effect of changes in posture and of graded exercise on stroke volume in man, J. Clin. Investigation, 39:1051-1061.

Webb, R. A., and Obrist, P. A., 1970, The physiological concomitants of reaction time performance as a function of preparatory interval series, Psychophysiology, 6:389-403.

Williams, F. M., Singh, B. N., Ambler, P. K., and Dorrington, R., 1976, The effects of propranolol, practolol and metoprolol on exercise-induced tachycardia in relation to plasma levels in man, Clin. & Exp. Pharmacol. & Physiol., 3:473-482.

Wood, D. M., and Obrist, P. A., 1964, Effects of controlled and uncontrolled respiration on the conditioned heart rate response in humans, J. Exp. Psychol., 68:221-229.

THE HIERARCHICAL ORDER OF CARDIOVASCULAR-RESPIRATORY COUPLING

F. Raschke

Institute of Occupational Physiology
and Rehabilitation Research
Robert-Koch-Str. 7a, D-3550 Marburg, West Germany

Cardiovascular and respiratory systems are coupled in the periphery in respect to the variables which they jointly control, such as metabolic transport and gas exchange. The physical properties of the common vascular bed (both large and small circulations which are in series) imply such coupling. Additionally afferents from cardiac (e.g., Koizumi et al., 1975), systemic arterial blood pressure (e.g., Eckberg and Orshan, 1977), and lung stretch receptors (e.g., Hainsworth, 1974) are linked in the common brainstem enabling coupling. Finally, there exists coordinated rhythmic activity of the regulating neuronal networks in the brainstem (Koepchen, 1977; Koepchen et al., 1981), resulting in various mutual interactions between the two systems.

One mode of interaction is respiratory sinus arrhythmia - the most striking indicator of coupling. Considerable agreement exists that in this case it is the respiratory rhythm (Koepchen and Thurau, 1959; Levy et al., 1966; Koepchen, 1977), or respiration-synchronous changes of systemic arterial baroreflex gating (Eckberg and Orshan, 1977; Melcher, 1980), lung inflation (e.g., Hainsworth, 1974), and venous return (Schlomka and Reindell, 1936; Weltz, 1941) which cause changes in heart rate.

Thus this kind of coupling mechanism is well described by the term "respiratory heart rate modulation". The amplitude of this modulation depends on tidal volume (e.g., Hirsch and Bishop, 1981a), breathing frequency (e.g., Angelone and Coulter, 1964), and altered inspired O_2 or CO_2 concentration (Hirsch and Bishop, 1981b). The phase of this modulation is strictly related to the phases of breathing pattern (cf. Angelone and Coulter, 1964; Kelman and Wann, 1970; Kitney, 1977; Raschke and Hildebrandt, 1979) with heart rate increasing during inspiration and decreasing during expiration when subjects are at rest.

The second mode of coupling is produced by a strict phase relation between the cardiac cycle and the onset of respiratory phases. This phenomenon has been first shown by Schoenlein (1895) in fish, and by Galli (1924) in man. Subsequently, extensive studies on this topic were carried out by Bucher and co-workers on the rabbit (e.g., Bucher et al., 1972). Until now there have been about 75 papers which describe this phenomenon in different species (for references, see Raschke, 1981). In mammals it has been stated that the onset of inspiratory or expiratory phase is phase-coupled or phase-coordinated to cardiovascular events. The mechanism of phase-coordination is described by means of a __triggering__ of respiratory onsets in relation to phases of the cardiac cycle.

Phase-coordination in humans has so far been studied in detail after graded physical load (Hildebrandt and Daumann, 1965), during night work with an inversion of the circadian rhythm (Engel et al., 1971), during anesthesia in children and adults (Engel and Hildebrandt, 1972), after caffeine intake (Engel and Hildebrandt, 1973), during night sleep (Storch and Hildebrandt, 1966; Raschke, 1981), and recently in the newborn (Hiebsch, 1984).

All the investigations in humans have shown that a marked phase-coordination mainly occurs during resting and recuperative conditions. On the other hand, such phase-coupling can be easily disturbed by even low levels of strain. Therefore it appears to be a particularly sensitive measure of the autonomic state.

Respiratory heart rate modulation (respiratory sinus arrhythmia, RSA) has been used in many studies as an indicator for the strain components of physical (e.g., Rohmert et al., 1973) and mental load (e.g., Mulder and Mulder, 1973; Hyndman and Gregory, 1975), and sleep staging (e.g., Engel, 1973; Bond et al., 1973). Because of the lack of investigations on phase-coordination in different sleep stages and with psychophysiological stressors, this paper gives the results of those experiments enabling a comparison of heart rate modulation (RSA) and phase-coordination under different conditions. The primary question has been the following: how is coupling realized in varying functional states which comprise an integral range of autonomic behavior? That is, our investigations took into account the waking state in relaxed supine and seated positions, the various sleep stages, and reactions to graded external stressors such as physical and mental load.

METHODS

The coupling mechanisms are described (a) by the amplitude of respiratory heart rate modulation (RSA) and (b) by the phase relationship between the R wave of the ECG and the following inspiratory onset (Figure 1). Respiratory heart rate modulation was assessed from epochs of instantaneous heart rate (HR) series (cardiotachogram) of 150 seconds. The conversion from RR interval into HR was used because instantaneous HR is normally distributed whereas RR interval times are not (Raschke, 1981); this thus enabled us to perform Fourier transformations. We established power density spectra via Fast Fourier Transformation using a lab computer (Plurimat-S/Intertechnique). The spectral density within the band of 8-30 cycles per min. was taken as an indicator of the amplitude of respiratory heart rate modulation. The square root of the respiratory peak's height gave the magnitude ΔHR (beats/min.). For comparison with studies on R-R interval variability (dimension in msec.), these ΔHR changes were reconverted and compared to the results of Engel (1973).

From recordings of the respiration curve using nasal thermistors, we computed the inspiratory onsets with a delay of less than 10 msec. with the aid of a computerized pattern recognition system (Raschke, 1982). The interval between the preceding R wave from the ECG and the following inspiratory onset (RI_i), and the RR_i interval upon inspiration onset were determined for each respiratory cycle as shown in Figure 1. Phase-coordination was defined according to von Holst (1939) in terms of relative coordination with statistical preference for distinct phases. Thus histograms with standardized number of inspiratory onsets were calculated. Chi-squared values of the distribution compared to an even distribution

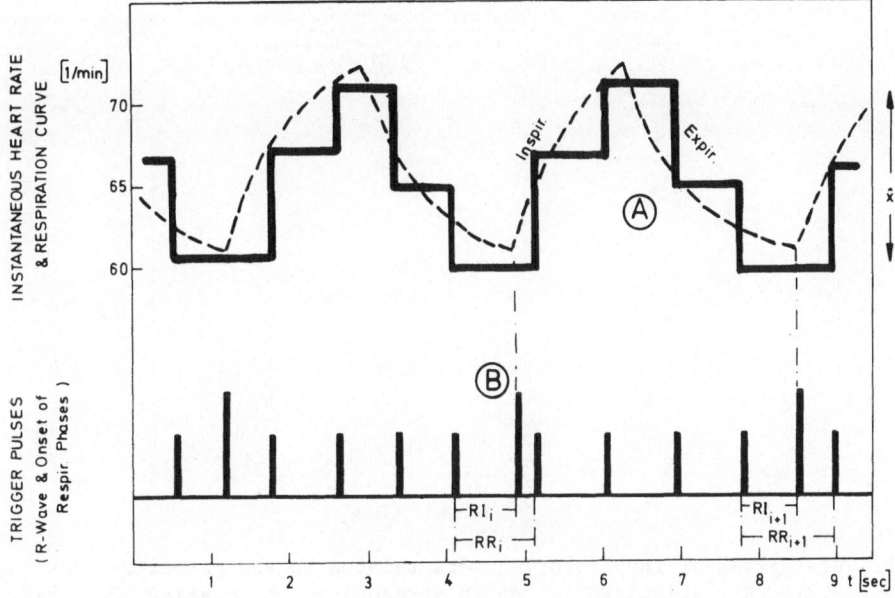

Fig. 1. Instantaneous heart rate (cardiotachogram) and respiration curve
above. Trigger pulses of ECG and exact inspiratory onset below.
Two modes of coupling are considered: A) Amplitude ($\hat{x}$) of
respiration synchronous heart rate modulation, B) Phase coordination between preceding R wave and inspiratory onset (RI_i).

served as an indicator of coupling rate. The subjects in our studies on
undisturbed night sleep were 16 healthy males, half untrained individuals,
half high performance athletes (Raschke, 1981).

In the second experiment on a multichoice reaction-time task (Wiener
Determinationsgerät - Dr Schuhfried), 5 men and 5 women participated. The
subjects were studied in relaxed supine (20 min.) and seated (5 min.)
position for baseline measurement. During the task, five different colored
lights were displayed in random order at 10 positions of a panel. The
answer was given by pressing one of five corresponding buttons on the
panel. The initial silent period was followed by an increasing load (10
min.) during which the signal speed was accelerated in steps of 1 min. from
38 to 120 signals/min. From the increasing load the individual's maximal
performance was determined in order to normalize the load. Fifty percent
of false, delayed, or missed responses were defined as maximal load.
Thereafter, 60, 80, or 100% of maximal load were given with constant speed
in random order labelled as B_1, B_2, B_3. Each load period (5 min) was
followed by 2 min. in between, or 6 min. rest in seated position at the end
of the experiment.

RESULTS

A typical pattern of phase-coordination from the record of a single
subject is shown in Figure 2. The x axis gives the standardized RR
interval, forming an even probability for each class. The 100% scale is
calculated from (RI_i x 100)/RR_i, divided into 20 ranges of 5% (cf. Figure
1). On the y axis the number of inspiratory onsets is plotted. The
histograms follow, from left to right, the sequence of the experiment
(increasing strain reordered). In supine relaxed position, a bimodal
distribution shows that in this case two preferred phases of the cardiac

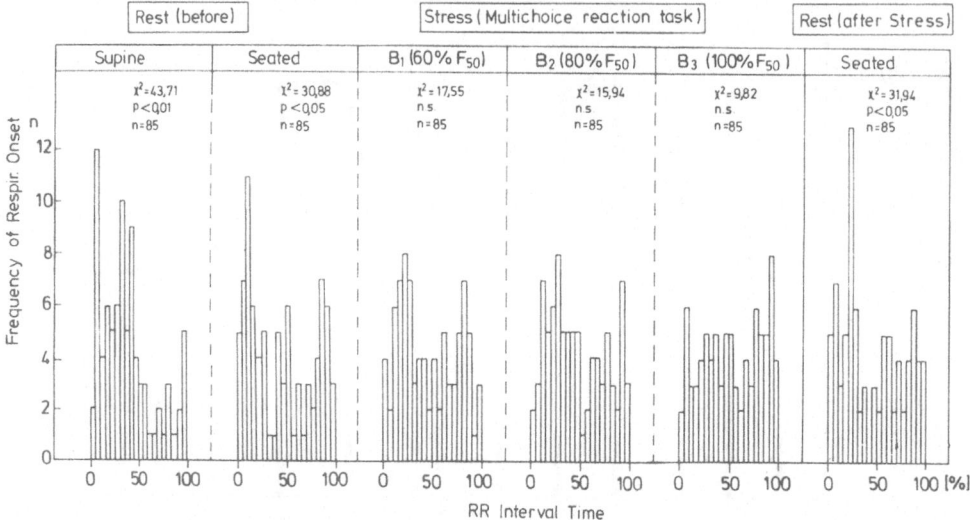

Fig. 2.   Histograms of inspiratory onsets related to the normalized cardiac
cycle (RI_i x 100)/RR_i given in percent) on the x axis. From left
to right subsequent sequences of the task are shown from a single
subject. χ^2 values indicate coupling rate.

cycle are associated with inspiratory onset. This pattern changes over
to a rather unimodal distribution in the seated position, both before and
after the task which shows a coupling preference for only one phase of the
cardiac cycle. During mental load, however, phase-coordination is considerably diminished at the low level (B_1), and completely lost at higher
levels (B_2 and B_3).

     The Chi-squared values given for each histogram indicate a quanti-
tative measure of coupling rate, showing that coordination is lost even at
the lowest level of strain. The Chi-squared values are not normally distributed. Therefore, we pooled these data for all subjects after logar-
ithmic transformation (log Chi-squared). In addition, the amplitude of
respiratory heart rate modulation was compared with coupling rate (log
Chi-squared), and mean heart rate. The results are shown in Figure 3.
Phase coupling at the top reveals the pattern already indicated in Figure
2, i.e., strongest coordination is found in the supine, less in the seated,
and no coordination at different load levels. In spite of this abrupt
breakdown of phase-coordination with a minor stressor, heart rate modulation decreases gradually, indicating a scaled strain response. Both
modes of coupling immediately return to the initial values subsequent to
load conditions, although there is a slight, but nonsignificant, reduction.
Mean heart rate at the bottom of the Figure shows no significant differences between resting conditions and task. Thus the indicated windows
refer to the typical sensitivity of cardiorespiratory response, so that
phase-coordination appears most sensitive to an external stressor, modulation shows moderate sensitivity, and mean heart rate is the least sensitive index.

     On the other hand, coordination is intensified during sleep as
compared to the waking supine position (Raschke, 1981). The strongest
degree of coupling was found in sleep stage 2 (light sleep), followed,
respectively, by stages 3 and 4 (deep sleep), stage 1 (light sleep), and
REM-sleep (dream sleep). The waking state at rest, therefore, represents
a medium intensity of coordination as related to sleep on the one side and
strain on the other.

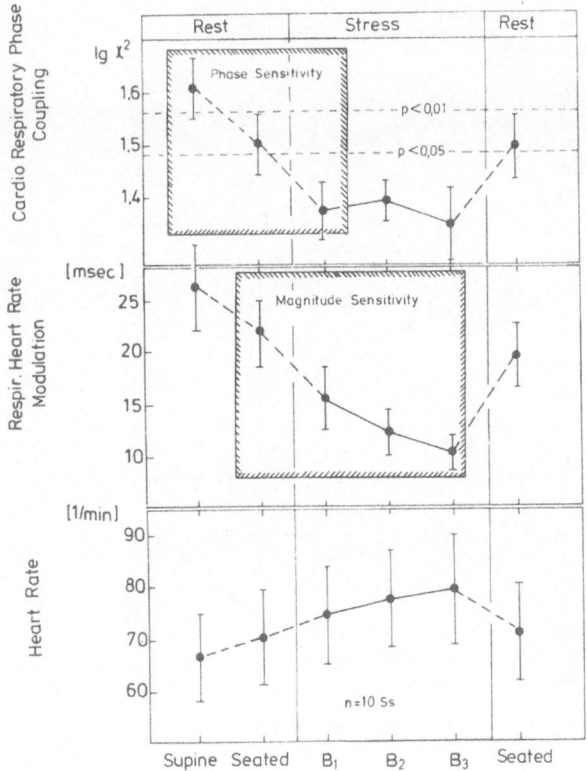

Fig. 3. Comparison of the modes of coupling during relaxed supine and
seated position and on a multichoice reaction time task with
increasing load (B_1, B_2, B_3). Cardio-respiratory phase coupling
above (coupling rate $\triangleq$ lg χ^2). For χ^2-calculation 85 respiratory
cycles were counted in each histogram. Mean of lg χ^2 of 10 Ss
with S.E. Respiratory heart rate modulation in the middle was
assessed from cardiotachograms of 150 sec via FFT, power and
amplitude density spectra of each sequence. Mean amplitude of
10 Ss with S.E. Mean heart rate of the Ss below. The windows
indicate the range of maximal slope of both modes of coupling.

Previous results from Hildebrandt and Daumann (1965) emphasize this
pattern for physical load on a bicycle ergometer. These authors showed, in
untrained subjects, that even the lowest physical work of 30 W led to a
breakdown of phase-coordination, with no return with up to 150 W.

The two modes of coupling are combined in Figure 4 (from Raschke and
Hildebrandt, 1982). This Figure comprises a wide variation in levels of
consciousness and strain. The windows refer to the range of maximal slope.
As can be clearly seen, the phase coupling above yields the highest selec-
tivity during rest and sleep, even changing monotonically with the x axis
inside the window. The maximal sensitivity of heart rate modulation in the
middle of the Figure shows marked decrease during slight work load (30 and
60 W). Eckoldt et al. (1980) have shown that heart rate modulation drops
below statistical significance at the endurance limit. At the bottom,
heart rate itself is represented by a well-known discrimination for the
physical load but only weak sensitivity to depth of sleep.

Comparing the different measurement parameters, a hierarchy of
regulating mechanisms is apparently produced by the autonomic system, in

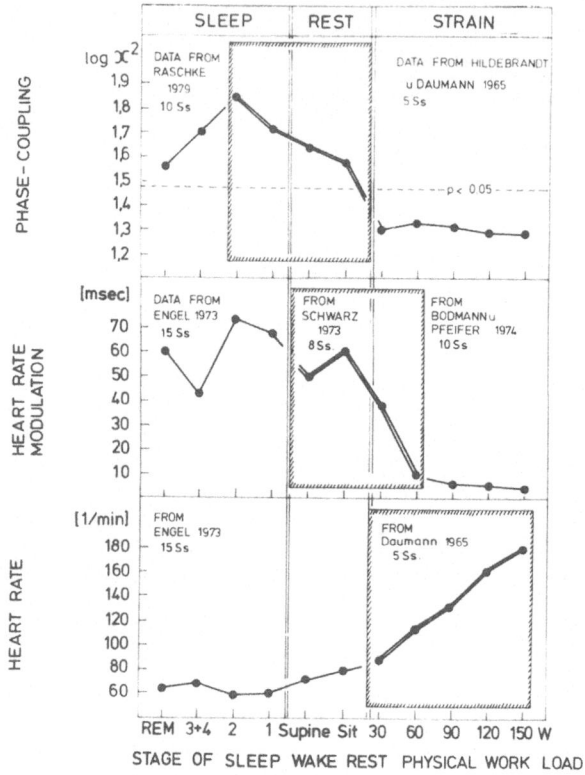

Fig. 4. Comparison of the modes of coupling in different sleep stages, the waking resting supine and seated position, and graded bicycle ergometer load (from Raschke and Hildebrandt, 1982). Phase coupling ($\lg \chi^2$) above, for methods cf. Figure 3. Heart rate modulation in the middle and mean heart rate below depicted from the literature. The windows refer to the maximal and monotonous change of the variables with x axis. They indicate the varying sensitivity of coupling depending on the functional state.

which the functional state requires various levels of integration. The indicators and their sensitivities essentially depend on the time window we apply to the physiological variables. An outline summarizing the results so far is given in Figure 5. The time windows are indicated from top to bottom with reference to the typical coupling mechanisms. In the panels below, the changes of mean heart rate and respiration rate are sketched with the range of their validity in different states shown at the top of the Figure. Sleep, training, and recovery produce a small decrease of mean rate, whereas strain components may produce a large increase. The second horizontal panel contains respiratory heart rate modulation (cardiotacho-grams). Its amplitude is larger, as shown in Figure 4, during sleep, and in well-trained subjects at rest (Schlomka and Reindell, 1936; Eckoldt et al., 1980). It decreases on strain, including even that strain produced by pathophysiological conditions as recently described, e.g., in diabetic man (Kitney et al., 1982; Pfeifer et al., 1982; Wieling et al., 1983) or patients with hypertension and coronary insufficiency (Eckoldt et al., 1980).

The upper panels give the typical pattern of phase-coordination as shown by our results. The Figure reveals a systematic order of cardio-respiratory coupling: increased magnitude of modulation and strong phase-

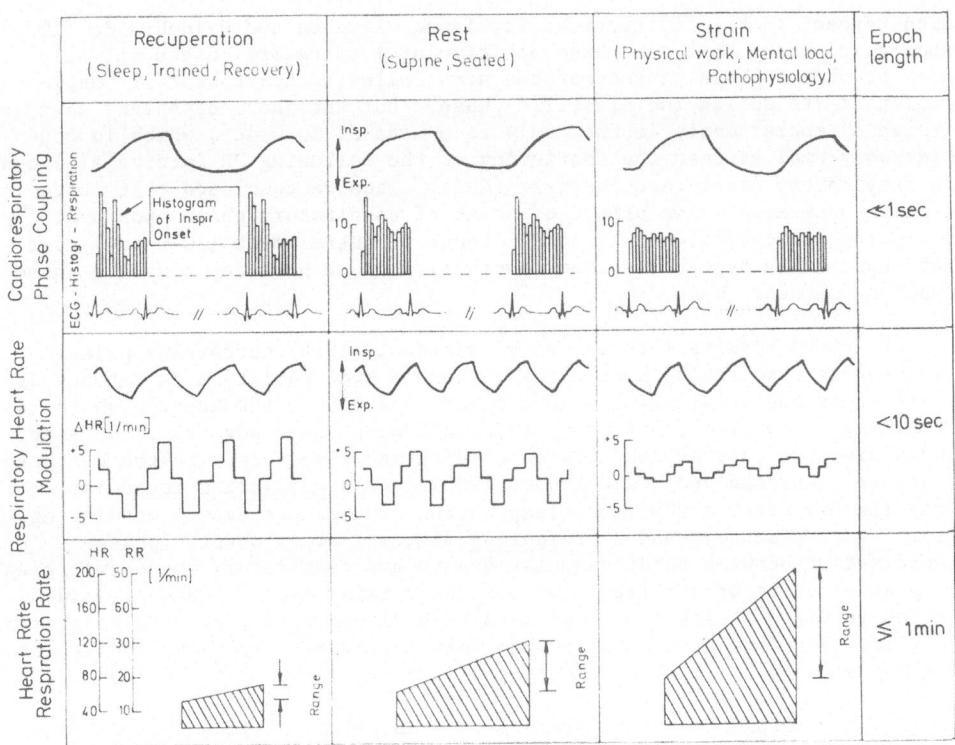

Fig. 5. Outline of the coupling mechanisms at different functional states.
Phase-coordination at the top (typical histograms of phase
coupling between heart beat and inspiratory onsets). Heart rate
modulation in the middle (cardiotachogram and respiration curve).
Typical range of mean respiration rate and heart rate below.
The resolution (epoch length) required for each mode of coupling
on the right. Each panel gives from left to right the typical
pattern of each variable for the transition from recuperation
(even trained Ss at rest) to strain.

coordination during sleep and recuperation, graded decrease of modulation
at medium strain components, and an abrupt loss of phase-coordination at
the lowest level of strain. Under high metabolic demands (elevated heart
rate and respiratory rate), both modes of coupling disappear completely.

DISCUSSION

Our investigations deal with a bidirectionality of cardiorespiratory
interaction. Thus the question of leading and following rhythms is of
great importance and has often been discussed. In the following brief
survey, different arguments are referred to with respect to the distinction
made in this paper between heart rate modulation and phase coupling.

A phase-coordination of respiratory onset to the following heart
beat(s) has been suggested, for example, by Weiss and Salzano (1971) and
Pessenhofer and Kenner (1975). But these authors did not consider the
investigations of Hinderling (1967), who has shown that in patients with
an implanted cardiac pacemaker, respiratory phases were coupled to the
artificial cardiac action. Subsequently, Bucher and Bucher (1977) showed
in the rabbit that even an artificial pulsatile blood infusion to the
carotid arteries entrained the respiratory phases (onset of expiration).

With respect to the bidirectionality issue, Raschke and Hildebrandt (1979) showed in humans that the phase position of inspiratory onsets actually does produce a phase advance of the next following heart beat if inspiration starts during the diastolic phase. But the phase-dependent advance (range of entrainment) amounts only to a mean of 30 msec., which is considerably smaller than the shortening of the following RR intervals(s) due to inspiratory heart rate increase .(RSA). Thus we concluded that there is a weak phase-modulating effect of onset of respiratory phase upon next following heart beat, but the small range of entrainment (30 msec.) does not support the hypothesis that inspiration onset produces complete phase coupling of heart beat.

Previous results (Stutte and Hildebrandt, 1966) concerning pulse-synchronous respiration have already shown a wide variation in latency of inspiratory onset following R-wave occurrence (400 - 600 msec.), which is much larger than the respiratory-induced R-wave phase advance of 30 msec. Therefore, the interaction between cardiac and respiratory rhythm has been separated (Raschke and Hildebrandt, 1982) into a _modulating_ mechanism (respiratory sinus arrhythmia, respiration-synchronous events modulating heart beat sequence), and a _triggering_ of respiratory onsets (phase-coordination between cardiovascular events and respiratory phase-switching, or phase-locking at distinct times of the cardiac cycle). Hence, modulation requires at least one complete respiratory cycle, whereas triggering only modifies the onset point of the next following respiratory phase after the R-wave.

We have found that cardiorespiratory coupling is linked to the functional state with a different timing sensitivity for the various experimental conditions. The responses to different situational stressors and dispositional traits have recently been reviewed by Grossman (1983), who made a distinction between phasic and nonphasic variables. The following considerations are limited to the phasic coupling mechanisms. As our results have shown, variations in cardiac triggering of respiratory onsets appear most sensitive to the application of external stressors, easily being disturbed by mental, emotional, and physical load. Respiratory heart rate modulation still occurs with such stressor stimuli, but is finally eliminated by elevated levels of strain with great energy expenditure. This leads to a highly specialized, nonphasic energy-producing behavior of the correcting unit with complete decoupling. Thus it seems that the degree of coupling mirrors the internal coherence between respiratory and cardiovascular systems. The mechanisms for RSA are well documented because numerous experiments have shown that it is mainly the intensity of vagal cardiac innervation (Katona and Jih, 1975; Eckoldt, 1983), which generates the magnitude of heart rate modulation. As indicated previously, the origin of these changes in vagal tone are manifold, but in any case, this type of coupling is much stronger than phase-coordination. With phase-coordination, respiratory phase-switching is more subtly related to cardiovascular events, but, nevertheless, in a statistical significant manner. The bimodal shape of the histograms accounts for at least two different cardiovascular events triggering respiratory phases. Stutte and Hildebrandt (1966), and Raschke (1981) have shown that even three (seldom more) phases of cardiac cycle are sometimes found. A multimodal genesis of respiratory phase-switching is known to exist (cf. for example, Paintal, 1980). In our research, we have shown the significance of afferents from the cardiovascular system, as compared to afferents from peripheral chemoreceptors or central chemosensitivity. Bucher and Bättig (1960) reported vagal cardiac afferents to be mainly responsible for the coupling mechanism, originating in the right atrium (Meier and Bucher, 1961). Therefore, phasic pressure and volume changes in the myocardium appear as important stimuli for phase-coordination (for autonomic system reactions to mechanical stretch of the atria, see, for example, Koizumi et al., 1975).

Another reflex mechanism might originate in systemic arterial baroreceptor afferents (according to the experiments of Bucher and Bucher, 1977). However, even an intracentral coordination (Koepchen et al., 1981) of cardiac and respiratory neuronal activity could account for the coupling mechanism.

The bivalent existence of two cardiac-cycle phases, which are preferred for inspiratory onset in the supine position, transformed into a one-phase coupling while seated (see Figure 2). Thus, the change with position indicates a systematically varying dominance of afferents or central gating. Former results showed that top performance athletes, during sleep, mainly manifested an inspiration onset starting during diastole, and expiratory onset starting at systole, whereas the untrained individuals only showed preference for a systolic coupling of inspiration onset (Raschke, 1982). These results may hint at the functional significance of phase-coordination, i.e., a rather economic filling and outflow mechanics of the heart in the trained individual, supported by exact respiratory timing. In these subjects maximal coherence of the two systems is realized, which is manifested by a greater amplitude of heart rate modulation as well as a close synchrony of cardiovascular and respiratory phases. The neuronal networks are highly phase-locked, revealing a stronger coherence during sleep as compared to the waking state. Increased internal coherence might be induced by a relative lack of interacting afferents from visual, tactile, locomotive, and somatic perception during sleep. On the other hand, we found that both modes of coupling, phase-coordination and heart rate modulation, are diminished or lost when elevated metabolic transport requires large, nonphasic energy production. Thus, the graded transition from a strong coherent, oscillatory level to an energy-producing tonic state seems to reflect the hierarchical integration of autonomic regulation.

REFERENCES

Angelone, A.,and Coulter, N. A., 1964, Respiratory sinus arrhythmia: a frequency dependent phenomenon, J. Appl. Physiol., 19:479.

Bond, W. C., Bohs, C., Ebey, J., and Wolf, S., 1973, Rhythmic heart rate variability (sinus arrhythmia) related to stages of sleep, Cond. Reflex, 8:98.

Bucher, K., and Bättig, P., 1960, Zur Bedeutung der Vagi für die pulssynchrone Atmung, Helv. Physiol. Pharmakol. Acta, 18:219.

Bucher, K., and Bucher, K. E., 1977, Cardio-respiratory synchronisms: synchrony with artificial circulation, Res. Exp. Med., 171:101.

Bucher, K., Schwitter, H., Hool-Zulauf, B., and Batschelet, E., 1972, Links between cardiac and respiratory rhythmicity, Res. Exp. Med., 157:281.

Eckberg, D. L., 1983, Human sinus arrhythmia as an index of vagal cardiac outflow, J. Appl. Physiol., 54:961.

Eckberg, D. L., and Orshan, C. R., 1977, Respiratory and baroreceptor reflex interactions in man, J. Clin. Invest., 59:780.

Eckoldt, K., Pfeifer, B., and Schubert, E., 1980, Sympathetic and parasympathetic innervation of the heart at rest and work in man as judged by heart rate and sinus arrhythmia, in: "Central Interaction between Respiratory and Cardiovascular Control Systems", H. P. Koepchen, S. M. Hilton and A. Trzebski, eds., Springer, Berlin, Heidelberg, New York.

Engel, P., Hildebrandt, G., and Pöllmann, L., 1971, Die Wirkung von Schlafunterbrechung und Nachtarbeit auf die Frequenz- und Phasenkoordination von Herzschlag und Atmung während des Schlafes, Arbeitsmed. Sozialmed. Arbeitshyg., 38:95.

Engel, P., and Hildebrandt, G., 1973, Über den Einfluß der Vigilanz auf die Phasenkopplung zwischen Herzschlag und Atmung, Psychol. Beiträge, 15:77.

Engel, P., Jaeger, A., and Hildebrandt, G., 1972, Über die Beeinflussung der Frequenz- und Phasenkoordination zwischen Herzschlag und Atmung durch verschiedene Narkotika, Arzneim.-Forsch. (Drug Res.), 22:1460.

Engel, R. R., 1973, Statistical analysis of heart rate and respiration during the different stages of human sleep, in: "The Nature of Sleep", U. Jovanovic, ed., Fischer, Stuttgart.

Galli, G., 1924, Deuxième contribution à l'étude des synchronismes cardio-respiratoires, Arch. Mal. Coeur, 17:208.

Grossman, P., 1983, Respiration, stress, and cardiovascular function, Psychophysiol., 20:284.

Hainsworth, R., 1974, Circulatory responses from lung inflation in anaestetized dogs, Am. J. Physiol., 226:247.

Hiebsch, W., 1984, Die Kopplung von Herzschlag und Atmung beim Neugeborenen – Untersuchungen zur Methodik der Kopplungsanalyse, M.D. Dissertation, Halle.

Hildebrandt, G., and Daumann, F. J., 1965, Die Koordination von Puls-und Atemrhythmus bei Arbeit, Int. Z. angew. Physiol., 21:27.

Hinderling, P., 1967, Weitere Charakterisierung von Synchronismen zwischen Kreislauf und Atmung, Helv. Physiol. Pharmacol. Acta, 25:24.

Hirsch, J. A., and Bishop, B., 1981a, Respiratory sinus arrhythmia in humans: how breathing pattern modulates heart rate, Am. J. Physiol., 241:H620.

Hirsch, J. A., and Bishop, B., 1981b, Respiratory sinus arrhythmia (RSA) in man: altered inspired O_2 and CO_2, in: "Adv. Physiol. Sci. vol. 9, Cardiovascular Physiology, Neural Control Mechanisms", A. G. B. Kovach, P. Sandor and A. Kollai, eds., Pergamon Press, London.

v. Holst, E., 1939, Die relative Koordination als Phänomen und als Methode zentralnervöser Funktionsanalyse, Erg. Physiol., 42:228.

Hyndman, B. W., and Gregory, J. R., 1975, Spectral analysis of sinus arrhythmia during mental loading, Ergonomics, 18:255.

Katona, P., and Jih, F., 1975, Respiratory sinus arrhythmia: noninvasive measure of parasympathetic cardiac control, J. Appl. Physiol., 39:801.

Kelman, G. R., and Wann, K. T., 1970, Studies on sinus arrhythmia, J. Physiol. (London), 213:59P.

Kitney, R. I., 1977, Magnitude and phase changes in heart rate variability and blood pressure during respiratory entrainment, J. Physiol. (London), 270:40P.

Kitney, R. I., Byrne, S., Edmonds, M. E., Watkins, P. J., and Roberts, V. C., 1982, Heart rate variability in the assessment of autonomic diabetic neuropathy, Automedica, 4:155.

Koepchen, H. P., 1977, Neurophysiologische Grundlagen der nervösen Steuerung der Herzfrequenz, insbesondere ihrer atemrhythmischen Schwankungen, Med. Sport, 17:136.

Koepchen, H. P., Klüssendorf, D., and Sommer, D., 1981, Neurophysiological background of central neural cardiovascular-respiratory coordination: basic remarks and experimental approach, J. Auton. Nerv. Syst., 3:335.

Koepchen, H. P., and Thurau, K., 1959, Über die Entstehungsbedingungen der atemsynchronen Schwankungen des Vagotonus (respiratorische Arrhythmie), Pflügers Arch., 269:10.

Koizumi, K., Ishikawa, T., Nishino, H., and McC. Brooks, C., 1975, Cardiac and autonomic reactions to stretch of the atria, Brain Res., 87:247

Levy, M. N., de Geest, H., and Zieske, H., 1966, Effects of respiratory center activity on the heart, Circ. Res., 18:67.

Meier, M., and Bucher, K., 1961, Zum Mechanismus der pulssynchronen Atmung. Beitrag zur Analyse der besonderen Rolle des linken Vagus, Arch. Int. Pharmacodyn., 131:348.

Melcher, A., 1980, Carotid baroreflex heart rate control during the active and the assisted breathing cycle in man, Acta Physiol. Scand., 108:165.

Mulder, G., and Mulder-Hajonides van der Meulen, W. R. E. H., 1973, Mental load and the measurement of heart rate variability, Ergonomics, 16:69.

Paintal, A. S., 1980, "Inputs" - Introduction, in: "Central Interaction between Respiratory and Cardiovascular Control Systems", H. P. Koepchen, S. M. Hilton, and A. Trzebski, eds., Springer, Berlin, Heidelberg, New York.

Pfeifer, M. A., Cook, D., Brodsky, J., Tice, D., Reenan, A., Swedine, S., and Halter, J. B., 1982, Quantitative evaluation of cardiac parasympathetic activity in normal and diabetic man, Diabetes, 31:339.

Pessenhofer, H., and Kenner, Th., 1975, Zur Methodik der kontinuierlichen Bestimmung der Phasenbeziehung zwischen Herzschlag und Atmung, Pflügers Arch., 355:77.

Raschke, F., 1981, Die Kopplung zwischen Herzschlag und Atmung - Untersuchungen zur Frequenz- und Phasenkoordination mit neuen Verfahren der automatischen Analyse, M.D. Dissertation, Univ. Marburg.

Raschke, F., 1982, Automatic pattern recognition of the onset of respiratory phases using thermistor techniques, in: "ISAM-Gent-1981", F. D. Stott, E. B. Raftery, D. L. Clement and S. L. Wright, eds., Academic Press, London, New York.

Raschke, F., and Hildebrandt, G., 1979, The mutual interaction between the RR-interval time and the onset of inspiration, Pflügers Arch., 382:R43.

Raschke, F., and Hildebrandt, G., 1982, Coupling of the cardiorespiratory control system by modulation and triggering, in: "Cardiovascular System Dynamics: Models and Measurements", Th. Kenner, R. Busse and H. Hinghofer-Szalkey, eds., Plenum Press, New York, London.

Rohmert, W., Laurig, W., Philipp, U., and Luczak, H., 1973, Heart rate variability and work-load measurement, Ergonomics, 16:33.

Schlomka, G., and Reindell, H., 1936, Untersuchungen über die physiologische Unregelmäßigkeit des Herzschlags, Z. Kreisl.-Forsch., 28:473.

Schoenlein, K., 1895, Beobachtungen über Blutkreislauf und Respiration bei einigen Fischen, Z. Biol., 32:511.

Schwarz, G., 1973, Über die Veränderungen der Herz- und Atemperiodenstreuung bei Tretarbeit mit verschiedenen Frequenzen und ihre Beziehung zum Trainingszustand, Ph.D. Dissertation, Univ. Marburg.

Storch, J., and Hildebrandt, G., 1966, Methodische Grundlagen zur Bestimmung der Puls-Atem-Kopplung beim Menschen und ihr Verhalten im Schlaf, Pflügers Arch., 289:R46.

Stutte, K. H., and Hildebrandt, G., 1966, Untersuchungen über die Koordination von Herzschlag und Atmung, Pflügers Arch., 289:R47.

Weiss, H. R., and Salzano, J., 1971, Control mechanism of whole number ratio of heart rate and breathing frequency, J. Appl. Physiol., 31:466.

Weltz, G. A., 1941, Atmungseinflüsse auf Füllung und Schlagzahl des Herzens, Arch. Kreisl.-Forsch., 8:1.

Wieling, W., Borst, C., v. Dongen-Torman, M. A., v. d. Hofstede, J. W., v. Brederode, J. F. M., Endert, E., and Dunning A. J., 1983, Relationship between impaired parasympathetic and sympathetic cardiovascular control in diabetes mellitus, Diabetologia, 24:422.

PATTERNS OF CARDIOVASCULAR-SOMATIC-RESPIRATORY INTERACTIONS

IN THE CONTINUOUS PERCEPTUAL-MOTOR TASK PARADIGM

Sven Svebak

University of Bergen, Norway

INTRODUCTION

This chapter summarizes a series of psychophysiological studies conducted in our laboratory over a number of years. This research has been primarily concerned with physiological correlates of extrinsic and intrinsic motivational factors during task performance. Extrinsic factors have centered around task difficulty and threat of aversive stimulation during the performance of continuous perceptual-motor tasks. Intrinsic motivational factors of importance in our experiments have been related to individual differences in propensity to seriousmindedness and type A behavior. Because we have been interested in patterns of motivationally dependent task responses across a range of physiological systems, we have simultaneously measured cardiovascular, respiratory and neuromuscular parameters in our studies. Our findings indicate that intrinsic and extrinsic motivational factors interact in specific ways under different conditions to produce physiological patterns of reactivity to continuous perceptual-motor tasks.

The continuous perceptual-motor task paradigm first achieved psychophysiological significance in the early literature on activation patterns. Illustrative of this approach are the mirror-tracking studies of Malmo (1965), which provided evidence of a monotonic increase in the level of cardiac, skeletal muscle and respiratory activation over the course of task performance. Terms like effort and involvement (task difficulty, liking, interest) were used by Malmo (1975) to explain the nature of the psychological moderator effects upon the slope of the physiological gradient curve. Malmo's paradigm, however, has largely come into disuse in the later activation research, perhaps partly due to the crudeness of the experimental tasks which he used.

In the last years, different versions of the currently more popular reaction-time task paradigm have, however, been used to explore the impact of attentional and motivational moderators upon cardiovascular (e.g., Obrist, Webb, Sutterer and Howard, 1970), somatic (e.g., Brunia, 1983) and event-related cortical potentials (see Loveless, 1983). In contrast to Malmo's findings of task-induced parallel increases in cardiac, somatic and respiratory activity, Obrist and co-workers have reported dissociation of cardiac and somatomotor systems in response to their reaction-time tasks (e.g., Obrist, 1976). The apparent difference in findings between Malmo and Obrist may not necessarily be due to the crude nature of Malmo's early tasks. Both teams addressed the correlates of effortful active coping, and discrepant findings may have been caused by paradigm-specific response characteristics. For example, the Obrist paradigm leaves the subject in a rather passive-attending state most of the time with interspersed phasic motor responses to GO-signals. In contrast, the continuous perceptual-motor task keeps the subject in a continuously active attending-responding state. This implies continuous information-processing of sensory input and coordination of motor responses and is likely to induce tonic activation. Our own paradigm in the last years has been based on Malmo's continuous perceptual-motor task approach.

The concept of effortful active coping has been crucial to the interpretation of results from experiments reported by the Obrist group (e.g., Light, 1981), and the term has incorporated task or context characteristics, rather than assessment of the psychological state of the performing individual by use of verbal report. The present research project investigated correlates of effort, but we have incorporated a distinction between information load and emotional load (Mulder and Mulder, 1980) utilizing, respectively, manipulations of task difficulty and threat of aversive consequences for inferior performance. We believe that our distinction between task difficulty (information load) and threat (emotional load) is more specific than is implied in the traditional reference to mental versus emotional workload.

Part of this research project has also included study of the differentiation between a seriousminded (telic) versus playful (paratelic) motivational approach to task performance. This terminology is taken from the recently developed reversal theory (Apter, 1982). The theory proposes differences between individuals in terms of a bias towards spending more time in the one state rather than in the opposite state. The Telic Dominance Scale (TDS) has been developed to assess empirically such differences among individuals in bias (dominance) toward a particular motivational state (see Murgatroyd, Rushton, Apter, and Ray, 1978). A state-measure (TSM) has also been constructed to assess state at any particular moment (see Svebak and Murgatroyd, 1984). Seriousmindedness is the essential feature of the telic state, and it is argued in the theory that a preference for planned behavioral sequences tends to go with the serious-minded state in order to assure goal achievement. In the paratelic state, tasks are performed for fun, as a joyful challenge or "just for the heck of it", rather than as a duty, and behavior tends to be more impulsive. Arousal is sought after in the paratelic state but is unpleasant and therefore avoided, if possible, in the telic state. In this way reversal theory deviates from optimal arousal theory and may therefore help to explain the old paradoxes of relations between arousal and hedonic tone. Reversal theory offers a phenomenology which appears to be related to the distinction between eustress and distress - a distinction where phasic (short-lasting) activation is taken to signify the former as opposed to a tonic (enduring) pattern of activation in the latter case (see Ursin, Murison, and Knardahl, 1983).

One recent part of the project has incorporated the Type A behavior pattern which is held to be one of the risk factors in the development of coronary heart disease (see, for example, Chesney, Eagleston and Rosenman, 1981). The psychometric data from our research have supported the view that seriousmindedness and Type A behavior (speed and impatience, hard-driving and competitiveness, job involvement) are orthogonal dimensions (Svebak and Apter, 1984). Hypothetically, these scales may, therefore, identify cardiovascular responders as those individuals who load highly on both measures.

METHODOLOGY

Our research program has included two versions of a continuous perceptual-motor task. In both cases duration has been set at 150 seconds like
that of the related tasks in the classical experiments (Malmo, 1965). One
version of the task is a single-person "ball-game" where the task for the
subjects is to control the movement of a "ball" by the operation of a knob
held between the thumb and index fingers of the active hand. The other
version of the task simulates "car-racing" and includes the operation of a
joy-stick to "drive" the subject's own "car" along a "road" without running
into other "cars" which appear along the "road".

Respiration has been measured by the use of two mercury-filled
silicone tubes which are strapped around the whole circumference of the
trunk. A calibration procedure is used for every silicone gauge and each
subject in order to assure precise measurement. (See Appendix 1 for a
documentation of the sensitivity and reliability of this technique.)

An "inspiratory volume index" (IVI) was calculated in some of the
experiments where respiration was measured via mercury strain-gauges at the
level of the armpits (thorax) as well as of the navel (abdomen). This
index is basically a correction of respiratory rate (RR: inspiration-
expiration cycles per minute) by multiplying it by the mean depth of inspiration as measured by the circumference increase for both trunk segments
across a consecutive set of respiratory cycles. The depth of inspiration
yielded a respiratory amplitude on the polygraph recording, and this
amplitude was scored as a percentage of the trunk circumference of the
actual segment. This relative amplitude helped to overcome the effect of
individual differences in trunk size across subjects. Svebak (1982) illustrated the effect of treatments upon the separate respiratory parameters of
RR, thorax-amplitude and abdomen-amplitude as well as upon the combined
scores calculated as the IVI. The latter scores appeared to offer the most
meaningful measure of the overall activity of the respiratory "pump".

Most of the experiments recorded EMG by the use of surface electrodes
located above the forearm flexor of the passive arm (which did not operate
the joy-stick). One experiment recorded EMG from the flexor as well as
extensor muscles of the upper right and left arm which both remained
passive throughout the performance of a perceptual-cognitive task.

Cardiovascular activity included heart rate, and pulse-transit time,
the latter held to index indirectly the systolic blood pressure changes:
the shorter the time lag the higher the systolic pressure.

The Effect of Task Difficulty

Two experiments (Svebak, Dalen and Storfjell, 1981) investigated the
effect of altered task difficulty upon the tonic changes in HR and passive
forearm flexor EMG over the course of task performance. The second experiment included measurement of respiration. Results from both experiments
showed a small overall effect of high task difficulty which included a
higher level of physiological activation than was seen in the easy version
of the task. Of greater interest was the difference in response patterns
between the cardiac and somatic measures. This difference was most distinct for the difficult version of the task: heart rate peaked early during
the performance period and approached the pre-baseline level towards the
end of the task. In contrast, EMG-scores were increasingly higher towards
the end of the task. Scores for respiration included RR, thorax-amplitude
and abdomen-amplitude; these were also low for the initial part of the
performance period as compared with the relatively higher scores calculated
for the final part of the task. In this way a tonic gradient pattern of

activation was apparent for both somatic and respiratory variables, but cardiac activation showed a different pattern of early peak response.

In light of the active coping which is called upon in this type of paradigm (to keep errors as few as possible), the cardiac-somatic coupling hypothesis of Obrist (1976) could not account for these results. Neither did the HR yield a pattern which indicated that its activation was under respiratory control due to a respiratory-induced loss of vagal influence upon the myocardium (see Grossman and Wientjes, 1985). The HR acceleration thus appeared to be under specific central nervous system control. On the other hand, the results for respiration gave rise to the hypothesis that respiratory activity does parallel the level of activity in the skeletal muscles as a task becomes increasingly demanding.

Moreover, these results did not support the old idea of a cardiac-somatic-respiratory gradient parallelism (Malmo, 1965) as a significant pattern of activation in the continuous perceptual-motor task paradigm. In light of the positive hedonic tone which was reflected in verbal reports of increased preference for the difficult version of the task, it was thought feasible that cardiac-somatic-respiratory parallelism would occur in this paradigm only provided that the task is performed within a state of mind which includes a negative hedonic tone. New experiments to address this hypothesis were performed which included the threat of aversive consequences for poor performance. It was expected that the addition of a threatening context to the task performance would be likely to induce a negative hedonic tone in the subject.

The Effect of a Threatening Context

One experiment manipulated threat of aversive electric shock for inferior performance in an otherwise constant task. Thus, emotional load was manipulated in a within-subject design. Heart rate, passive forearm flexor EMG and respiratory activity were measured before, during and after task performance using a counterbalanced order of the threat and no-threat treatments.

Results did not lend support to the idea of a cardiac-somatic-respiratory gradient pattern of activation when the task was performed within a threatening context. Instead, initial HR peak-responses (Figure 1) as well as late EMG peak-responses (Figure 2) were higher with the threat contingency. This meant that the discrepancy between the HR and EMG activation patterns was amplified, rather than attenuated, by the introduction of a threatening context to the task performance.

Respiratory parameters were combined into IVI-scores (Figure 3), and results confirmed earlier findings (Svebak et al., 1981) of a parallel pattern of respiratory-somatic activation during task performance in the absence of threat. For the threat-treatment, in contrast, the IVI-scores reflected a marked initial activation which was similar to that seen with HR. It seems, therefore, that a parallel pattern of cardiac and respiratory activation occurs when our task is performed within a threatening context. When threat of aversive consequences is not present, performance causes a parallel respiratory-somatic pattern of activation.

With regard to performance measures, error scores were significantly reduced when the task was performed within the threatening context. It has been argued elsewhere (Svebak, 1982) that altered error scores reflect altered effort, provided a task remains the same. The experiment reported by Svebak (1982) tested the hypothesis that a threatening context may alter patterns of cardiac-somatic respiratory interaction more dramatically when the task performed is perceived by the subject both as effort-demanding and

222

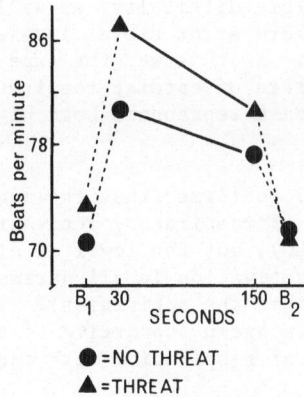

Fig. 1. Changes in heart rate over the course of continuous perceptual-motor task performance with and without threat of aversive consequences for inferior performance. Pre- and post-baseline levels are included.

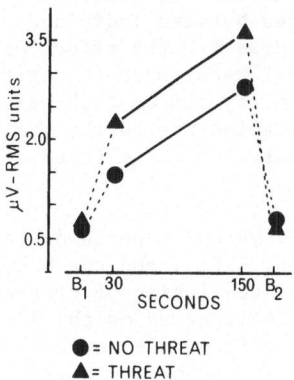

Fig. 2. Tonic changes in the electromyographic activity (integrals for 10-second epochs) of the passive forearm flexor muscle for two context contingencies to task performance.

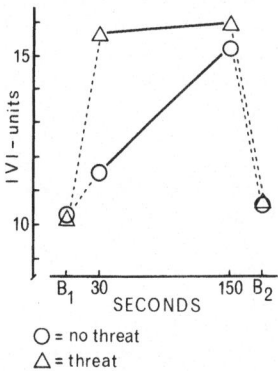

Fig. 3. The effect of a threatening context to task performance upon inspiratory volume index (IVI) scores. (The IVI is taken to reflect the overall activity of the respiratory "pump".)

as a difficult one. Therefore difficulty, as well as threat, was manipulated in this experiment where error scores indexed altered effort due to
the manipulation of threat. In this way the experiment explored the possibility that a parallel pattern of cardiac-respiratory activation is particularly marked when our task represents both high information load and
high emotional load.

Results (Svebak, 1982) confirmed that the manipulation of threat is
significant to the pattern of respiratory activation (initial peak-like for
HR or late peak-like for EMG), but the level of difficulty appeared significant to the degree of activation in all parameters (i.e., the more
difficult the task, the higher the activation). The reduced error scores
in the threat treatment were again supportive of a significant role for
effort in the coordination of respiration with cardiac activation.

Verbal reports for "interest" and "liking" indicated that the hedonic
tone was not significantly altered by the treatments. In this way the
verbal reports gave rise to the hypothesis that there may not be a uniform
effect of an extrinsic threat upon hedonic tone which subjects attribute to
the task: a threat may make the task appear as more interesting and even
exciting to one subject, whereas it causes the task to become less
interesting and even anxiety-provoking to another subject. Group means for
scores reflecting such verbal reports (interest, liking) will not reflect
these qualitative differences between individuals in effects of extrinsic
threat upon hedonic tone. However, the effect of threat may be more consistently reflected in verbal reports on the perception of one's own motivational state rather than in reports on task perception; and the altered
pattern of respiratory activation due to the manipulation of threat may
thus be a more systematic correlate of altered self-perception than of
altered task-perception.

One experiment included verbal reports on task- and self-perception
(Svebak, Storfjell and Dalen, 1982), and the subjects were again exposed to
a threat versus no-threat constellation of treatments. Verbal reports for
self-perception were essentially based on the distinction between the telic
(seriousminded) and paratelic (playful) motivational states as outlined in
the introductory section. Scores for items relating to task perception
(difficulty, interest, liking) failed to reflect the threat manipulation,
but scores for items associated with self-perception indicated that the
subjects were, on the average, significantly more seriousminded, planning
oriented and worked-up, as well as more achievement-motivated, in the
threat versus the no-threat treatment. On the other hand, scores for the
cardiac, somatic and respiratory variables again documented the cardiac-
respiratory activation parallelism for threat and the respiratory-somatic
response parallelism within a neutral context. Hence, the verbal reports
shed new light on the psychological significance of the altered pattern of
respiratory activation as a function of a threatening context.

We assume that effort can be also high when a task is performed just
for fun in the playful state (like is often seen in sports) and not only
when it is performed in the seriousminded state. Results for effort and
seriousmindedness were confounded in the data reported by Svebak et al.
(1982). A part of our research project developed an approach which permitted the effects of high effort upon activation to be studied, both as
correlates within a seriousminded and a playful motivational approach to
the task performance. Significant to this approach was the assumption that
seriousmindedness and playfulness may be relatively stable characteristics
of different individuals and both characteristics may be approaches to the
performance of a particular task, threat and effort not withstanding. The
next section of this chapter describes the effect of such moderator variables upon task-induced cardiac-somatic-respiratory interactions.

The concept of emotional load is particularly oriented towards unpleasant emotions. It muddles the obvious distinction between pleasant and unpleasant emotional experiences like anxiety and joy. The felt level of arousal may be equally high in both cases. The distinction between the telic (seriousminded, planning oriented) and paratelic (playful, spontaneous) motivational states (see below) incorporates a state-specific experience of high felt arousal as unpleasant anxiety in the telic state and as pleasant excitement in the paratelic state (Apter, 1982).

We have recruited subjects to form extreme groups reflecting a distinction between seriousminded and playful state-dominance. Responses to the telic state measure (TSM) confirmed that subjects maintained their dominant state also in the experimental situation. In contrast, scores on felt level of arousal and number of errors did not distinguish between the two groups. Physiological measures indicated that the tonic EMG gradient of the passive forearm flexor is a correlate of effortful active coping in the telic state (or in the telic state-dominant individual: Svebak, 1984); these data also showed a high thoracic respiratory amplitude in the telic state-dominant subjects during task performance. Structured interviews on everyday life-style strongly corroborated the external validity of these laboratory findings. The subject groups did not, however, yield significant differences in tonic heart rate over the course of the perceptual-motor task performance. (A more detailed account, including case illustrations on everyday life-styles, has been reported by Svebak and Murgatroyd, 1985.)

Other telic/paratelic extreme-group experiments have recorded EMG activity from the flexor muscle of both forearms, and effort has been manipulated by the use of a threatening context during the task performance. (At this point "effort" should be regarded as the appropriate concept because error scores have been consistently reduced by the threat of having electric shocks as punishment for inferior performance. The nonspecific concept of "emotional load" is not favored because verbal reports have failed to yield a systematic effect of threat upon changes in hedonic tone.) Results from these experiments lend support to the hypothesis that the tonic gradient of EMG activation in the passive forearm is a correlate of effort in the telic state. The high phasic EMG response amplitude of the active forearm flexor, due to acute changes in the position of the joy-stick, is a correlate of effort in the paratelic state. (See Svebak, 1983, and 1984, for more detailed presentations.)

Results for HR and respiration support the hypothesis that threat of electric shock provokes a substantial initial parallel cardiac-respiratory activation, provided that the subject expends effort in the telic state and experiences a negative hedonic tone. The role of the playful state in the pyramidal control of skeletal muscle responding, and the association of seriousmindedness with extrapyramidal somatic responding, point towards a complex regulatory system for cardiac-somatic-respiratory interactions. (See Svebak, 1986, for details.)

More recent results have strengthened the hypothesis of an association between the telic state and non-intended (extrapyramidal) tonic increase in muscle tension. Data were obtained from a perceptual-cognitive task which permitted both arms to remain passive. Again the EMG gradient was marked when the task was performed in the telic state under distress (effort and negative hedonic tone), and this pattern emerged for recordings from the biceps and triceps of the right and left upper arms. The subjects were recruited by the use of a stratified sample criterion; extreme-group recruitment was not used here. (A preliminary report of these data was given by Rimehaug and Svebak, 1984.)

Svebak and Apter (1984) documented orthogonality for responses given to the TDS and the student version of the JAS used to measure Type A behavior (see above). In light of the moderate success for JAS-scores as predictors of cardiovascular responsiveness including coronary heart disease (e.g., Chesney et al., 1981), the high HR response to threat in our telic state-dominant subjects gave rise to the idea that the seriousminded subgroup among Type A individuals might respond with the highest cardiovascular activation in the continuous perceptual-motor task paradigm. A recent experiment in our laboratory (performed in collaboration with Arne Öhman and Helge Nordby) made use of a factorial extreme-group design (Type A/telic etc.), and results for HR and pulse-transit time (see above) yielded significant support to this idea: the highest HR scores and lowest pulse transit-time scores were obtained from the individuals characterized by a combination of seriousmindedness and Type A behavior. There was no systematic relationship between response patterns for the cardiovascular measures and those for passive forearm flexor EMG.

CONCLUSION - A TENTATIVE CENTRALIST PERSPECTIVE

Pribram and McGuiness (1975) have described the functions of two major central regulatory systems: the arousal system produces a phasic response to sensory input and the activation system maintains a tonic readiness for motor action. They also suggested that an effort system is responsible for the coordination of the arousal and activation systems in active motor responding. Our findings show qualitatively different physiological response patterns which relate to a distinction between playful and seriousminded approaches to effortful active coping. The predominance of phasic motor responses in the playful state and of tonic motor responses in the seriousminded state indicate a central role for the arousal system in the former and for the activation system in the latter.

Apparently, when the effort system was coordinated with the activation system (the seriousminded state), cardiac-respiratory acceleration had a short rise-time and was substantial in the continuous perceptual-motor task performance. The extrapyramidal activation of skeletal muscles was also marked although the rise-time was relatively long. In light of the trivial physical workload which is involved in this paradigm, the cardiac-respiratory activation appears to have surpassed the altered demand for O_2 due to increased metabolism during task performance (see the concept of "additional heart rate"; Strømme, Wikeby, Blix and Ursin, 1978). A secondary effect of this constellation of effort with activation appeared to be the amplification of the negative hedonic tone (e.g., anxiety) which may serve to alarm the individual and mobilize coping skills. On the other hand, activation without much effort brought respiration in parallel with the ongoing extrapyramidal activity.

When the effort system appeared to have been predominantly coordinated with the arousal system (the playful state), motor discharge was channeled primarily through the pyramidal pathway to the skeletal muscles, and cardiac and respiratory activity reflected the active stimulus-related physical workload. Probably, the constellation of the arousal and effort systems is a logical substrate of the playful version of Type A behavior, whilst the constellation of the activation and effort systems is a substrate of the seriousminded version of the Type A behavior pattern.

Acknowledgements

The research which has been reviewed in this chapter was supported by grants from various sources including the British Council, the Norwegian Research Council for Social Science and the Humanities, and the Meltzer Foundation at the University of Bergen.

REFERENCES

Apter, M. J., 1982, "The Experience of Motivation: The Theory of Psychological Reversals", Academic Press, London.

Brunia, C. H. M., 1983, Motor preparation changes in amplitude of achilles tendon reflexes during a fixed foreperiod of one second, Psychophysiology, 20:658-664.

Chesney, M. A., Eagleston, J. R., and Rosenman, R. H., 1981, Type A behavior: Assessment and intervention, in: "Medical Psychology: Contributions to Behavioral Medicine", C. K. Prokop and L. A. Bradley, eds., pp. 19-36, Academic Press, New York.

Grossman, P., and Wientjes, K., 1985, Respiratory-cardiac coordination as an index of cardiac functioning, in: "Cardiovascular Psychophysiology: Theory and Methods", J. Orlbeke, G. Mulder and L. van Doornen, eds., pp. 451-464, Plenum Press, New York.

Light, K. C., 1981, Cardiovascular responses to effortful active coping: Implications for the role of stress in hypertension development, Psychophysiology, 18:216-225.

Loveless, N. E., 1983, Event-related brain potentials and human performance, in: "Physiological Correlates of Human Behavior, Vol 2: Attention and Performance", pp. 79-97, Academic Press, London.

Malmo, R. B., 1965, "On Emotions Needs and our Archaic Brain", Holt, Rinehart and Winston, New York.

Mulder, G., and Mulder, L. J. M., 1980, Coping with mental workload, in: "Coping and Health", S. Levine and H. Ursin, eds., pp. 233-258, Plenum Press, New York.

Murgatroyd, S., Rushton, C., Apter, M. J., and Ray, C., 1978, The development of the Telic Dominance Scale, J. Pers. Ass., 42:519-528.

Obrist, P. A., 1976, The cardiovascular-behavioral interaction - As it appears today, Psychophysiology, 13:95-107.

Obrist, P. A., Webb, R. A., Sutterer, J. R., and Howard, J. L., 1970, The cardiac-somatic relationship: Some reformulations, Psychophysiology, 6:569-587.

Pribram, K. H., and McGuinness, D., 1975, Arousal, activation and effort in the control of attention, Psychol. Rev., 82:116-149.

Rimehaug, T., and Svebak, S., 1984, Right and left upper arm flexor and extensor EMG-activity during cognitive-perceptual task performance: The significance of telic state and hedonic tone, Bull. Br. Psychol. Ass., 37:A46.

Strømme, S. B., Wikeby, P. C., Blix, A. S., and Ursin, H., 1978, Additional heart rate, in: "Psychobiology of Stress: A Study of Coping Men", H. Ursin, E. Baade and S. Levine, eds., pp. 83-89, Academic Press, New York.

Svebak, S., 1982, The effect of task difficulty and threat of aversive electric shock upon tonic physiological changes, Biol. Psychol., 14:113-128.

Svebak, S., 1983, The effect of information load, emotional load and motivational state upon tonic physiological activation, in: "Biological and Psychological Basis of Psychosomatic Disease", H. Ursin and R. Murison, eds., pp. 61-73, Pergamon Press, Oxford.

Svebak, S., 1984, Active forearm flexor tension patterns in the continuous perceptual-motor task paradigm: The significance of motivation, Internat. J. Psychophysiol., 2:167-176.

Svebak, S., Cardiac and somatic activation in the continuous perceptual-motor task: The significance of threat and serious-mindedness, Internat. J. Psychophysiol., 3:155-162.

Svebak, S., and Apter, M. J., 1984, Type A behavior and its relation to seriousmindedness (Telic dominance), Scand. J. Psychol., 25:161-167.

Svebak, S., Dalen, K., and Storfjell, O., 1981, The psychological significance of task-induced tonic changes in somatic and autonomic activity, Psychophysiology, 18:403-409.

Svebak, S., and Murgatroyd, S., 1985, Telic dominance: A multimethod validation of reversal theory constructs., J. Pers. Soc. Psychol., 48:107-116.

Svebak, S., Storfjell, O., and Dalen, K., 1982, The effect of a threatening context upon motivation and task-induced physiological changes, Br. J. Psychol., 73:505-512.

Ursin, H., Murison, R., and Knardahl, S., 1983, Conclusion: Sustained activation and disease, in: "Biological and psychological basis of psychosomatic disease", H. Ursin and R. Murison, eds., pp. 269-277, Pergamon Press, Oxford.

It has been a widespread assumption about the mercury-filled strain gauge technique that the signal is contaminated by marked DC-shifts over a recording period of several minutes. In Figure 4 I have included 3 examples of such Hg-gauge recordings. The upper part of that Figure illustrates the stability of a signal from a 51 cm long non-stretched gauge. The middle part is based upon the use of a 71 cm gauge, and the lower tracing is from a 96 cm Hg-gauge. They all operated with a 25-35% fraction added to their non-stretched length which means they were designed for trunk-circumferences of around 66, 92, and 120 cm respectively. The tracings show no evidence of DC-components, and they illustrate that calibration is maintained within the nearest millimeter after a 20-minute recording period of stable stretching. The recalibration (stepwise

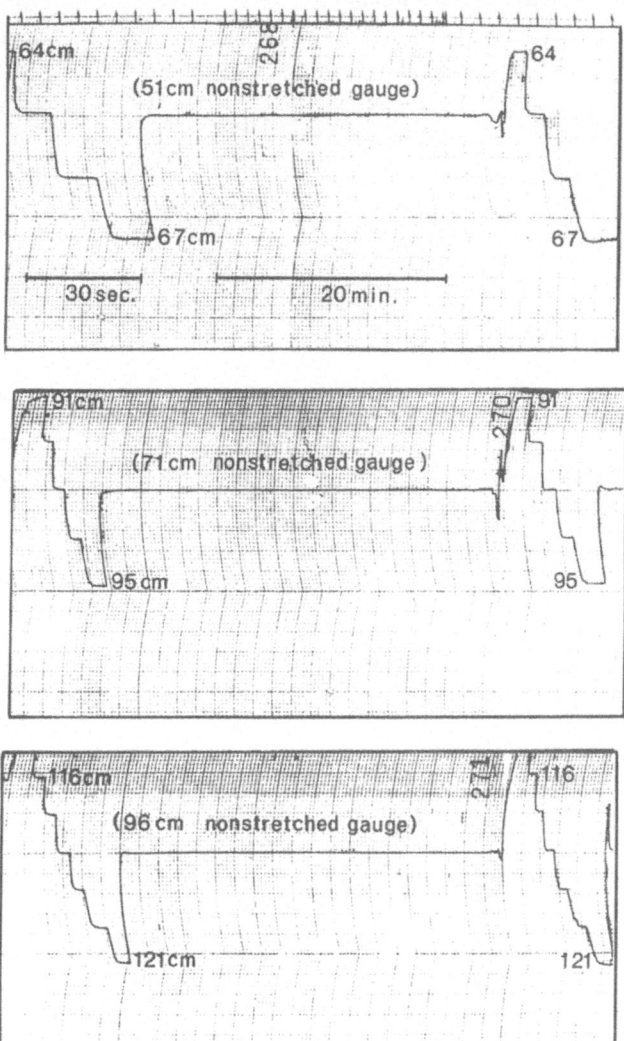

Fig. 4.   Three illustrations of the stability and sensitivity of signals derived from mercury-filled strain gauges where the DC-component has not been filtered out. The calibration of the gauges before and after a 20 minute-period, of constant stretching is included to document that the scale is maintained.

stretching of the gauge by adding 1 cm at each step) was performed by a
trained person who was blind to the polygraph tracings and who, therefore,
started and ended the whole procedure of stepwise stretching upon command
from another person watching the polygraph. When calibration is included
in experimental applications of this Hg-gauge technique, it permits that
trunk circumference changes can be scored as fractions of the trunk
circumference level. This correction procedure eliminates effects of
difference in trunk size in between-subject/same trunk level or thoracic/
abdominal disparity where such anatomical differences between subjects are
of no interest to the researcher.

These strain gauges have been made in our laboratory. They represent
a modified version of those used by the late Arthur Shapiro at the
Downstate Medical Center, New York, in the 1960s. It was brought to the
University of Bergen by Bjørn Christiansen, and a detailed documentation is
available upon request to the author.

BIOFEEDBACK AND SELF-REGULATION

BIOFEEDBACK-ASSISTED HEART RATE DECELERATION:
SPECIFICITY OF CARDIOVASCULAR AND METABOLIC
EFFECTS IN NORMAL AND HIGH RISK SUBJECTS

Catherine M. Stoney, Alan W. Langer,
James R. Sutterer and Paul D. Gelling*

Behavioral Physiology Laboratory, Department of Psychology
Syracuse University, 101 Stevens Place, Syracuse
New York 13210, USA
*Department of Bioelectronics and Computer Sciences
State University of New York, Upstate Medical Center
Syracuse, New York 13210, USA

An important theoretical issue in cardiovascular psychophysiology is whether biofeedback-assisted alterations in heart rate (HR) reflect only changes in cardiac function, are mediated indirectly by changes in somatic or respiratory responses, or reflect a common central nervous system integration of cardiac-somatic activity. In this connection, the first position was advanced by Miller and collaborators (Miller and DiCara, 1967; Miller and Banuazizi, 1968; DiCara and Miller, 1968), who argued that operant control of HR could be obtained in the absence of somatic mediation. This series of studies, employing the curarized preparation, putatively demonstrated that appreciable bidirectional HR changes could be conditioned independent of somatomotor activity. On the other hand, Obrist (1981) and others have been concerned with the common central coupling of cardiac and somatic processes during both classical (Obrist, 1968) and operant HR conditioning procedures. In an early classical aversive conditioning study with humans, a strong relationship between the magnitude and direction of phasic HR and somatomotor activity was noted (Obrist, 1968). Similarly, concomitant changes in HR and somatic activity were found during an operant conditioning paradigm that employed visual binary HR feedback for both HR acceleration and deceleration and a shock avoidance contingency (Obrist, Galosy, Lawler, Gaebelein, Howard and Shanks, 1975). These findings are consonant with the hypothesis that such voluntary HR changes covary in a consistent and positive manner with somatic-metabolic activity. This is further substantiated in animal studies where oxygen consumption ($\dot{V}O_2$) was used as an index of metabolic (somatic) activity. Brener, Phillips and Connally (1977) found high correlations between HR activity and both ambulation and $\dot{V}O_2$ in rats during operant conditioning of both HR acceleration and deceleration. Further evidence, though indirect, suggesting that operantly conditioned HR changes are metabolically linked has been reported by Gliner, Horvath and Wolfe (1975). In this study, large and significant decreases in HR were obtained in curarized rats subjected to an aversive shock avoidance operant conditioning paradigm. Although $\dot{V}O_2$ was not measured in this experiment, the fact that HR decreases were associated with a fall in cardiac output suggests that the effect was probably related to a decrease in $\dot{V}O_2$, since under most physiologic conditions cardiac output typically covaries with oxygen utilization.

Thus, even with the curarized preparation operantly conditioned decreases in HR produce significant alterations in tissue perfusion and, hence, oxygen delivery.

Of related interest to the above studies investigating the somatic alterations that occur with voluntary changes in HR are studies concerned with the mediation of cardiac functioning by respiratory responses. For example, Levenson (1976), employing bidirectional binary HR feedback, found reliable cardiac and respiratory rate decreases from baseline during periods of attempted HR decrease. In a second experiment, capitalizing on a between-subjects design, he showed significant slowing in both cardiac and respiratory rates when subjects attempted to decrease HR, whereas HR increase trials produced both reliably faster heart and respiratory rates. In contrast, Holmes, Solomon and Buchsbaum (1979) found that the indirect control of respiration (varying depth and rate) was related to biofeedback-based HR increases, but not decreases. In a more comprehensive second study (Holmes, Solomon, Frost and Morrow, 1980), subjects were first instructed to either increase or decrease HR with biofeedback, while their respiratory patterns were recorded. Following this phase of the experiment, subjects were asked to pace their previously recorded respiratory activity, while HR was assessed. Results indicated that the HR obtained while subjects were practicing paced respiration were similar to those obtained during biofeedback, thus indicating that the HR changes occurring during biofeedback were mediated by changes in respiration. A more direct test of the effect of respiratory modulation on operant conditioning of HR in humans has been reported by Vandercar, Feldstein and Soloman (1977), who found that direct control of respiratory rate and tidal volume vitiated attempts to produce cardiac acceleration and deceleration. Overall, the above findings strongly suggest that voluntary HR changes are at least in part dependent upon cardiac-somatic and respiratory integration.

Recently, our laboratory has focused on attempting to elucidate the metabolic, pulmonary, and hemodynamic concomitants of biofeedback-induced HR reductions in healthy, normal subjects (Langer, Stoney, Charlton and McCubbin, 1983). Therefore, the aim of the present study was to determine if a biofeedback-based decrease in HR would be associated with a corresponding change in $\dot{V}O_2$, and similarly, if $\dot{V}O_2$ could be reduced through feedback, whether the pattern would include a deceleration in HR.

STUDY ONE

Method

Subjects. Subjects were 80 randomly-selected healthy male volunteers from an introductory psychology class at Syracuse University. Participation was in partial fulfillment of course credit. All subjects were initially screened to rule out any present or recurrent medical or psychological problems, and to obtain written informed consent. Subjects were randomly assigned to one of four treatment groups (20 subjects per group), with groups receiving instructions either to lower HR with the use of a visual, analog biofeedback meter (HRFB), to decrease HR with merely the instructions to do so (HRDI), to lower $\dot{V}O_2$ with feedback (O2FB), or to sit quietly (CONTROL). All groups were comparable in age, height and weight.

Apparatus. All physiological variables were monitored non-invasively and calculated, stored and displayed in real time by a microcomputerized DEC LSI-11/23 system, running under the RT/11 operating system. Subjects respired through a 2-way non-rebreathing valve during all phases of the experiment. Heart rate (HR), oxygen consumption ($\dot{V}O_2$), carbon dioxide production ($\dot{V}CO_2$), minute ventilation ($\dot{V}_E$), were calculated on a breath-by-

breath basis. Systolic (SBP) and diastolic (DBP) blood pressure was monitored every two minutes with an ultrasonic-based blood pressure monitoring
device (Roche Arteriosonde 1030). A complete system description is available elsewhere (Langer, Hutcheson, Charlton, McCubbin, Obrist, and Stoney,
1985). Feedback for HR and $\dot{V}O_2$ was accomplished by processing the digital
values for these variables through a digital-to-analog converter. Proportional, visual feedback was given on the basis of the running (approximately two minute), updated average of either HR or $\dot{V}O_2$ and the corresponding real-time breath value.

Procedure. All subjects were habituated to the physiological recording apparatus for an initial 15-min session. Approximately one week later,
they returned for one session of either HR feedback (HRFB), $\dot{V}O_2$ feedback
(O2FB), HR deceleration with instructions only (HRDI) or rest (CONTROL).
This session consisted of providing all subjects with instructions specific
to their treatment group, followed by a 10-min baseline, a 10-min period
during which subjects either attempted to reduce the appropriate physiological variable (with or without metered feedback) or sat quietly, and a
10-min recovery period. At the conclusion of this session, subjects were
asked to rate, on a 10-point Likert scale, the degree of relaxation (1 =
most relaxed) they experienced during the session.

All physiological variables (HR, $\dot{V}O_2$, $\dot{V}CO_2$, $\dot{V}_E$, SPB and DBP) were
reduced to one-minute averages for each subject. These data were then
averaged across subjects by treatment group (HRFB, O2FB, HRDI, and
CONTROL). The first 5-min of baseline (rest) were discarded on the basis
that subjects were adapting to the apparatus during this period. Four
minutes were selected a priori for statistical analysis; min-4 was selected
as being representative of the baseline period, min-7 and 15 as representative of the feedback, HR deceleration or rest period, and min-25 as
representative of the recovery period. A 4 (Treatment (HRFB vs. O2FB vs.
HRDI vs. CONTROL)) x 4 (Time (min-4 vs. min-7 vs. min-15 vs. min-25)) ANOVA
for repeated measures was performed on each of these variables separately.
Post-hoc tests were analyzed by Tukey's Honestly Significant Difference
test statistic (Kirk, 1968). Subjective data of the relaxation question
were analyzed by the Mann-Whitney U test statistic.

Results

The ANOVA for HR indicated a significant effect for treatment group
($F(3,77) = 2.81$, $p < 0.04$). Post-hoc tests demonstrated that the HRFB,
HRDI, and O2FB groups all showed reliably ($p < 0.05$) lower HR throughout
the entire session as compared to the CONTROL group. There were no significant differences among the HRFB, HRDI, and O2FB groups in HR (see Table
1). The absolute HR levels for these three groups was typically about 66
bpm and approximated a steady-state condition throughout all phases of the
session (rest, transition, physiological reduction and recovery periods).
The CONTROL group, on the other hand, demonstrated a similar steady-state,
with an average HR of about 73 bpm.

The pattern of response for all groups in $\dot{V}O_2$ is also shown in Table
1. The ANOVA generated no significant time or treatment effects, indicating that none of the groups were different with respect to $\dot{V}O_2$. However,
it is clear that these metabolic patterns tend to follow the pattern for
HR. The $\dot{V}O_2$ levels approximated a steady-state, ranging from the values of
the HRFB group (0.240 L/min) to the values exhibited by the CONTROL group
(0.289 L/min).

ANOVAs on all of the other respiratory and hemodynamic measures ($\dot{V}CO_2$,
$\dot{V}_E$, SBP and DBP) demonstrated no differential effects among the four groups
during rest (baseline), the task period or during recovery. All of these

Table 1. Average Heart Rate (HR) and Oxygen Consumption (VO_2) (±SEM) for baseline (min-4), transition (min-7), feedback or rest (min-15) and recovery (min-25).

	HR					$\dot{V}O_2$			
	min-4	min-7	min-15	min-25		min-4	min-7	min-15	min-25
HRFB	67.57 ±2.8	65.45 ±2.6	65.01 ±2.4	65.42 ±2.7		.257 ±.011	.248 ±.013	.246 ±.013	.247 ±.013
O2FB	68.33 ±2.3	66.60 ±2.2	65.21 ±1.9	64.83 ±2.4		.274 ±.011	.256 ±.012	.256 ±.009	.266 ±.012
HRDI	65.87 ±1.9	66.09 ±2.2	64.48 ±2.0	65.59 ±1.7		.284 ±.011	.275 ±.011	.260 ±.010	.240 ±.015
CONTROL	73.80 ±2.1	72.67 ±2.2	72.28 ±2.0	73.44 ±2.3		.276 ±.012	.276 ±.012	.278 ±.014	.289 ±.015

measures approximated a steady-state throughout the entire session, with all values falling within normal ranges for resting, healthy males.

The Mann-Whitney U test on the subjective relaxation data indicated no significant differences among any of the groups in how relaxed they rated themselves throughout the session.

Discussion

These results suggest that the instructions to reduce HR (with or without the use of visual analog biofeedback) or $\dot{V}O_2$ (with feedback) results in a reliable reduction in HR. Because the availability of metered feedback did not produce further decreases from the instructions-only group, and because the $\dot{V}O_2$ feedback group exhibited HR reductions similar to the HRFB group, these appear to be effects that are not specific to the type of feedback presented or the actual availability of feedback.

The ability of the instructions-only subjects (HRDI) to effect HR control in the absence of actual feedback information about cardiac functioning is not a unique finding (Blanchard and Young, 1973; Bergman and Johnson, 1972), especially for HR slowing (Levenson, 1976, 1979; Young and Blanchard, 1974; Bouchard and Granger, 1977). The present results are consistent with the data presented by Cuthbert, Kristeller, Simons, Hodes and Lang (1981), who found not only that HR and EMG feedback produced both small and similar HR reductions, but also that a group that was merely instructed to reduce HR was as successful in HR deceleration as both feedback groups. Similar effects for instructions-only groups have been found for other cardiodeceleratory tasks (Twentyman, Malloy and Green, 1979). In addition, it has been shown (Gatchel, 1974; Lang and Twentyman, 1974; Twentyman et al., 1979) that increasing the amount of cardiac information presented to subjects does little to improve performance on a biofeedback-assisted cardiac deceleration task.

The lack of metabolic and ventilatory alterations in the HRFB and HRDI groups argues for these effects eliciting cardiac reductions that are somewhat specific to the system being modified. However, it should be noted that there was a definite trend for the HRFB group to demonstrate lower $\dot{V}O_2$ values than the control group (see Table 1). Thus, these HR effects appear not to be completely independent of somatomotor activity, as reflected by the lower, albeit nonsignificant levels in $\dot{V}O_2$. In addition, no respiratory parameters were significantly altered with either the feedback or instruction-only groups. In contrast, both Levenson (1976) and Vandercar et al. (1977) noted that the respiratory rate during HR deceleratory feedback was significantly reduced. It is relevant to note that our visual display provides HR feedback on a breath-by-breath basis so that HR variations due to sinus arrhythmias are not a component feature of the information HR feedback subjects obtain in order to alter HR. Interestingly, the O2FB group did demonstrate a somewhat general physiological response, since they significantly altered HR, even though they were given feedback on $\dot{V}O_2$. The lack of physiological specificity after only one session of feedback training has been suggested by Brener (1981) to be most often found during acquisition of control.

STUDY TWO

Individual Differences

Large between-subject variability has prompted numerous investigators to explore those factors that may predispose some individuals to greater HR controllability than that demonstrated by most subjects. In this connection, it is commonly reported that greater physiologic reductions can be noted in biofeedback subjects who have elevated base levels than in those who have normal or low resting physiological levels (Furedy and Klajner, 1978; Stephens, Harris, Brady and Shaffer, 1975; Twentyman et al., 1979). It has therefore been postulated that the differential responses for clinical and normal populations may be attributable to an initial values (Cuthbert et al., 1981; Wilder, 1967) or floor (Williamson and Blanchard, 1979) effect. This concept has led Schwartz (1975) to expand the motor skills model of the achievement of autonomic control to include the idea that control of visceral systems cannot supercede the biological constraints of that system. This hypothesis suggests that biofeedback techniques to reduce physiologic activity from elevated levels in clinical and normal populations may not only be feasible, but may in fact result in more robust attenuations than those seen in normal resting individuals who exhibit relatively low resting levels of physiological activity.

Attempts to train normal subjects in HR decelerations have therefore included efforts to circumvent the problem of floor effects. Training subjects with initially high HR levels has resulted in somewhat larger magnitude HR reductions. For instance, Stephens et al. (1975) found that normal subjects with high resting heart rates and/or high HR variability, were best able to reduce HR with biofeedback. Further, it has been reliably demonstrated that biofeedback-induced HR decreases can be elicited during both static (Clemens and Shattock, 1979) and dynamic (Goldstein, Ross, and Brady, 1977; Persky and Engel, 1980) exercise challenge, with little or no decrement in exercise performance. In addition, Sirota, Schwartz and Shapiro (1974, 1976) have demonstrated phasic HR control in anticipation of an aversive stimulus in subjects given HR feedback to both accelerate and decelerate HR, with these subjects appearing to exhibit tonic HR control over successive trials. Also, Riley and Furedy (1981) have demonstrated successful phasic HR decelerations with feedback in subjects with task-induced (muscle-tensing task) elevated baseline HR. However, Harris, Katkin, Lick and Habberfield (1976) studied the effects of paced respiration on the modification of HR and electrodermal responses to a painful stressor. They found that subjects who were instructed to pace their respiratory patterns to a rate based on 4 seconds of inspiration and 4 seconds of expiration had HR values similar to a control group that was not instructed to alter ventilatory responses. Giving visual feedback of pulse transit time (TT), Steptoe and associates have demonstrated the ability of subjects to control TT during an auditory choice reaction time task (Steptoe, 1978), as well as during stressful cognitive tasks (Steptoe and Ross, 1982). Interestingly, the latter study also found that the voluntary control of TT was especially prominent among the most cardio-vascularly-reactive subjects.

In further exploring the individual differences widely noted in bio-feedback HR reduction studies, we reasoned that in individuals for whom an elevated cardiovascular response to stress is commonly noted, these tech-niques may be especially effective. A clinically relevant dimension of individual differences which has been shown to be directly related to potentiating cardiovascular responses to behavioral stress is the Type A coronary-prone behavior pattern (see Matthews, 1982, for a review).

Although the specific mechanism that mediates the relationship between the Type A coronary-prone behavior pattern and the development of CHD has not been empirically identified, many reports have postulated that Type As have an excessive sympathetic nervous system reactivity to psychological stress (Eliot, Buell and Dembroski, 1982; Krantz and Durel, 1983). In this light, a variety of overt behavioral, cardiovascular and other autonomic measures in asymptomatic Type A individuals have been assessed. Studies measuring basal levels of HR, SBP and DBP typically report similarity among healthy Type A and B individuals (Manuck and Garland, 1979; Contrada, Glass, Krakoff, Krantz, Kehoe, Isecke, Collins and Elting, 1982; Stern and Elder, 1982; Glass, Krakoff, Contrada, Hilton, Kehoe, Mannucci, Collins, Snow and Elting, 1980). Recently, several investigations have noted wide-ranging differential physiological response patterns between Type A and Type B individuals subjected to aversive (stressful) behavioral tasks. Responses in HR (Dembroski, MacDougall and Shields, 1977; Contrada et al., 1982), SBP (Manuck and Garland, 1979; Lawler, Allen, Critcher and Standard, 1981), plasma levels of catecholamines (Friedman, Byers, Diamant and Rosenman, 1975; Glass et al., 1980), and serum cholesterol and cortisol levels (Williams, Lane, Kuhn, Melosh, White and Schanberg, 1982; Lovallo and Pishkin, 1980) have been observed that are of a greater magnitude in Type A subjects than those exhibited by Type B subjects. On the basis of these findings, many of these authors have suggested that Type A subjects are more sympathetically reactive during times of psychological stress than their Type B counterparts. As with the overt display of Type A behavior patterns, these physiologic responses are most prominent under those specific situations that these individuals evaluate as stressful or chal-lenging (Matthews, 1982).

Thus, given the association between the Type A behavior pattern and the exaggerated physiologic response to behavioral stress which putatively plays a mediating role in cardiovascular pathology, we propose that the direct modification of physiological rather than overt behavioral responses would be a potentially viable method for reducing the risk of CHD in these individuals. Therefore, the present study explored the ability of healthy, asymptomatic Type A and Type B college males to effect visceral (HR) con-trol using the same biofeedback procedure described in experiment one. In addition, the efficacy of this type of biofeedback to modify cardiovascular and pulmonary reactions to a stressful, behavioral task was explored (Stoney, Langer and Sutterer, 1983) in both Type A and Type B subjects.

Method

Subjects. A large population of undergraduates were administered the Jenkins Activity Survey (JAS) for college students. Forty-eight healthy, asymptomatic males were selected for participation in this experiment. Twenty-four scored in the upper 10% on the JAS (mean = 12.5), and were therefore considered to be highly developed Type As, and twenty-four scored in the lower 10% on the JAS (mean = 2.9), and were typed as well-developed Type Bs. All subjects refrained from eating, drinking and smoking for three hours prior to participation, and were 24 hours drug-free.

Apparatus. The physiological recording apparatus for study two was as described in the previous experiment. In addition, breath-by-breath partial pressures of end-tidal oxygen ($P_{ET}O_2$) and carbon dioxide ($P_{ET}CO_2$) were analyzed. Also, a DEC PDP-8e minicomputer working under the OS8 operating system and connected to a SKED interface (Snapper) provided experimental control for the aversive reaction time (RT) task.

Procedure. All subjects participated in two sessions, spaced approximately one week apart. Both sessions consisted of continuous recordings of a 5-min baseline period, a 10-min biofeedback or rest, and RT task period, and a 10-min recovery period. During session one, one-half of the Type A subjects (n = 12) and one-half of the Type B subjects (n = 12) were trained on the HR biofeedback task as described in the previous experiment. The other Type A (n = 12) and Type B (n = 12) subjects were instructed to sit quietly during this session, and therefore served as the control groups. During session two, all subjects participated in a 10-min unsignalled shock-avoidance reaction time stress task. This paradigm, modified from the Obrist et al. (1978) procedure, requires subjects to respond to a series of 25 randomly spaced 1 kHz tones by depressing a telegraph key as quickly as possible. In a given block of trials, the first occurrence of a reaction time that is slower than the previous response results in a 1 mA constant current shock to the leg. All subjects received four shocks. The two groups that had previously been trained in HR biofeedback were again given breath-by-breath feedback and instructed to reduce HR during the aversive RT task. The control groups were instructed only on the nature of the RT task itself. At the completion of each session, all subjects were asked to rate, on a 10-point Likert scale, the relative degree of relaxation (1 = most relaxed), stress (1 = least stressed) and, after the RT task, pain from shocks received (1 = least pain) that they experienced.

All physiological variables were reduced to one minute averages for each subject and session, and the individual data were averaged across subjects by group (Type A or Type B), task (biofeedback or rest) and session (one and two). One minute was selected a priori as representative of each of the three time periods. They were min-4 for baseline, min-14 for the biofeedback or rest and RT period, and min-25 for recovery. The HR value of the breaths on which shock was administered was deleted to prevent artifactual contamination of the HR data.

For the biofeedback session, a 2 (Type A vs. Type B) x 2 (biofeedback vs. rest) ANOVA was performed separately on the baseline and recovery scores for each physiologic (HR, SBP, DBP, $\dot{V}O_2$, $\dot{V}CO_2$, $P_{ET}O_2$, $P_{ET}CO_2$, and $\dot{V}_E$) variable. There were no significant differences among the four groups during baseline for any of these variables, so that additional analyses on the change from baseline was deemed appropriate. Therefore, all reported analyses result from a 2 (Type A vs. Type B) x 2 (biofeedback vs. rest) ANOVA on the difference from min-4 to min-14 for each variable.

For session two, the ANOVAs on the baseline and recovery scores for HR, SBP, DBP, $\dot{V}O_2$, $\dot{V}CO_2$, $P_{ET}O_2$, and $P_{ET}O_2$ demonstrated no reliable differences among the groups during baseline or recovery. Therefore, the reported analyses are generated from a 2 (Type A vs. Type B) x 2 (biofeedback and RT vs. RT only) ANOVA on the change scores from min-4 (baseline) to min-14 (stress) for each dependent measure. There was, interestingly, a significant effect for $\dot{V}_E$ at baseline min-4, indicating that the Type A subjects had a significantly elevated minute ventilation during baseline from the Type B subjects.

Results

Session One. The average min-by-min HR for all four groups during session one is illustrated in Figure 1. Clearly, there is a definite trend for the magnitude of the difference between the Type A feedback and resting control groups to be greater than the Type B feedback and control groups. The peak response noted at about min-16 for both of the feedback groups is reflective of an increase in somatic activity when the feedback task is over. The ANOVA on the change from baseline scores revealed a significant decrease in HR for both feedback groups ($F(1,44) = 4.04$, $p < 0.05$), although there was no effect for the Type A/B dimension. Interestingly, the analysis of the HR values at recovery showed that these feedback effects were sustained when the feedback was no longer available ($F(1,44) = 5.03$, $p < 0.03$). No other physiological parameters differentiated the groups during session one.

Session Two. The ANOVA on the change scores for HR during session two revealed a significant effect for feedback $F(1,44) = 5.54$, $p < 0.02$. Figure 2 (upper panel) illustrates the magnitude of these effects, demonstrating that the attenuation of the HR response of the Type A biofeedback subjects (mean = 68 bpm) was quite large relative to the Type A control group (mean = 80 bpm). In contrast, the difference in the HR response between the Type B feedback group (mean = 72 bpm) and the Type B control group (mean = 74 bpm) was much smaller. Interestingly, the marked tachycardia elicited by the Type A control group was not reflected in any changes from the other groups in $\dot{V}O_2$ ($p > 0.1$), suggesting that this cardiac effect was not metabolically warranted (Figure 2, lower panel).

Figure 3 (upper panel) depicts the ventilatory response ($\dot{V}_E$) of the four groups during the RT session (session two). Again, it is quite clear that the Type A control group was ventilating more than the other groups. The ANOVA on the change from baseline scores indicated a significant effect for feedback, $F(1,44) = 7.74$, $p < 0.008$, indicating a significant attenuation in the $\dot{V}_E$ for both Type A and Type B feedback groups as compared to control groups. As previously noted, during baseline min-4, $\dot{V}_E$ was greater in Type A subjects than both Type B groups. The data for $P_{ET}CO_2$, in conjunction with the $\dot{V}_E$ response, shows that both control groups showed a gradual decline in $P_{ET}CO_2$, consistent with the $\dot{V}_E$ response noted in these subjects (Figure 3, lower panel). In contrast, both feedback groups maintained a relative steady state during the RT stress task. During recovery, there was no further decline in $P_{ET}CO_2$ for the control groups, and a new

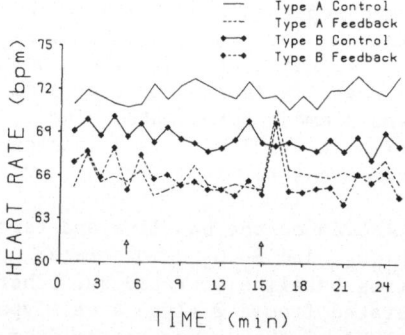

Fig. 1. Average min-by-min HR during 5-min rest, 10-min biofeedback (lines with symbols) or rest (lines without symbols), and 10-min of recovery. The solid lines designate Type A subjects and the dashed lines indicate Type B subjects.

240

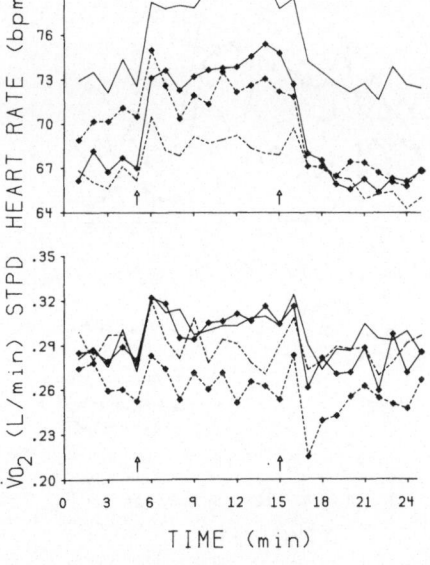

Fig. 2. Average min-by-min HR (upper panel) and $\dot{V}O_2$ (lower panel) during 5-min rest, 10-min reaction time with (lines with symbols) or without (lines without symbols) biofeedback, and 10-min of recovery. The solid lines designate Type A subjects and the dashed lines indicate Type B subjects.

steady state was established, a pattern that appears to be closely linked with the ventilatory pattern exhibited by these subjects.

The ANOVA on the change scores for $\dot{V}CO_2$ demonstrated a reliable effect for biofeedback, $F(1,44) = 5.3$, $p < 0.03$, suggesting that biofeedback has the capacity to significantly attenuate the $\dot{V}CO_2$ response to behavioral stress for both Type A and Type B subjects. Figure 4 (upper panel) describes these effects. The lower panel of Figure 4 details the pattern of responses in $P_{ET}O_2$ noted in all four groups. The ANOVA failed to produce any significant effects for feedback ($p > 0.1$), as well as any differences in the Type A/B dimension ($p > 0.1$).

The pattern of response in SBP is noted in Figure 5 (upper panel). The pressor response evident in the two control groups (Type A and B) appears to be most prominently decreased in the Type A feedback group. The ANOVA on the change scores for SBP indicated a significant effect for feedback, $F(1,44) = 5.20$, $p < 0.03$. In contrast, there were no reliable effects for DBP, illustrated in Figure 5 (lower panel), although there is a mild trend for both feedback groups to display a lower DBP response during RT than both control groups.

Mann-Whiney U tests on the subjective ratings of the degree of relaxation, stress and pain experienced during this session demonstrated no significant differences between any of the groups. Analysis of the RT scores themselves indicated that there were no differences between the Type A feedback and control groups, although there was a significant decrease in RT scores in the Type B control group compared to the Type B feedback group.

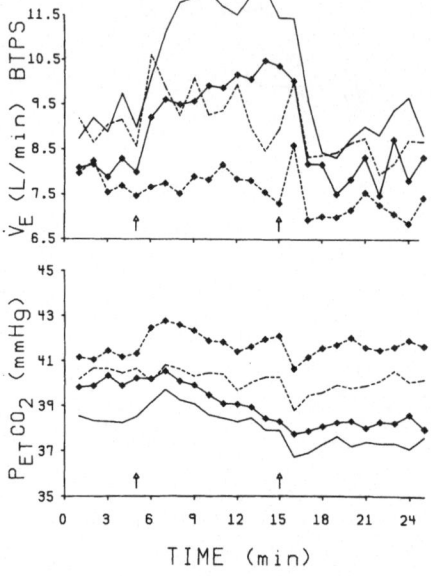

Fig. 3. Average min-by-min $\dot{V}_E$ (upper panel) and $P_{ET}CO_2$ (lower panel) during 5-min rest, 10-min of reaction time or reaction time plus biofeedback, and 10-min of recovery. Symbols and lines are as noted in Figure 2.

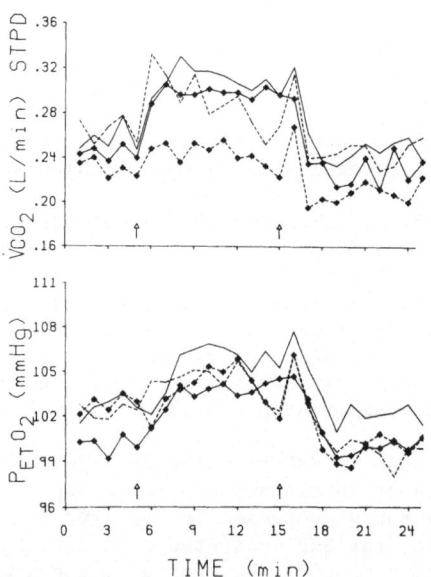

Fig. 4. Average min-by-min $\dot{V}CO_2$ (upper panel) and $P_{ET}O_2$ (lower panel) during 5-min of rest, 10-min of reaction time or reaction time plus biofeedback, and 10-min of recovery. Symbols and lines are as noted in Figure 2.

Discussion

The results of session one clearly demonstrate biofeedback-assisted HR reductions from normal, steady-state levels in healthy Type A and Type B males. These data, in conjunction with the lack of significant alterations

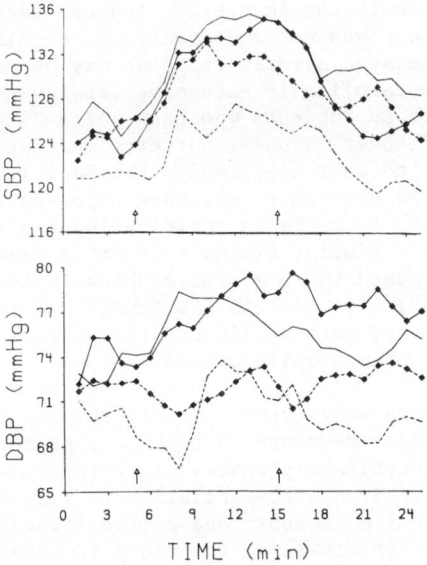

Fig. 5. Systolic (upper panel) and diastolic (lower panel) blood pressure
         during 5-min of rest, 10-min of reaction time or reaction time
         with biofeedback, and 10-min of recovery, based on 1-min averages.
         Symbols and lines are as noted in Figure 2.

in $\dot{V}O_2$, $\dot{V}CO_2$, $\dot{V}_E$, SBP and DBP, are in agreement with the results of experiment one.   Further, although there appears to be a certain cardiac
specificity in this response, the overall HR changes in resting individuals
are of a relatively small magnitude.   The relevance of these results to
therapeutic applications lies in the fact that Type A coronary-prone individuals are as able as their Type B counterparts to exert cardiac control.
To date, only one study has investigated the efficacy of biofeedback techniques with healthy Type A subjects at rest (Stern and Elder, 1982).   These
authors found the ability of Type A subjects to reduce HR with auditory
feedback to be partially dependent on the relative degree of challenge
provided by instructions.

     The data from the RT task session (session two) indicates that HR
biofeedback is successful in blunting the tachycardia elicited by a behavioral stress task.   In addition, it is clear that the most robust attenuations in HR were demonstrated by the Type A feedback group.   The large,
though non-significant difference in baseline HR values for the Type A
control and feedback groups are most likely explained by the Type A
controls exhibiting an anticipatory HR response to stress prior to the
onset of RT.   Moreover, this difference may also be related to the possibility that the Type A feedback group may be exhibiting cardiac control
prior to the onset of feedback, similar to the pattern noted in experiment
one.   The successful attenuation of the SBP response in the two feedback
groups clearly demonstrates the generalizability of HR biofeedback to blunt
cardiovascular responses to behavioral stress.   This alteration in blood
pressure reactivity is consistent with the feedback-assisted TT increases
during RT noted by Steptoe (Steptoe, 1978; Steptoe and Ross, 1982), because
TT has been found to be highly inversely correlated with SBP (Steptoe,
1978).   Further, these data are in agreement with other studies that have
shown feedback-assisted attenuations in cardiovascular reactions to behavioral stressors (DeGood and Adams, 1976; Victor, Mainardi and Shapiro,
1978), and extends the findings of these authors to include the demonstration of voluntary control during an aversive behavioral task in the
Type A coronary-prone individual.

Interestingly, the fact that the stress-induced tachycardia elicited in the Type A control group was not accompanied by an alteration in $\dot{V}O_2$ suggests that this exaggerated cardiac response may be metabolically unwarranted. A similar, metabolically excessive cardiovascular effect has been clearly demonstrated in subjects who show large HR reactivity to a psychological stressor (Langer, Stoney, Sutterer and Obrist, see this volume; Turner, Carroll and Courtney, 1983). In addition, in a recent study, Gliner, Bunnell and Horvath (1982) have reported an overall cardiac and metabolic dissociation in subjects anticipating a stressful public speaking task. Finally, a similar tissue (systemic) overperfusion has also been reported in dogs exposed to an aversive shock avoidance task (Langer, Obrist and McCubbin, 1979), in which it was found that the HR and cardiac output changes that occurred during this behavioral task, relative to exercise, were in excess of metabolic demand.

The increase in minute ventilation seen in the Type A control group was accompanied by a gradual decrease in $P_{ET}CO_2$, a pattern which suggests a tendency towards a hyperventilatory state. In this connection, there are few studies that have described overventilation in normal subjects. However, Suess, Alexander, Smith, Sweeney and Marion (1980) noted a decrease in $P_{ET}CO_2$ and an increase in breathing frequency in normal subjects during an aversive behavioral task, and suggested that such a pattern was indicative of hyperventilation. In addition, they postulated that the prominent between-subject variability in these pulmonary measures may be in part due to personality variables. Although these variables were not identified, the present data indicate that the Type A/B dimension may be highly relevant in this respect. The present study, moreover, shows that such an increase in ventilation can be effectively modified by cardiac biofeedback, again demonstrating that HR biofeedback can produce a generalized reduction in stress-induced cardiopulmonary adjustments.

Therefore, this study provides good evidence to suggest that Type A subjects exposed to psychological stress without feedback exhibit a physiological pattern of enhanced pulmonary ventilation and cardiovascular reactivity that is probably sympathetically-mediated. In addition, this cardiac response to stress appears to be metabolically inappropriate. Empirical support for the position that the Type A coronary-prone individual may display enhanced cardiovascular reactivity to stress that is mediated by sympathetic influences comes from a recent model that postulates that the Type A pattern is itself an overt behavioral reflection of sympathetic nervous system reactivity, which is a result of genetic or conditioned influences (Krantz and Durel, 1983). From a more theoretical standpoint, a compelling hypothesis for the mechanism underlying the connection between behavior patterns and the risk of CHD has been recently suggested, and expanded to include the coronary-prone individual (Schneiderman, 1983). This model posits that elevations of blood pressure and increased catecholaminergic release, as a result of stress-induced elevations in sympathetic nervous system activity, can induce direct endothelial wall damage and thereby cause increased plaque formation at the site of damage. More indirect damage occurs when the catecholamine release helps to mobilize free fatty acids from adipose tissue. In the absence of metabolic demand, these free fatty acids are hydrolized to triglycerides, and a portion of them are converted to low density lipoproteins, which have been strongly implicated in the development of CHD (Eder, 1982). This proposed mechanism is further supported by the positive association between behaviorally-induced sympathetic nervous system reactivity and the subsequent development of cardiovascular pathology which has been demonstrated in a number of animal studies (Miller and Mallov, 1977; Corley, Shick, Mauck, Clark and Barber, 1977; Henry, Ely, Stephens, Ratcliffe, Santisteban and Shapiro, 1971). Unfortunately, however, such a mechanism in human populations has not been empirically tested. It is clear that future research should be directed at this critical epidemiological question, most especially in relation to those populations (e.g., Type A) at risk for the development of cardiovascular pathology.

Finally, the type of biofeedback employed in this study is at least as effective with Type A coronary-prone individuals as with their Type B counterparts. In this connection, a few studies have investigated the clinical utility of bifeedback techniques in the treatment and management of a variety of psychophysiological disorders (Blanchard and Miller, 1977), with reports of differing degrees of therapeutic gains (Blanchard and Abel, 1976; Basmajian, 1981; Glasgow, Gaarder and Engel, 1982). Although there exists little or no evidence to show that biofeedback can be successfully employed to modify pulmonary dysfunction, several researchers (Engel and Bleecker, 1974; Pickering and Gorham, 1975; Pickering and Miller, 1977; Kristt and Engel, 1975; Benson, Shapiro, Tursky and Schwartz, 1971) have reported successful modifications of the frequency and severity of cardio-vascular symptoms using cardiovascular biofeedback paradigms. However, it is important to note that the bulk of these investigations typically attempt to attenuate abnormally elevated cardiac and hemodynamic levels in patients with already well-established disease. Unfortunately, the clini-cal utility of these procedures is somewhat compromised by the fact that decreases in resting levels of cardiovascular activity, while frequently statistically significant, are seldom clinically meaningful. The present study has demonstrated successful reductions of stress-induced cardio-pulmonary and hemodynamic responses to the normal range in individuals who are asymptomatic, including some who are at high risk for the future devel-opment of cardiovascular disease. Therefore, if the cardiopulmonary and hemodynamic consequences of behavioral stress are relevant features in the initiation and/or progression of various cardiovascular pathophysiologies, the application of biofeedback to blunt these responses may hold consider-able promise as an effective behavioral preventative technique. Obviously, whether such a promise is fulfilled will critically await the outcome of well-controlled longitudinal studies.

Acknowledgements

This research was supported in part by NIH grants HL-28938 and BSRG-S07 RR077068-18.

REFERENCES

Basmajian, J. V., 1981, Biofeedback in rehabilitation: A review of principles and practices, Arch. Phys. Med. & Rehab., 62:469-475.
Benson, H., Shapiro, D., Tursky, B., and Schwartz, G. E., 1971, Decreased
systolic blood pressure through operant conditioning techniques in
patients with essential hypertension, Science, 173:740-742.
Bergman, J. S., and Johnson, H. J., 1972, Sources of information which
affect training and raising of heart rate, Psychophysiology, 9:30-
39.
Blanchard, E. B., and Abel, G. G., 1976, An experimental case study of the
biofeedback treatment of a rape-induced psychophysiological cardiovascular disorder, Behavior Therapy, 7:113-119.
Blanchard, E. B., and Miller, S. T., 1977, Psychological treatment of
cardiovascular disease, Arch. Gen. Psychi., 34:1402-1413.
Blanchard, E. B., and Young, L. D., 1973, Self-control of cardiac functioning: A promise as yet unfulfilled, Psychol. Bull., 79:145-163.
Bouchard, M., and Granger, L., 1977, The role of instructions versus
instructions plus feedback in voluntary heart rate slowing, Psychophysiology, 14:475-482.

Brener, J., Phillips, K., and Connally, S. R., 1977, Oxygen consumption and ambulation during operant conditioning of heart rate increases and decreases in rats, Psychophysiology, 14:483-491.

Brener, J., 1981, Control of internal activities, Brit. Med. J., 37:169-174.

Clemens, W. J., and Shattock, J. R., 1979, Voluntary heart rate control during static muscular effort, Psychophysiology, 16:323-327.

Contrada, R. J., Glass, D. C., Krakoff, L. R., Krantz, D. S., Kehoe, K., Isecke, W., Collins, C., and Elting, E., 1982, Effects of control over aversive stimulation and Type A behavior on cardiovascular and plasma catecholamine responses, Psychophysiology, 19:408-419.

Corley, K. C., Shiel, P. O'M., Mauck, H. P., Clark, L. S., and Barber, J. V., 1977, Myocardial degeneration and cardiac arrest in squirrel monkeys: Psysiologicol and psychological correlation, Psychophysiology, 14:322-328.

Cuthbert, B., Kristeller, J., Simons, R., Hodes, R., and Lang, P. J., 1981, Strategies of arousal control: Biofeedback, mediation and motivation, J. Exp. Psychol., 110:518-546.

DeGood, D. E., and Adams, A. S., 1976, Control of cardiac responses under aversive stimulation, Biofeedback & Self-Regulation, 1:373-385.

Dembroski, T. M., MacDougall,, J. M., Shields, J. L., 1977, Physiological reactions to social challenge in persons evidencing the Type A coronary-prone behavior pattern, J. Human Stress, 3:270-279.

DiCara, L. V., and Miller, N. E., 1968, Changes in heart rate learned by curarized rats as avoidance responses, J. Comp. & Physiol. Psychol., 65:8-12.

Eder, H. A., 1982, Lipoproteins as risk factors for coronary heart disease, Bull. New York Acad. Med., 58:219-228.

Eliot, R. S., Buell, J. C., and Dembroski, T. M., 1982, Bio-behavioural perspectives on coronary heart disease, hypertension and sudden cardiac death, Acta Med. Scand., 660:203-213.

Engel, B. T., and Bleecker, E. R., 1974, Application of operant conditioning techniques to the control of cardiac arrhythmias, in: "Cardiovascular Psychophysiology", P. A. Obrist, A. H. Black, J. Brener, and L. V. DiCara, eds., Aldine, Chicago.

Friedman, H., Byers, S. D., Diamant, J., and Rosenman, R. H., 1975, Plasma catecholamine response of coronary-prone subjects (Type A) to a specific challenge, Metabolism, 24:205-210.

Furedy, J. J., and Klajner, F., 1978, Imaginational Pavlovian conditioning of large magnitude cardiac decelerations with tilt as US, Psychophysiology, 15:538-543.

Gatchel, R. J., 1974, Frequency of feedback and learned heart rate control, J. Exp. Psychology, 103:274-283.

Glasgow, M. S., Gaarder, K. R., and Engel, B. T., 1982, Behavioral treatment of high blood pressure II. Acute and sustained effects of relaxation and systolic blood pressure biofeedback, Psychosomatic Med., 44:155-170.

Glass, D. C., Krakoff, L. R., Contrada, R., Hilton, W. F., Kehoe, K., Mannucci, E. G., Collins, C., Snow, B., and Elting, E., 1980, Effect of harassment and competition upon cardiovascular and plasma catecholamine responses in Type A and Type B individuals, Psychophysiology, 17:453-463.

Gliner, J. A., Bunnell, D. E., and Horvath, S. M., 1982, Hemodynamic and metabolic changes prior to speech performance, Physiol. Psychol., 10:108-113.

Gliner, J. A., Horvath, S. M., and Wolfe, R. R., 1975, Operant conditioning of heart rate in curarized rats: Hemodynamic changes, Am. J. Physiol., 228:870-874.

Goldstein, D. S., Ross, R. S., and Brady, J. V., 1977, Biofeedback rate training during exercise, Biofeedback & Self-Regulation, 2:107-125.

Harris, V. A., Katkin, E. S., Lick, J. R., and Habberfield, T., 1976, Paced respiration as a technique for the modification of autonomic response to stress, Psychophysiology, 13:386-391.

Henry, J. P., Ely, D. L., Stephens, P. M., Ratcliffe, H. L., Santisteban, G. A., and Shapiro, A. P., 1971, The role of psychosocial factors in the development of arteriosclerosis in CBA mice, Atherosclerosis, 14:203-218.

Holmes, D. S., Solomon, S., and Buchsbaum, H. K., 1979, Utility of voluntary control of respiration and biofeedback for increasing and decreasing heart rate, Psychophysiology, 16:432-437.

Holmes, D. S., Solomon, S., Frost, R. O., and Morrow, E. F., 1980, Influence of respiratory patterns on the increases and decreases in heart rates in heart rate biofeedback training, J. Psychosomatic Res., 24:147-153.

Kirk, R. E., 1968, "Experimental Design: Procedures for the Behavioral Sciences", Wadsworth Publishing, California.

Krantz, D. S., and Durel, L. A., 1983, Psychobiological substrates of the Type A behavior pattern, Health Psychology, 2:393-411.

Kristt, D. A., and Engel, B. T., 1975, Learned control of blood pressure in patients with high blood pressure, Circulation, 51:370-378.

Lang, P. J., and Twentyman, C. T., 1974, Learning to control heart rate: Binary vs. analogue feedback, Psychophysiology, 11:616-629.

Langer, A. W., Obrist, P. A., and McCubbin, J. A., 1979, Hemodynamic and metabolic adjustments during exercise and shock avoidance in dogs, Am. J. Physiol: Heart & Circ. Physiol., 5:H225-H230.

Langer, A. W., Stoney, C. M., Charlton, J. C., and McCubbin, J. A., 1983, The efficacy of biofeedback training to reduce heart rate or oxygen consumption: Specificity of cardiac and pulmonary responses, Psychophysiology, 20:455-456.

Langer, A. W., Hutcheson, J. S., Charlton, J. D., McCubbin, J. A., Obrist, P. A., and Stoney, C. M., 1985, On-line minicomputerized measurement of cardiopulmonary function on a breath-by-breath basis, Psychophysiology, 22:50-58.

Lawler, K. A., Allen, M. R., Critcher, E. C., Standard, B. A., 1981, The relationship of physiological responses to the coronary-prone pattern in children, J. Behav. Med., 4:203-216.

Levenson, R. W., 1976, Feedback effects and respiratory involvement in voluntary heart control of heart rate, Psychophysiology, 13:108-114.

Levenson, R. W., 1979, Cardiac-respiratory-somatic relationships and feedback effects in a multiple session heart rate control experiment, Psychophysiology, 16:367-373.

Lovallo, W., and Pishkin, V., 1980, A physiological comparison of Type A and B men exposed to failure and uncontrollable noise, Psychophysiology, 17:29-39.

Manuck, S., and Garland, F. N., 1979, Coronary-prone behavior pattern, task incentive and cardiovascular response, Psychophysiology, 16:136-142.

Matthews, K. A., 1982, Psychological perspectives on the Type A behavior pattern, Psychol. Bull., 91:293-323.

Miller, D. G., and Mallov, S., 1977, The quantitative determination of stress-induced myocardial damage in rats, Pharmacol., Biochem. & Behavior., 7:139-145.

Miller, N. E., and Banuazizi, A., 1968, Instrumental learning by curarized rats of specific visceral response, intestinal or cardiac, J. Comp. & Physiol. Psychol., 65:1-7.

Miller, N. E., and DiCara, L., 1967, Instrumental learning of heart rate changes in curarized rats: Shaping and specificity to discriminative stimulus, J. Comp. & Physio. Psychol., 63:12-19.

Obrist, P. A., 1968, Heart rate and somatic-motor coupling during classical aversive conditioning in humans, J. Exp. Psychol., 77:180-193.

Obrist, P. A., 1981, "Cardiovascular Psychophysiology: A Perspective", Plenum Press, New York.

Obrist, P. A., Gaebelein, C. J., Teller, E. S., Langer, A. W., Grignolo, A., Light, K. C., and McCubbin, J. A., 1978, The relationship among heart rate, carotid dP/dt, and blood pressure in humans as a function of the type of stress, Psychophysiology, 15:102-115.

Obrist, P. A., Galosy, R. A., Lawler, J. E., Gaebelein, C. J., Howard, J. L., and Shanks, E. M., 1975, Operant conditioning of heart rate: Somatic correlates, Psychophysiology, 12:445-455.

Perski, A., and Engel, B. T., 1980, The role of behavioral conditioning in the cardiovascular adjustment to exercise, Biofeedback & Self-Regulation, 5:91-104.

Pickering, T., and Gorham, G., 1975, Learned heart-rate control by a patient with a ventricular parasystolic rhythm, Lancet, 1:252-253.

Pickering, T. G., and Miller, N. E., 1977, Learned voluntary control of heart rate and rhythm in two subjects with premature ventricular contractions, Brit. Heart J., 39:152-159.

Riley, D. M., and Furedy, J. J., 1981, Effects of instructions and contingency of reinforcement on the operant conditioning of human phasic heart rate change, Psychophysiology, 18:75-81.

Schneiderman, N., 1983, Behavior, autonomic function and animal models of cardiovascular pathology, in: "Biobehavioral Bases of Coronary Heart Disease", T. M. Dembroski, T. H. Schmidt, and G. Blumchen, eds., Karger, New York.

Schwartz, G. E., 1975, Biofeedback, self-regulation, and the patterning of physiological processes, Am. Scientist, 63:314-324.

Sirota, A. D., Schwartz, G. E., and Shapiro, D., 1974, Voluntary control of human heart rate: Effect on reaction to aversive stimulation, J. Abnormal Psychol., 83:261-267.

Sirota, A. D., Schwartz, G. E., and Shapiro, D., 1976, Voluntary control of human heart rate: Effect on reaction to aversive stimulation: A replication and extension, J. Abnormal Psychol., 85:473-477.

Stephens, J. H., Harris, A. H., Brady, J. V., and Shaffer, J. W., 1975, Psychological and physiological variables associated with large magnitude voluntary heart rate changes, Psychophysiology, 12:381-387.

Steptoe, A., 1978, The regulation of blood pressure reactions to taxing conditions using pulse transit time feedback and relaxation, Psychophysiology, 15:429-438.

Steptoe, A., and Ross, A., 1982, Voluntary control of cardiovascular reactions to demanding tasks, Biofeedback & Self-Regulation, 7:149-166.

Stern, G. S., and Elder, R. D., 1982, The role of changing incentives in feedback-assisted heart rate reduction for coronary prone adult males, Biofeedback & Self-Regulation, 7:53-69.

Stoney, C. M., Langer, A. W., and Sutterer, J. R., 1983, A comparison of feedback-assisted cardiodeceleration in Type A and B male college students: Modification of stress-induced cardiac and metabolic adjustments, Psychophysiology, 20:472-473.

Suess, W. M., Alexander, A. B., Smith, D. D., Sweeney, H. W., and Marion, R. J., 1980, The effects of psychological stress on respiration: A preliminary study of anxiety and hyperventilation, Psychophysiology, 17:535-540.

Turner, J. R., Carroll, D., and Courtney, H., 1983, Cardiac and metabolic responses to "space invaders": An instance of metabolically-exaggerated cardiac adjustment?, Psychophysiology, 20:544-549.

Twentyman, C. T., Malloy, P. F., and Green, A. S., 1979, Instructed heart rate control in a high heart rate population, J. Behavioral Med., 2:251-261.

Vandercar, D. H., Feldstein, M. A., and Soloman, H., 1977, Instrumental conditioning of human heart rate during free and controlled respiration, Bio. Psychol., 5:221-231.

Victor, R., Mainardi, A., and Shapiro, D., 1978, Effects of biofeedback and voluntary control procedures on heart rate and perception of pain during the cold pressor test, Psychosomatic Med., 40:216-225.

Wilder, J., 1967, "Stimulus and Response: The Law of Initial Value", John Wright and Sons, Bristol, England.

Williams, R. B., Lane, J. D., Kuhn, C. M., Melosh, W., White, A. D., and Schanberg, S. M., 1982, Type A behavior and elevated physiological and hemodynamic responses to cognitive tasks, Science, 218:483-485.

Williamson, D. A., and Blanchard, E. B., 1979, Heart rate and blood pressure feedback: A review of the recent experimental literature, Biofeedback & Self-Regulation, 4:1-34.

Young, L. D., and Blanchard, E. B., 1974, Effects of auditory feedback of varying information content on the self-control of heart rate, J. Gen. Psychol., 91:61-68.

THE USE OF FEEDBACK TO REDUCE THE

CARDIOVASCULAR RESPONSE TO EXERCISE

D. W. Johnston, C.R. Lo and G.V. Marie

University of Oxford

Ever since the earliest studies of cardiovascular feedback (e.g., Engel and Hansen, 1967; Brener and Hothersall, 1967) and during the brief flowering of interest in the operant control of autonomic responses in lower animals (Miller, 1969), three questions have dominated empirical, non-therapeutic studies of biofeedback-aided learning or control. These are the following:

1. Is voluntary control of autonomically innervated systems possible?
2. Does biofeedback aid such control?
3. If achieved, is this control direct and specific to the systems being fed back or part of an overall pattern of nervous and metabolic adjustments?

Other questions have, of course, been asked at various times, such as whether biofeedback should be considered as motor skill learning (Lang, 1975; Johnston and Lethem, 1981), operant conditioning (Black, Cott and Pavloski, 1977) or perhaps no learning at all (Johnston, 1977a). These questions, however, have not excited as much interest nor are they as fundamental as the three highlighted above. We do not propose to review the extensive literature on these issues (see, for example, Yates, 1980, or Williamson and Blanchard, 1979) but assume that there would be general agreement with our claim, at least, with respect to the cardiovascular system, that (1) humans can control cardiovascular responses voluntarily; (2) biofeedback seldom aids such control, at least if the goal is the reduction of cardiovascular activity; and (3) such control is not specific but is part of an overall pattern of respiratory, motor and, probably, metabolic adjustments (e.g., Obrist et al., 1975; Brener, 1974; Johnston, 1977b). Occasional rather tentative claims of specificity are made (e.g., Manuck, 1976) but have not been convincingly demonstrated. These conclusions are based, to a large extent, on studies of healthy volunteers at rest in benign environments, and the answers obtained might well be different in active or aroused subjects. It is easy to see that control could be more difficult if the subjects were alert or frightened since they might be distracted or overloaded with complex information. Alternatively, the limits set by the low levels of heart rate and blood pressure typically obtained in the laboratory may be removed in aroused subjects and effects that were previously hidden might become apparent. Different training methods might well be appropriate in different circumstances: for example, biofeedback might be incompatible with demanding cognitive tasks, and purely verbal methods, that may require less information processing, could be more effective under these circumstances. Furthermore, specific cardiovascular control might be possible if the links between metabolism and cardiovascular activity are diminished by very demanding but just possible tasks (as Obrist, 1981, has claimed).

In this paper we wish to present a series of studies on biofeedback-aided cardiovascular self-control during dynamic and static exercise. These studies were not primarily directed at the questions we have outlined above but instead were part of an examination of the possible use of cardiovascular biofeedback in the management of angina pectoris (Johnston, 1982; Johnston and Lo, 1983), but they do bear directly on the questions posed. Physical exercise offers a convenient technique for exploring these issues. It reliably produces changes in cardiovascular parameters that are less prone to habituation than those induced by psychological techniques and produces substantial changes without imposing excessive information processing demands on the subject. In addition, since both cardiovascular and somatic activity are heightened by exercise, the methodological, if not physiological, opportunities for disassociation may thereby be increased.

In our studies, we have examined cardiovascular self-control during both dynamic and static exercise. We were influenced in our decision to study this phenomenon both because of the classical view that these two types of exercise differ in their hemodynamic effects and in the mechanisms likely to be involved in the production of these effects (e.g., Tuttle and Horvath, 1957). Dynamic exercise is usually seen as producing large elevations in cardiac output, heart rate, oxygen consumption and systolic blood pressure, with little or no change or even decreases in diastolic blood pressure and peripheral resistance. The increases in cardiac output, heart rate and oxygen consumption are closely linked to each other and to the work being carried out by the subject. Static exercise, in contrast, produces much less marked increases in cardiac output, heart rate, oxygen consumption and systolic blood pressure and more marked increases in diastolic blood pressure and peripheral resistance. The cardiovascular changes are less clearly linked to oxygen consumption and, until recently, were thought to be independent of the muscle mass involved in the exercise, and determined by the most vigorously contracting muscle group, independent of size.

The picture has, in recent years, become much more complex. Blomquist et al. (1981) presented data suggesting that at least part of the difference between dynamic and static exercise may be due to the differing muscle masses involved in typical experiments, dynamic exercise normally using much larger muscles than static exercise. Mitchell et al. (1981) and Seals et al. (1983) have disputed the claim of Lind and McNichol (1967) and others that the cardiovascular response to static exercise is independent of muscle mass and have shown that larger muscles produce larger responses. The picture has been further complicated by the findings of Petrofsky and Lind (1980) that the cardiovascular response to static exercise is also determined by the composition of the muscle, muscles that contain a higher percentage of fast twitch fibers producing larger cardiovascular responses. These complexities need to be born in mind when the results of the self-control studies are evaluated.

CARDIOVASCULAR BIOFEEDBACK DURING DYNAMIC EXERCISE

Prior to and during the period in which we conducted our studies, two reports appeared on the effects of heart rate biofeedback during dynamic exercise. Goldstein et al. (1977) reported that heart rate feedback during exercise on a treadmill led to reliable lowering of both heart rate and systolic blood pressure in feedback subjects when compared to a mixed group of subjects who variously had either exercise training alone or both exercise and instructions to lower heart rate and blood pressure. Surprisingly, subjects who had initially exercised without biofeedback, failed to benefit from feedback when they later received it. Perski and Engel (1980), in a similar study of subjects exercising on a bicycle ergometer, reported that the five subjects receiving heart rate feedback, reliably reduced their heart rate but not their systolic blood pressure compared to five subjects who simply exercised. In this study exercise-only subjects did benefit when they went on to receive biofeedback. With respect to the three questions posed in the introduction, it appears reasonably convincing that question 1 can be answered in the affirmative, human subjects can reduce heart rate, at least, while exercising. These two studies did not focus closely on the other two issues. Our experiments seek to cast further light on all three questions.

In our first study (Lo and Johnston, 1984a) we compared feedback of heart period (interbeat interval, IBI) with verbal instructions exhorting the subject to attempt to lower both heart rate and blood pressure while exercising at a constant workload on a simple bicycle ergometer. Because of our interest in the treatment of patients with angina pectoris, we also included a condition in which subjects received feedback of a composite variable that correlates highly with the rate pressure product (RPP), a measure conventionally used in cardiology as an indirect index of myocardial oxygen consumption and hence closely related to the onset of pain in angina. The RPP (heart rate multiplied by systolic blood pressure) correlates over 0.9 with the product of IBI and pulse transit time, the latter being a moderately strong correlate of systolic blood pressure (Marie et al., 1984). We therefore provided one group of subjects with IBI x pulse transit time feedback. Pulse transit time was taken as the time between the R-wave of the ECG and the arrival of the peripheral pulse at the wrist. This measure is conventionally abbreviated to RPI. Three groups of twelve healthy volunteers received four sessions of visual analogue feedback of either IBI, product (IBI x RPI) or verbal instructions. On each session five 6-minute feedback trials were provided. Figures 1 and 2 show the mean alterations in IBI and RPI from an 8-minute exercise baseline at the start of each session, i.e., subjects who did not change their performance during feedback trials would score zero on this measure. The results are very similar on both IBI and RPI. There was very little difference between the three conditions on the first session, but on subsequent sessions, subjects receiving product feedback increased both IBI and RPI (i.e., lowered heart rate and, probably, SBP) by reliably greater amounts than did instruction-only subjects. These findings are, therefore, broadly in line with those of Goldstein et al. and Perski and Engel, and extend their studies by suggesting that biofeedback is particularly effective in aiding cardiovascular control when compared to purely verbal methods, that were totally ineffective. It should be noted that subjects receiving purely verbal instructions appeared to deteriorate somewhat after the first session of training. This deterioration, although not statistically significant, may suggest that part of the power of feedback is motivational and may, therefore be achieved by other techniques.

In the second study (Lo and Johnston, 1984b) the cardiovascular effects of product feedback during dynamic exercise was compared with exercise alone or with relaxation instructions given during exercise. The latter were based on Benson's analysis of the relaxation response (Benson et al., 1974). Steptoe and Ross (1982) have shown that such relaxation instructions attenuate the pressor response to arousing cognitive tasks and, at the very least, may serve to increase subject compliance and motivation so that they persist with their attempts to lower heart rate and blood pressure. In most respects, the design of this study was similar to

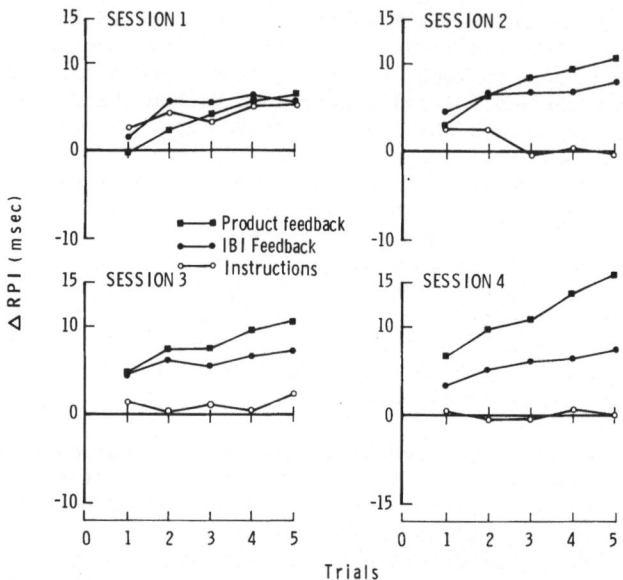

Fig. 1. Change in RPI from an exercise baseline in subjects exercising
on a bicycle ergometer.

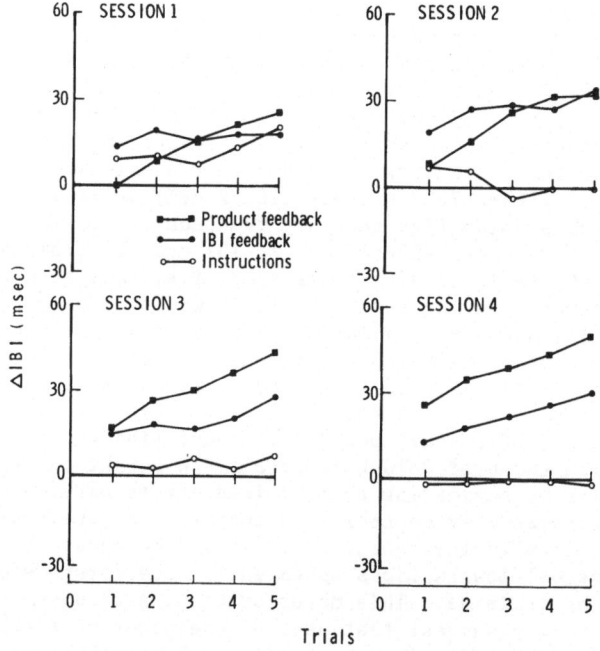

Fig. 2. Change in IBI from an exercise baseline in subjects exercising on
a bicycle ergometer.

the previous one, except that on each session six feedback trials were
provided, and on two of the sessions, feedback was provided while the
subjects were not exercising (the result of the latter sessions will not
be presented). In addition to IBI and RPI, respiration rate and a correlate of respiratory amplitude were measured using a bellows placed around
the lower chest. As before, there were twelve subjects in each group. As

can be seen from Figures 3 and 4, subjects receiving product feedback
lengthened IBI and RPI significantly more than either relaxation or
exercise-only subjects. The latter did not differ from each other or
from baseline. Taken together, these two experiments demonstrate that
cardiovascular feedback can reduce the cardiovascular response to dynamic
exercise while neither relaxation training, verbal instructions or exercise
itself had any such effect.

The issue of the specificity of biofeedback-aided learning was studied
by examining the changes in respiratory rate and amplitude. Respiratory
rate was reliably and consistently slowed in subjects receiving product
feedback so that compared to an exercise baseline, their intercycle time
was increased by 1633 msecs, whereas relaxation subjects only increased by
a non-significant 193 msecs and exercise alone by 39 msecs. That is,
respiration rate slowed in the feedback subjects from approximately 20
cycles per minute to 15 cycles per minute while exercising. There were no
consistent changes that differentiated training conditions on the amplitude
measure. It therefore appears that feedback during exercise, as with
feedback in the resting state, is associated with an overall pattern of
physiological change and is not specific to the system being fed back.

CARDIOVASCULAR CONTROL DURING STATIC EXERCISE

Clemens and Shattock (1979) have reported that subjects can both
increase and decrease heart rate with the aid of feedback while carrying
out a voluntary hand grip. It is not known whether feedback is necessary
for this control. We examined an analogous issue by comparing the effects
of RPI feedback with verbal instructions in subjects attempting to control
their blood pressure during a brief 50% maximum voluntary contraction using
a hand dynamometer (Marie, 1982).

We used essentially the same design in three studies with broadly
similar results and in this paper we shall report only on the final and
most comprehensive of these studies. Two groups of twelve volunteers

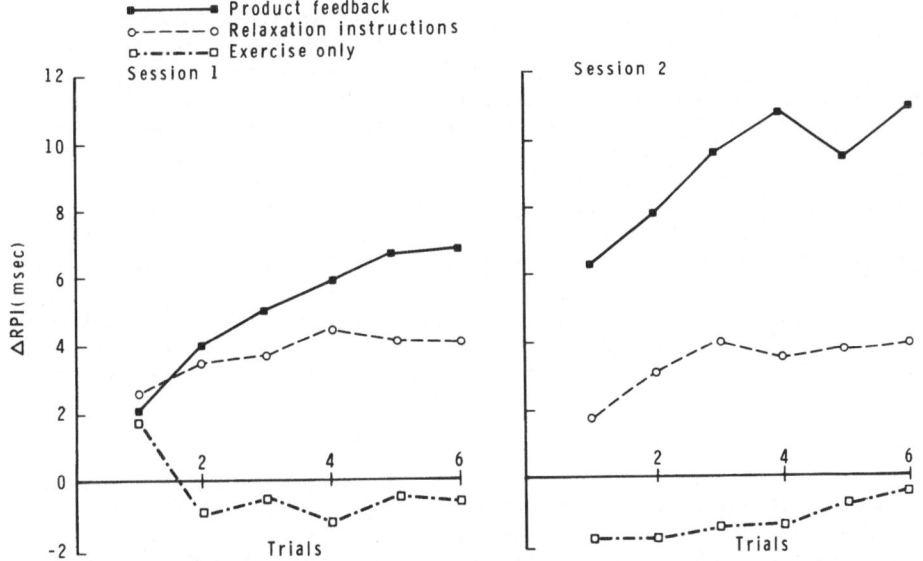

Fig. 3. Change in RPI from an exercise baseline in subjects exercising on
          a bicycle ergometer.

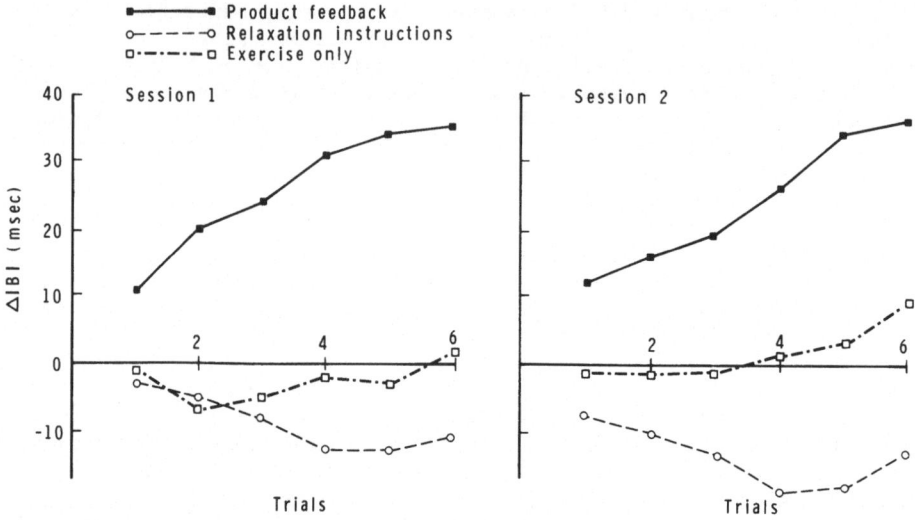

Fig. 4. Change in IBI from an exercise baseline in subjects exercising on a bicycle ergometer.

attempted to lower blood pressure during a 50% MVC of 30 seconds duration. Feedback subjects received a complex form of RPI feedback in which the current RPI was displayed as an illuminated spot on a video display unit (VDU). This spot varied along the vertical axis depending on the length of the RPI. Over a 30-second period each successive RPI appeared as a point on a graph-like display that built up from left to right across the screen, the previous RPI's remaining visible. Every 30 seconds the screen cleared and the display started to build up again from the left. The subject, therefore, had available his current RPI and a record of his previous performance. This display is quite different from that used either in the studies of dynamic exercise, where a conventional speedometer-like display was used, or, indeed, in any of our previous biofeedback studies. The feedback was provided during exercise and for the following 60-second recovery period. The subjects received four sessions of feedback training, and on each session they received ten training trials, on five of which they carried out the static exercise, the other five being conventional self-control trials carried out at rest. Subjects in the no-feedback condition were simply instructed to attempt to reduce the blood pressure rise caused by exercise and to speed the recovery as much as possible but given no further instructions. Subjects in this condition also watched a non-informative VDU display resembling that seen by feedback subjects. Previous research in our laboratory has shown (Steptoe, 1977) that part of the effects of biofeedback in lowering cardiovascular activity are masked by the arousing effects of the feedback display. This can be allowed for by requiring non-feedback subjects to attend to a similar display. The results, for both IBI and RPI, in the form of changes from a rest period at the start of each session, are shown in Figure 5. It is readily apparent that there is no substantial difference between the feedback and instruction-only conditions, either during the exercise or the recovery period.

Two other experiments have also failed to demonstrate any convincing feedback effect during static exercise (Marie, 1982). However, detailed examination of the pattern of results of the feedback subjects in these studies shows a slightly unusual picture, since feedback subjects apparently perform slightly better than no-feedback subjects for 30 seconds, then the difference disappears and then reappears again. This may be just

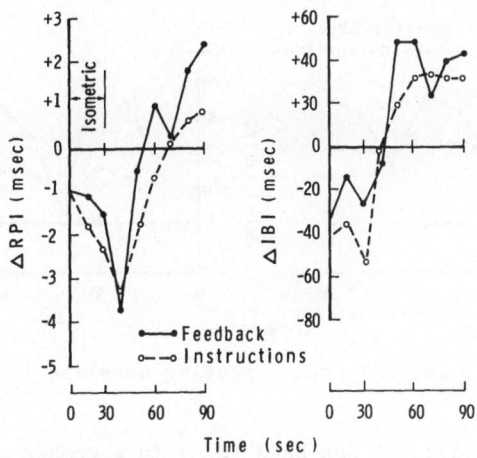

Fig. 5. Change in RPI and IBI from a resting baseline in subjects carrying
out and recovering from contracting a hand dynamometer at 50% MVC
for 30 seconds.

change variation, but, in fact, exactly the same pattern is seen in a much
clearer form during the trials without exercise (see Figure 6) and is
plausibly explained by reference to the feedback display. It will be
recalled that in the static exercise studies this display built up for
30 seconds and was cleared during which time there was a brief gap and a
message was displayed on the screen instructing subjects to continue to
control their blood pressure. The apparent development and loss of control, seen in Figure 6, is almost certainly due to subjects displaying
control when the feedback display was present and either losing or or
relinquishing it during the period when the screen was cleared. The same
pattern is seen in an attenuated form during the exercise trials. It is,
therefore, possible that there is a slight feedback effect during static
exercise.

     Such minutia aside, it is reasonable to conclude that we have provided
no evidence that control of the cardiovascular system during static exercise is aided by biofeedback. Since no other physiological systems were
measured in this experiment, it is not possible to comment directly on the
likely mechanisms for this effect. It would almost certainly be infor-
mative to record respiration during the 30 second period; subjects may
well have slowed their breathing or, indeed, held their breath for part of
the time. Furthermore, we failed to include in any of our experiments a
static exercise-only condition, and, therefore, we are unable to comment on
whether control is possible during such exercise. Clemens and Shattock
have claimed that subjects are able to reduce the heart rate response to
static exercise. This question could benefit from further exploration
since in Clemens and Shattock's study, the use of voluntary control was
confounded with practise at the exercise. If the response to such exercise
reduces with repetition, the apparent effect of voluntary control in reducing the heart rate response will be inflated.

     In discussing these findings we would like to focus on the following
issues:

1. Is the effect of feedback during dynamic exercise different from the
   effect found in other circumstances?
2. Why is feedback ineffective during static exercise?
3. What are the mechanisms undering the effectiveness of feedback during
   dynamic exercise?

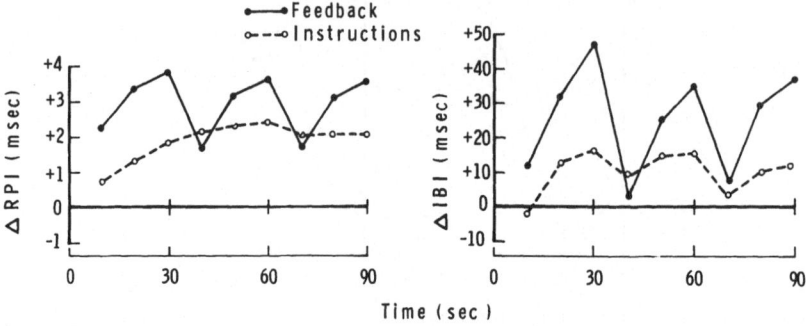

Fig. 6.   Change in RPI and IBI from a resting baseline in subjects at rest.

As we stated earlier, it has been found in a number of studies that
cardiovascular feedback in resting subjects is no more effective in the
lowering of heart rate and blood pressure than other methods that do not
use feedback. This conclusion should be qualified by pointing out that
two studies, Steptoe (1977) and this study by Marie, just described and
illustrated in Figure 6, have both shown effects of feedback in resting
subjects when controls for the arousing effects of the feedback display
were incorporated. The first possibility to consider, therefore, is simply
that exercise, by arousing the subject, minimises the arousing effect of
the feedback display and hence enables the underlying feedback effect to
appear. It is difficult to refute this argument without specific studies,
but the size of the advantage obtained by feedback when arousal is controlled for appears to be different from that obtained during exercise.
Compare, for example, Figure 6 and Figures 3 and 4; feedback only confers
an advantage of 2 or 3 msecs RPI in the resting subjects but anything up
to 15 msecs in those exercising. It is acknowledged that it is difficult
to compare directly studies with such different training procedures, length
of trials, and other features, but it does appear that feedback during
exercise does confer a greater advantage on subjects than is conferred by
controlling for the arousing effects of display alone.

The second possibility is that the elevated baselines which are produced by dynamic exercise, eliminate baseline effects that otherwise reduce
the effects of feedback at rest, and hence larger effects can be demonstrated. In the second dynamic exercise study (Lo and Johnston, 1984b), we
included a rest condition, and the changes produced by feedback at rest and
during dynamic exercise were not greatly different; the difference lay in
the advantage conferred by feedback over the alternative procedures during
exercise. The latter were essentially ineffective and did not enable the
subjects to control their cardiovascular responses to exercise to any
significant extent, whereas at rest they were moderately successful. This,
therefore, raises as a real possibility the proposition that cardiovascular
feedback during dynamic exercise does have unique effects that are not
displayed under all other circumstances. This proposition will be discussed more fully after the findings with static exercise have been considered.

Reduction of the cardiovascular response to static exercise was not
aided by biofeedback to any significant extent. Doubtless there are many
possible explanations for this apparent difference between dynamic and
static exercise. For example, the amount of training offered in our static
exercise studies was much less than those offered in dynamic exercise
(because of the difficulty of repeatedly carrying out a static exercise at
50% MVC). Furthermore, during static exercise, the trials were of shorter
duration, the feedback was unusual, and the cardiovascular changes were a

complex variation in levels over a 90-second trial. This may have made the discrimination of successful control strategies difficult. It is also possible that the static exercise imposed greater information-processing demands on the subject or was more distracting than the rather simple cycling exercise used for studying dynamic exercise. (It is certainly the case that the static exercise was subjectively more demanding.) Few of these possibilities can be excluded on the basis of the currently available information, but it is likely that at least part of the explanation lies in the nature of the cardiovascular effects of static exercise and not in the learning parameters.

As we indicated in the introduction, it was held for some time that the cardiovascular response to static exercise is dependent on the vigor of the contraction in the most vigorously contracting muscle group and not on the total muscle mass involved. Since the 50% MVC involved in the hand grip in this experiment certainly involves the most vigorous contraction of the subjects' muscles in this experiment (there being no reason why they should, and many reasons why they should not, be carrying out a more vigorous contraction in some other muscle group), it can be argued that minor reductions in the activity of other muscles not involved in the static exercise would have little or no cardiovascular effects. If alterations in muscular activity are a mechanism for cardiovascular self-control, as seem very likely, then static exercise may offer few such possibilities. However, as we have seen, it is now held that the muscle mass involved in the static exercise does effect the cardiovascular response, thereby allowing the possibility that reductions in muscle activity in muscles irrelevant to the isometric exercise, could lower the pressor responses by lowering the total muscle mass involved. We doubt whether this is a probable explanation of our results.

The original experiments, such as those by Lind and McNicol (1967), showing the independence of the pressor response from muscle mass compared, for example, isometric exercise with one forearm with exercise involving both forearms. The latter did not produce a greater cardiovascular response. The more recent studies showing the effects of mass on muscle tension have compared widely different muscle masses such as hand grip with a complex lifting exercise involving both legs, arms and trunk (Seals et al., 1983). The muscles involved in our experiments are much more akin to that studied by Lind and McNicol than the more recent researchers, and, therefore, it is likely that the response to static exercise in our experiments is independent of any variation in the muscle mass involved. Therefore, it is improbable that minor reductions in irrelevant muscles that were at or near rest would have an effect on the cardiovascular response. We would, therefore, maintain that in our static exercise studies the reduction of irrelevant muscular activity, which is a likely mechanism of cardiovascular self-control, is not available to any significant extent and so such self-control is either impossible or very slight - too slight to be aided by feedback.

Let us finally return to the mechanisms of control during dynamic exercise. Since we favor a muscular and metabolic explanation for our failure to find effects during the static exercise, it is hardly surprising that we also favor a somatic explanation of our positive findings during dynamic exercise. The cardiovascular effects of dynamic exercise are directly related to the work load and oxygen consumption that subjects incur in carrying out these exercises. It is very likely, particularly in the untrained subjects, that many irrelevant muscles are involved when exercising on a treadmill or a bicycle ergometer and the same work load could be maintained with reduced oxygen consumption if subjects learn to suppress activity in these irrelevant muscles. We did not have the facilities to measure oxygen consumption in our experiments but the slowed respiration rate observed is certainly consistent with the position that subjects learned to work more efficiently with the aid of feedback. We are, therefore, proposing that cardiovascular feedback can be effective when there is significant irrelevant muscular activity, the reduction of which reduces heart rate and blood pressure. At rest in benign environments, irrelevant muscular activity is slight, and so feedback offers only a very limited possibility of control (one that may be obscured by the arousing effects of the feedback display). During static exercise of the type we have studied, the irrelevant muscles may not affect the cardiovascular response, and, therefore, cannot be used to reduce it. In dynamic exercise, in contrast, there is, we are arguing, a considerable amount of irrelevant muscular activity that can be controlled and hence reduce the cardiovascular response to that exercise.

REFERENCES

Benson, H., Beary, J. F., and Carol, M. P., 1974, The relaxation response, Psychiatry, 37:37-46.

Black, A. H., Cott, A., and Pavloski, R., 1977, The operant learning theory approach to biofeedback training, in: "Biofeedback, Theory and Research", G. E. Schwartz and J. Beatty, eds., pp. 89-127, Academic Press, New York.

Blomquist, C. G., Lewis, S. F., Taylor, W. F., and Graham, R. M., 1981, Similarity of the hemodynamic responses to static and dynamic exercise of small muscle groups, Circ. Res., 48:187-192.

Brener, J., 1974, A general model of voluntary control applied to the phenomena of learned cardiovascular change, in: "Cardiovascular Psychophysiology - Current Issues in Response Mechanisms, Biofeedback and Methodology", P. A. Obrist, A. H. Black, J. Brener and L. V. Di Cara, eds., pp. 365-391, Aldine, Chicago.

Brener, J., and Hothersall, D., 1967, Paced respiration and heart rate control, Psychophysiology, 4:1-6.

Clemens, W. J., and Shattock, R. J., 1979, Voluntary heart rate control during static muscular effort, Psychophysiology, 16:327-332.

Engel, B. T., and Hansen, S. P., 1967, Operant conditioning of heart rate slowing, Psychophysiology, 4:83-89.

Goldstein, D. S., Ross, R. S., and Brady, J. V., 1977, Biofeedback heart rate training during exercise, Biofeedback & Self-Regulation, 2:107-126.

Johnston, D. W., 1977a, Biofeedback, verbal instructions and the motor skills analogy, in: "Biofeedback and Behavior", J. Beatty and H. Legewie, eds., pp. 331-341, Plenum, New York.

Johnston, D. W., 1977b, Feedback and instructional effects in the voluntary control of digital pulse amplitudes, Biol. Psychol., 5:159-171.

Johnston, D. W., 1982, The behavioral treatment of the symptoms of ischaemic heart disease, in: "The Behavioral Treatment of Disease", R. Surwit, R. Williams and A. Steptoe, eds., pp. 115-127, Plenum, New York.

Johnston, D. W., and Lethem, J., 1981, The production of specific decreases in interbeat interval and the motor skills analogy, Psychophysiology, 18:288-300.

Johnston, D. W., and Lo, C. R., 1983, The effects of cardiovascular feedback and relaxation on angina pectoris, Behavioral Psychotherapy, 11:257-264.

Lang, P. J., 1975, Acquisition of heart rate control: method theory and clinical implications, in: "Clinical Applications of Psychophysiology", D. C. Fowles, ed., pp. 167-191, Columbia University Press, New York.

Lind, A. R., and McNicol, G. W., 1967, Circulatory responses to sustained hand-grip contractions performed during other exercise, both rhythmic and static, J. Physiol. (London), 192:595-607.

Lo, C. R., and Johnston, D. W., 1984a, Cardiovascular feedback during
    dynamic exercise, Psychophysiology, 21:199-206.
Lo, C. R., and Johnston, D. W., 1984b, The self-control of the cardio-
    vascular response to exercise using feedback of the product of
    interbeat interval and pulse transit time, Psychosomatic Medicine,
    46:115-125.
Manuck, S. B., 1976, The voluntary control of heart rate under differential
    somatic constraint, Biofeedback & Self-Regulation, 1:273-284.
Marie, G. V., 1982, Voluntary control of cardiovascular activity during
    rest and physical exercise. Thesis submitted for D.Phil., Oxford
    University.
Marie, G. V., Lo, C. R., Van Jones, J., and Johnston, D. W., 1984, The
    relationship between arterial blood pressure and pulse transit time
    during dynamic and static exercise, Psychophysiology, 21:521-527.
Miller, N. E., 1969, Learning of visceral and glandular response, Science,
    163:434-445.
Mitchell, J. H., Schibye, B., Payne, F. C., and Saltin, B., 1981, Response
    of arterial blood pressure to static exercise in relation to muscle
    mass, force development, and electromyographic activity, Circ. Res.,
    170-175.
Obrist, P. A., 1981, Cardiovascular Psychophysiology: a perspective,
    Plenum, New York.
Obrist, P. A., Galosy, R. A., Lawler, J. E., Gaebelein, C. J., Howard, J.
    L., and Shanks, E. M., 1975, Operant conditioning of heart rate:
    somatic correlates, Psychophysiology, 12:445-455.
Perski, A., and Engel, B. T., 1980, The role of behavioral conditioning in
    the cardiovascular adjustment to exercise, Biofeedback & Self-
    Regulation, 5:91-104.
Petrofsky, J. S., and Lind, A. R., 1980, The blood pressure response during
    isometric exercise in fast and slow twitch skeletal muscles in the
    cat, European J. Appl. Physiol. & Occup. Physiol., 44:223-230.
Seals, D. R., Washburn, R. A., Hanson, P. G., Painter, P. L., and Nagle, F.
    J., 1983, Increased cardiovascular response to static contraction of
    larger muscle groups, J. Appl. Physiol., 54:434-437.
Steptoe, A., 1977, Voluntary blood pressure reductions measured with pulse
    transit time: training conditions and reactions to mental work,
    Psychophysiology, 14:492-498.
Steptoe, A., and Ross, A., 1982, Voluntary control of cardiovascular
    reactions to demanding tasks, Biofeedback & Self-Regulation,
    7:149-166.
Tuttle, W. W., and Horvath, S. M., 1957, Comparison of the effects of
    static and dynamic work on blood pressure and heart rate, J. Appl.
    Physiology, 10:294-296.
Williamson, D. A., and Blanchard, E. B., 1979, Heart rate and blood
    pressure feedback: 1. A review of the recent experimental
    literature, Biofeedback & Self-Regulation, 4:1-34.
Yates, A. J., 1980, Biofeedback and the modification of behavior, Plenum,
    New York.

SPECTRAL ANALYSIS OF BIOFEEDBACK INDUCED HEART RATE

DECREASES IN SINUS TACHYCARDIA

Kees HL Janssen* and Rob Beckering

Tilburg University
TNO Soesterberg

Self-control of heart rate has been one of the most extensively studied areas in biofeedback research. Overall, the impression nowadays is that when given exteroceptive feedback of cardiac activity, most subjects can gain control to some extent over their heart rate. In this Chapter, we will first give an outline of the role that respiratory and somatic factors have played in human heart rate feedback research. We will then discuss what impact this has had on the development of heart rate feedback as a tool in clinical practice, and more specifically, its application for sinus tachycardia. Furthermore, background information is given on symptoms, etiology, and conventional therapy of sinus tachycardia. Subsequently we will present some recent findings on application of heart rate feedback for this arrhythmia from our own laboratory. Lastly, we will show how the application of spectral analysis may contribute towards unravelling some of the neuro-physiological mechanisms involved in sinus tachycardia and its treatment with heart rate feedback.

RESPIRATORY AND SOMATIC FACTORS IN EXPERIMENTAL HEART RATE FEEDBACK

Of any single factor that has been suggested to be of influence for the efficacy of heart rate feedback training, somatic influences appear to be capable of producing the most significant heart rate changes. Within somatic mediation, respiratory influences have received far more attention than effects due to muscular changes (Williamson and Blanchard, 1979; McCanne and Sandman, 1976). This is understandable since it has been known for some time that there are sizable cyclic variations in heart rate that occur in phase with respiration: respiratory sinus arrhythmia (RSA). Moreover, it has been demonstrated several times that alterations in respiratory patterns can cause appreciable changes in heart rate (Davis and Neilson, 1967; Sroufe, 1971; Johns, 1970). In the emerging area of heart rate feedback, an important question to be answered was whether subjects could learn to control their heart rate directly, obviously underscoring the necessity to control for respiration. This often was done through some sort of pacing procedure, but instructed variations and correlational techniques were also applied (Holmes et al., 1980). The results of these studies with controlled procedures were that subjects could still acquire

---

* In fond memory of my mother.

control of heart rate, but with smaller effects as compared to free respiration. Obrist and his colleagues have convincingly demonstrated that
the fewer the constraints on subjects, the better their ability to change
heart rate (Obrist, 1976; Obrist, Galosy, Lawler, Gaebelein, Howard and
Shanks, 1975). As constraints were added to respiration and skeletal
muscle manoevers, smaller changes could be reached. However, even in the
most restricted condition, subjects could still reliably show some control
of heart rate. Furthermore, since the amount of control was of limited
magnitude even in the free respiration condition, serious doubts were
raised as to the practical usefulness of heart rate feedback per se. This
was especially true for biofeedback assisted heart rate deceleration where
'overall' positive results have not been as numerous or of the same magnitude as with heart rate acceleration. This has brought about the bizarre
situation of heart rate feedback being perhaps the most intensively re-
searched biofeedback area in experimental psychology, in which evidence on
parameters relevant to outcome of training continues to be built up, but
without resulting in the development of significant clinical applications.

CLINICAL HEART RATE FEEDBACK: THE CASE OF SINUS TACHYCARDIA

This paradoxical situation probably could have been circumvented if
in discussing the magnitude of treatment effects on heart rate, there had
been greater consideration of the biological limits of the cardiovascular
system, i.e., the range of its possible variations which contribute towards
the healthy homeostatic functioning of the organism. The subjects in most
of these feedback studies have been young (college age) and free of
disease. Since the normal resting heart rate is usually about 70 beats
per minute (bpm), the potential range of change to be expected for heart
rate acceleration and deceleration would be on the order of 100 bpm and
15 bpm respectively (Cheatle and Weiss, 1982). Thus as for deceleration
effects, the observed magnitude of effect should always be evaluated
against this limited range in which decreases in heart rate can still be
said to be biologically meaningful. Also, since clinical populations may
have resting heart rates that may well differ from 70 bpm, no definite
inferences on the therapeutic potential of heart rate feedback can be made
from these studies with nonclinical populations.

This point becomes especially pungent if one considers the several
reports that demonstrate the potential of learned deceleration of heart
rate for sinus tachycardia (Engel and Bleecker, 1974; Scott, Blanchard,
Edmundson and Young, 1973; Vaitl, 1975; Janssen, 1983). Sinus tachycardia
refers to an abnormally increased heart rate in which the rhythm still
generates from the sinoatrial node. Hence the electrocardiogram has normal
QRS complexes, except that the heart rate is considerably higher than
normal. Three independent general causes of tachycardia are increased body
temperature, toxic conditions of the heart, and stimulation of the heart by
the autonomic nerves (Guyton, 1981). In healthy individuals, sinus tachycardia occurs as an adaptation mechanism for adjusting cardiac output to
the demands of the organism, e.g., in physical exercise or emotion (Robles
de Medina et al., 1980), or in congitive-informational tasks (Mulder and
Mulder, 1981). In cases of chronic or recurrent sinus tachycardia, if
differential diagnosis excludes organic pathology, psychosocial and psychodynamic factors can be found to be involved. Symptoms that often accompany
the tachycardia include strong precordial pulsation, respiratory distress,
chest symptoms, and jerking pulse (Garnier, 1981). Thus tachycardia may
constitute a frightening, burdensome and taxing experience to the person,
and one way for it to persist is when its interpretation (or cognitive
attribution) induces a state of anxiety in the subject. The physiological
changes thus brought about will intensify the cardiac sensations, and this
will anchor the subject to his interpretations and anxiety, i.e., a vicious
circle as described by Liebhart (1974).

Besides a discomfort in itself, sinus tachycardia may also add considerably to risk of later hypertension. Although not all patients with borderline hypertension will later develop sustained hypertension (Julius, 1977), there is some evidence that when borderline hypertension and tachycardia are combined, the risk for later hypertension is particularly high (Paffenbarger et al., 1968). This finding seems to confirm the results of an earlier study by Levi et al. (1945), which also established that tachycardia during youth, even without blood pressure elevation, carried an excessive risk for future hypertension. Instigated by such epidemiological findings, Manuck and Proietti (1982) have extrapolated from their experiments on high heart rate reactors with a parental history of hypertension, that these subjects may be among those most likely to develop hypertension in later life. The same inference was made by Light and Obrist (1980) when they observed that subjects with both marginally elevated casual systolic pressure and high heart rate reactivity to stress, had by far the highest incidence of parental hypertension. Steptoe et al. (1984) report on evidence suggesting more directly that exaggerated cardiac responsiveness to active challenges may be characteristic of the prehypertensive profile. Lastly with monkeys, an association has been found between heart rate reactivity under stress and the development of atherosclerosis (Manuck et al., 1983).

Treatment of sinus tachycardia commonly is with beta-adrenergic blocking agents. Many of these are associated with undesirable side-effects. For example propranolol may cause or worsen heart block or cardiac failure (Winkle et al., 1975). Another effect may be irreversible reduction of glomurelar filtration rate, which would limit beta blocker use for patients with pre-existing renal insufficiency (Bauer and Brooks, 1979). Other side-effects include fatigue, depression, nausea, diarrhea, hyperglycemia and hyperosmolar coma (Winkle et al., 1975). While not all beta-blocking agents require as much caution as propranolol, one general side-effect they share is the induction of bronchospasm, which renders them unsuitable for patients who besides their tachycardia display asthmatic symptoms.

HEART RATE FEEDBACK FOR SINUS TACHYCARDIA: SOME RECENT FINDINGS

From the foregoing discussion, it seems possible that self-control procedures, such as heart rate feedback could contribute to the treatment of sinus tachycardia. Unfortunately, much of what we know about this application of heart rate feedback derives from case studies, a fairly low level of inference (Engel and Bleecker, 1974); Scott et al., 1973; Vaitl, 1975; Blanchard and Abel, 1976; Janssen, 1983). The main problem with these case studies is that we cannot be sure to what extent they are representative for the entire population of psychosomatic sinus tachycardia. Therefore, in our laboratory we designed a group outcome study in an attempt to establish a higher level of inference for this application of heart rate feedback. After cardiological examination, seven patients with elevated heart rate and related symptoms were diagnosed as having psychosomatic sinus tachycardia (Table 1). After two baseline recording sessions, treatment consisted of twelve heart rate feedback sessions twice weekly, in which the subject trained to lower heart rate with analogue visual and auditory signals. Three months after treatment, patients returned for a follow-up session. Patients charted their complaints every four hours throughout baseline and treatment period, and again two weeks prior to the follow-up session. The results of this study are reported elsewhere in detail (Janssen and Berger, 1985), but in summary their analysis reveals the following: as a group there is a clear improvement over treatment in terms of charted subjective complaints. Likewise, significant decreases in heart rate values were observed, although for three patients, running baseline values remained constant. The latter patients

Table 1. Patient Characteristics upon Intake. History (Hst) Refers to Earliest Documented Tachycardia as Established by Medical Examination and Persistence of Complaint and Symptoms

Age	m/f	Hst	Medication	Symptoms	Smoking	Alcohol	Other Usage
A 37	f	1yr	4*isoptin80/d 4*inderal10/d	fear of faint; visus disturbance + tinnitus during, precordial pulsation after effort; incid. PVC's	–	–	–
B 51	m	7mo	–	respiratory distress, precordial symptoms after effort	–	–	–
C 55	m	5yr	–	precordial pulsations, dyspnoe, anxiety, incid. PVC's, nightmares with tachycardia	–	–	–
D 27	m	1yr	–	incid. tension headache disturbed sleep, high heart rate reactor	20cgts/d	some	–
E 40	f	6mo*	–	palpitations, disturbed sleep, feels agitated, irritated	–	–	–
F 18	f	4yr	–	early fatigue, rest after effort worsens tachycardia causing panic, incid. migraine	–	–	–
G 23	f	2yr	2*Lopressor 50/d	disturbed sleep, rest after effort worsens tachycardia, tingling hands + feet, headaches	–	–	–

*Intermittent palpitations occurred since early adulthood.

did attain, however, considerable in-session control of their heart rate, and going by the charting of their complaints, two of them definitely improved with therapy. For all patients as a group, effects of treatment on heart rate and on complaint endured at follow-up (Figure 1).

The clinical usefulness of heart rate feedback was further supported by significant changes in neuroticism and neurosomatization, and by patients' reports of positive effects of treatment on their life situation. What subsequently intrigued us was which processes might have been at work in this treatment to explain these effects. Several alternative explanations can be raised for the effects obtained. One is that nonspecific factors have been involved that could not be eliminated because of the design of the study. Going by verbal comments of the patients, the novelty of the treatment applied must have influenced them somehow in the charting of their complaints. Also habituation may have had its contribution, as two baseline sessions may not have been sufficient to become at ease in the artificial situation of a recording baseline session. On the other hand,

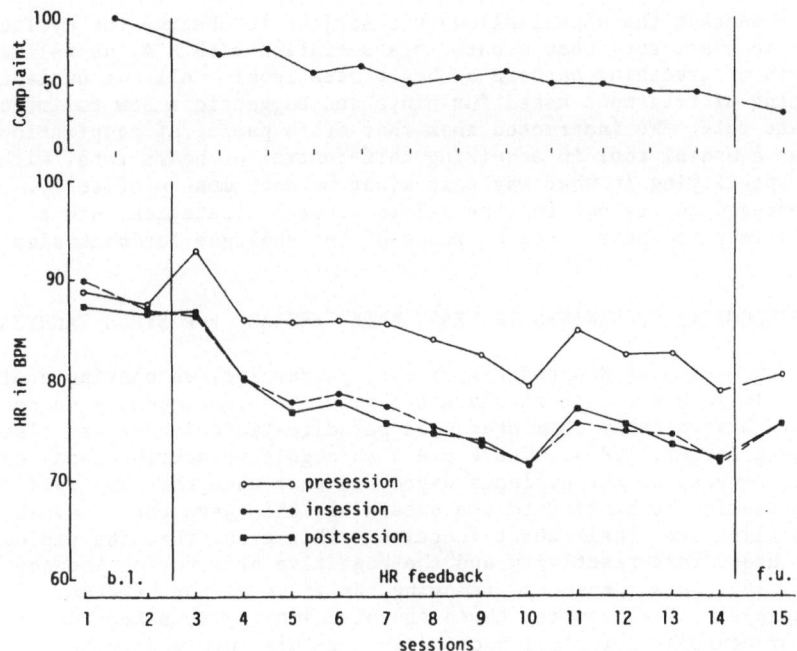

Fig. 1. Effects of heart rate feedback averaged for 7 sinus tachycardia
patients. Upper panel shows results for subjective complaint,
expressed as percentage of baseline score. Lower panel gives
average heart rate values (bpm) of three recording trials of
3 min in each session: pre-session, beginning of session without
feedback signals; in-session, during session with feedback
signals; post-session, end of session without feedback signals.

specific factors may still have been at work in this treatment along with
nonspecific factors. Specificity is suggested by the finding for heart
rate data of a significant Sessions x Trials interaction, indicating that
at end of treatment with the aid of feedback signals patients were able to
attain considerably lower in-session levels of heart rate as compared to
without signals during baseline.

It is noteworthy here to look at earlier reports on clinical heart
rate feedback, where compared to the twelve sessions as employed in our
study extensive training periods were required: Engel and Bleecker (1974)
21 sessions, Scott et al. (1973) 19 sessions. Importantly, in contrast to
the analogue signals (visual and auditory) in our study, binary feedback
signals were employed in these studies, and this does not allow the subject
to observe directly the possible interdependence of heart rate with somatic
and respiratory activity. Following the experimental tradition of establishing operant conditioning of heart rate without any mediation (e.g.,
Miller, 1969), early studies on heart rate feedback with humans merely
considered somatic and respiratory activity as nuisance variables. In
clinical trials of heart rate feedback in order to eliminate these factors,
not only were the feedback signals employed binary, but also the subject
was instructed that the response being monitored was not related to respiration nor to muscle tension. This attitude of methodological rigor,
although laudable in itself, seriously hampered the development of heart
rate feedback towards clinical maturity. Only later has it become clear
that with analogue signals the effects of heart rate feedback are superior
to those obtained with binary signals (Blanchard and Epstein, 1978; Colgan,
1977). It is not mere speculation that the decisive factor in this dif-

ference is whether the signal allows the subject to observe the cyclic variation in heart rate that occurs in association with RSA, as well as the effects of breathing pattern on heart rate level. All our patients in beginning of treatment asked for hints and suggestions how to influence their heart rate. We instructed them that often pacing of respiration had proven a useful tool in acquiring self-control of heart rate, without, however, specifiying in what way this might be done most profitably. They were encouraged to try out for themselves several strategies, and to monitor the effects on heart rate by means of the analogue feedback signals.

NEUROPHYSIOLOGICAL MECHANISMS IN HEART RATE FEEDBACK FOR SINUS TACHYCARDIA

The assumption of RSA and respiratory patterning, as playing a significant role in heart rate feedback training, has consequences on several levels. We have already commented upon paradigmatic consequences elsewhere (Janssen and Berger, 1985). There are also cognitive-attributional consequences: several of our patients expressed that when they observed the close association of heart rate and breathing, this gave them a sense of controllability over their heart function. This means that the vicious circle of heart rate reactivity and the cognitive attribution thereof (Liebhart, 1974) was opened up, removing, as it were, the keystone of the symptom complex. Furthermore, there are also implications for our understanding of neurophysiological mechanisms possibly involved in heart rate feedback. One major hiatus here concerns the relative importance of both division of the autonomic nervous system in the human learning of heart rate control through biofeedback. However, there have been studies of Pavlovian heart rate conditioning (Obrist et al., 1965) and clinical studies of patients with complete heart block (Engel, 1972) suggesting that parasympathetic innervation may play the more important role in learned control of heart rate in humans. In order to establish whether this also applies to situations where self-control of heart rate is acquired through biofeedback, what is clearly needed is a noninvasive technique. Invasive techniques applied to either branch of the autonomic nervous system could result in compensatory adjustment through feedback mechanisms in the cardiovascular system (Matyas and King, 1976). Blockade of either branch by chemical techniques would implicitly do injustice to the possibility of interactive control by the two branches. This is undesirable in view of empirical evidence suggesting the existence of nonadditive interaction effects in vagal and sympathetic heart rate regulation (Levy, 1971). Still, in contrast to the wide variety of noninvasive tests available for sympathetic function (e.g., Campese et al., 1980), only surgical interventions in animals or pharmacological manoeuvers (atropine) in humans have been available until recently to investigate parasympathetic control of heart rate.

The advent of power spectre technique for the analysis of heart rate fluctuations has provided a quantitative, noninvasive tool for the assessment of short-term cardiovascular control systems. Sayers (1973) and later Chess et al. (1975) showed that in addition to the well-known fluctuations in heart rate associated with the respiratory cycle, there are periodic fluctuations at still lower frequencies. Accordingly the power spectre of heart rate fluctuations contains not only a peak centered around the respiratory frequency (0.15 to 0.50 Hz), but also a low-frequency peak and a mid-frequency peak, that might relate to cyclic fluctuations in thermo-regulation and to baroreceptor regulation of blood-pressure, respectively (Hyndman, 1974; Kitney, 1972). The respiratory peak typically is related to RSA fluctuations. Although both parasympathetic and sympathetic divisions are assumed to play a significant role in RSA, vagal effects appear to be dominant (Anrep et al., 1936; Chess et al., 1975; Grossman and Wientjes, this volume; Katona and Jih, 1975; Levy et al., 1966; Porges, this volume). Katona and Jih (1975) established the existence of a linear and powerful relationship between variations in heart rate associated with spontaneous respiration, and degree of parasympathetic heart rate control. With spectral analysis, RSA can be measured by the integration of the heart rate power spectre in the respiration frequency band (V). This measure has indeed been found reliably to follow induced changes in cardiovagal tone (McCabe et al., 1979; Yongue et al., 1980).

In our group of sinus tachycardia patients, we have tried to elucidate the status of autonomic regulation of heart rate, and more specifically, whether with heart rate feedback there would be any shift in vagal regulation of heart rate. The vehicle for this attempt was RSA, as measured by the energy in the respiratory band of the heart rate power spectre. Thus there were two aspects to this effort: first to assess RSA level during baseline and to compare this with existing knowledge on associations between RSA and heart rate level in normals and in other clinical populations. Secondly we were interested to see how heart rate feedback would affect RSA, and also to what extent these possible influences on RSA would be associated with the treatment effects. These effects on RSA were taken as indexing changes in cardiovagal tone. Thus if the parasympathetic branch is responsible for improvement in heart rate control during feedback training, then heart rate changes over sessions should be paralleled by changes in RSA.

Level of RSA was measured by the energy in the respiratory band of the heart rate power spectre (0.15 to 0.50 Hz). Spectral densities were computed with a modified version of a program designed by Mulder (1979). The major modifications were:

- bandwidth for computation of spectral densities increased to 1.0 Hz so as to avoid boundary effects around 0.50 Hz;
- sample frequency raised to 2.5 Hz;
- convolution window set at 250 to allow more adequate interpolation of IBI's;
- tapering of first and last 10% of data so as to better fulfil preconditions of stationarity and ergodicity;
- detrending by deduction of overall average instead of moving average filter; this yields a more even transmission characteristic, especially in the low frequency area.

The latter modification was most essential for our purpose, since our subjects, besides being instructed not to alter their breathing within a recording trial, were allowed to breathe freely according to how they felt would best serve their purpose. Thus shifts in peak frequencies in the respiratory band would be very likely to occur over treatment. With an uneven transmission characteristic, this would have precluded the possibility to compare RSA levels at baseline and at end of treatment.

In this way spectral densities were computed from 0.01 to 1.00 Hz by 0.01 Hz. This was done for the second session (baseline), the ninth session (mid-treatment), and session 14 (end of treatment). For brevity we will give graphical representations of the first and the latter only (Figure 2). What is interesting in these figures first of all is the shape of the power spectres at baseline, because this might reveal something of how modulation of heart rate in these patients takes place before treatment. As has been described before, generally a heart rate spectre shows peaks at three separate frequencies, supposedly corresponding with temperature, blood-pressure, and respiratory modulations of heart rate. What is surprising in these plots at baseline is the complete or near-complete absence of energy in the respiratory band in subjects B, C, D and E. It is of additional interest that in these subjects the same pattern reliably

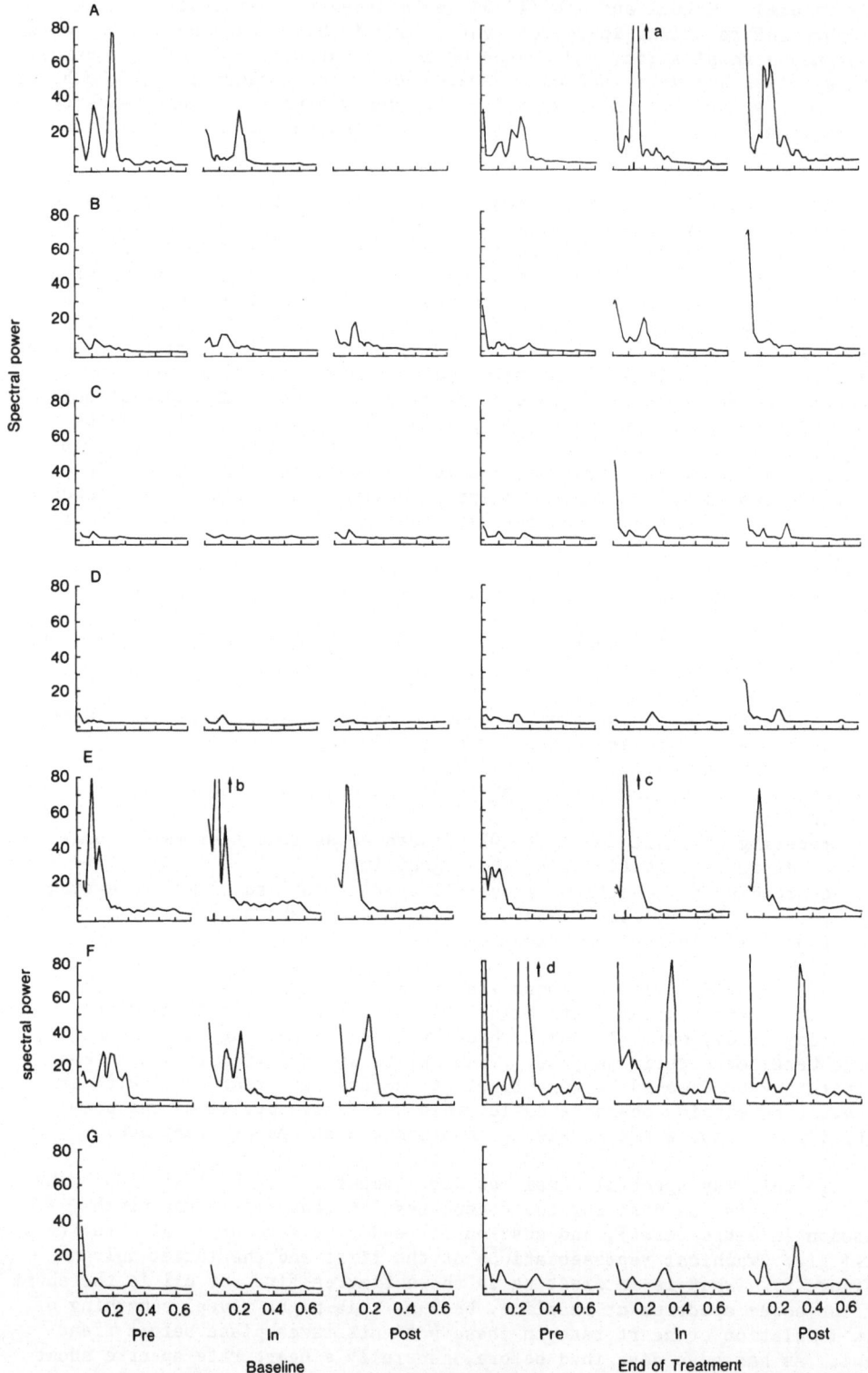

Fig. 2. Power spectra of heart rate computed for each patient during pre-,
in-, and post-session recording trials of session 2 (baseline)
and session 14 (end of treatment). (a = 147; b = 160; c = 127;
d = 185).

emerges in all three recordings at baseline. This would indicate that
variations in these subjects in heart rate are not strongly related to
respiratory cycle. Furthermore, heart rate variations seem to occur more
or less randomly, as there is also little energy below 0.15 Hz in the plots
of these subjects. RSA appears to have increased in several of the subjects towards end of treatment.

To better evaluate these data, the energy in the respiratory band was
calculated per subject per recording. These values are presented as RSA
in Table 2, together with concomitant IBI average values. There are wide
intersubject differences as to RSA levels. Therefore to further analyze
these data we expressed the values at end of treatment as percentage of
baseline values. With simple t-tests we determined the probability that
these percentages would deviate from 100%. This proved to be the case for
the in-session recordings ($p < 0.05$), whereas for post-session recording
the effect was just beyond the range of significance. Results for pre-
session values were clearly insignificant.

Finally, we explored the association between heart rate changes over
treatment and concomitant changes in RSA, also including data from the
ninth session, i.e., halfway treatment. Given the idiosyncratic nature of
RSA as a parameter, besides correlations across subjects for each recording
separately, we also computed correlations across trials per subject (Table
3). With Fisher's z-transformation, the average correlation within subjects was 0.65 ($p < 0.05$), whereas across subjects the average correlation
was 0.57.

Table 2. Spectral Densities in Respiratory Band (.15-.50 Hz) and Inter-
          beat Intervals per Patient per Recording Trial in Session 2
          (Baseline), 9 (Midtreatment), and 14 (End of Treatment).
          Incidental PVC's in Subject A Precluded Reliable Computation
          of Spectral Densities in 2 Recording Trials

		pre		in		post	
		RSA	IBI	RSA	IBI	RSA	IBI
A	2	11.084	800	5.036	776	----	773
	9	----	822	12.216	894	----	849
	14	6.316	813	9.157	858	11.007	888
B	2	1.260	633	1.215	659	1.926	667
	9	2.147	722	2.454	822	2.313	854
	14	1.125	734	3.700	802	1.508	820
C	2	.206	703	.198	726	.201	728
	9	1.196	797	3.414	906	3.205	917
	14	.577	789	1.405	831	1.119	853
D	2	.314	609	.168	576	.138	568
	9	.268	732	.393	769	3.046	786
	14	.714	743	.882	809	1.155	792
E	2	2.577	666	6.145	663	1.986	657
	9	.631	601	.678	709	.640	703
	14	.845	625	2.347	704	2.628	693
F	2	7.695	693	6.431	716	9.289	726
	9	7.931	837	10.079	913	7.298	923
	14	33.433	865	13.393	938	13.500	948
G	2	.989	748	1.175	754	1.884	766
	9	.341	644	2.410	758	1.575	750
	14	1.520	797	2.275	880	2.980	911

Table 3. Correlations Between Spectral Energy in Respiratory Band and
          Interbeat Intervals. Upper Panel: per Subject Across 3
          Recording Trials of Sessions 2, 9 and 14. Lower Panel: per
          Trial of Same Sessions Across Subjects

Subjects:	A	B	C	D	E	F	G
r(HR*RSA)	.68	.54	.93	.56	.09	.28	.85

Sessions:	Baseline			Midtreatment			Endtreatment		
Trials:	pre	in	post	pre	in	post	pre	in	post
r(HR*RSA)	.64	.30	.36	.69	.76	.69	.63	.65	.61

DISCUSSION

These results illustrate how spectral analysis may contribute towards
our understanding of cardiovascular-respiratory integration in patients
with sinus tachycardia. The virtual absence of RSA during baseline in four
of our patients indicates a dissociation of heart rate and respiration that
may bear significant health risks for them. Of course age and heart rate
level may provide some explanation for these results, as both are known to
be inversely related to RSA in normals (Jennet and McKillop, 1971; Hellman
and Stacy, 1976). However, the present results on RSA go far beyond what
could be expected from these factors on the basis of other studies (Roscoe,
1980; Levy et al., 1966; McCrady et al., 1966; Davies, 1975). Moreover,
such findings have been observed in various populations with cardiovascular
problems (Grossman and Wientjes, 1985). More specifically reduction of RSA
is known to occur in borderline and established hypertension (Eckholdt et
al., 1976; Johnston, 1980), sick sinus syndrome and other sinus node disorders (Grassman and Blomquist, 1977; Hinkle et al., 1972), and mitral
stenosis and coronary insufficiency (Eckholdt et al., 1980). Although the
physiological mechanisms that underlie the disturbed RSA in these disorders
may differ (e.g., several reflex mechanisms or direct interaction of respiratory and cardiovascular medullary centers), parasympathetic efferents
are thought to be primarily responsible for mediating these effects upon
the sinoatrial node (Katona and Jih, 1975). Parasympathetic cardiac control has been found to be reduced in cardiac disease states in general
(Eckberg et al., 1971). Conversely, evidence has been offered to suggest
that vagal stimulation may provide a protective mechanism in acute myocardial infarction (Goldstein et al., 1973; Myers et al., 1974). Also
when parasympathetic input is removed by vagotomy, the enhanced sympathetic
activity may lead to an electrical instability of the myocardium and
eventually cardiac arrest (Lown et al., 1977).

RSA appears in this group as a highly idiosyncratic but stable phenomenon. Thus it lends itself to wide individual differences, rendering its
use as a statistic somewhat problematic at present. This might explain
that under all three conditions (pre-, in- and post-recordings) there is an
increase in RSA over treatment, however with statistical significance only
for the in-recordings, i.e., when the subjects had the feedback signals at
their disposal. This may relate, once again, to the point that the analogue feedback signals allowed the subjects to monitor the respiratory
effects on RSA. This led them to experiment with various breathing patterns so as to enhance RSA. Idiosyncracy seems also involved in the extent
to which heart rate changes are paralleled by changes in RSA. On the
average, changes in both parameters are well correlated, but individual
correlations range from 0.086 to 0.927. A low correlation is understand-

able when, over treatment, changes in heart rate are minimal as can be observed with subject E. Still significant decreases in heart rate seem possible sometimes without being firmly tied to concomitant changes in RSA as occurred in subject F. Generally, however, there appears to be a substantial within-subject association between these two measures over treatment.

Thus the present results lend support to the view that decreases in heart rate in a biofeedback paradigm are vagally mediated. This adds to other more indirect evidence in support of this view. T-wave amplitude has been suggested to index sympathetic input to the sinoatrial node (Furedy and Heslegrave, 1983). Thus Matyas and King (1976) found a T-wave difference between acceleratory and deceleratory heart rate feedback trials in normal subjects, which unlike heart rate differences did not improve with trial repetition. From this they inferred that the improvement in heart rate control was vagally mediated. However, such inference should be valued against the objections recently raised against this use of T-wave amplitude (e.g., Obrist, 1981). Other indirect evidence comes from patients with heart block where supraventricular tissue can show learned control of rhythm, but the innervated ventricle cannot learn rate control (Engel, 1972). This becomes meaningful in light of the abundant parasympathetic, as well as sympathetic, innervation of the sinoatrial and atrioventricular nodes (the ventricles are supplied mainly by sympathetic nerves and by far fewer parasympathetic fibers; Guyton, 1983; however, also see Levy, 1984).

The latter evidence and findings on Pavlovian heart rate conditioning (Obrist, 1965), together with our results, support the notion that, in humans, learned control of heart rate, in general, is essentially related to the parasympathetic division of the autonomic nervous system. Yet, even then we must be careful here. RSA is not yet completely understood. Various interactions between peripheral and central mechanisms independently contribute to the phenomenon (Grossman, 1983). For example, de Boer (1985) has recently shown how blood pressure-mediated responses may be of influence. Moreover, it still is open to discussion how RSA is best quantified to yield an optimal index of cardiovagal tone (Grossman and Wientjes, this volume). The choice, for this purpose, of RSA, in itself seems appropriate however, as the vagus exerts the major control over cardiac chronotropic effects (Porges, this volume). Also the response time of the parasympathetic branch is much shorter than that of the sympathetic branch (Lumbers et al., 1978; Levy et al., 1966). Moreover, in the latter study sympathetic firing was found to be more variable during the respiratory cycle than vagal activity. Therefore, only the parasympathetic nervous system reacts rapidly enough to mediate high-frequency modulations of heart rate corresponding to the mid- and high-frequency peaks of the spectre (Akselrod et al., 1981).

In conclusion, our results would justify further attempts towards clinical application of heart rate feedback. With spectral analysis we found a virtual absence of respiratory sinus arrhythmia in four of our sinus tachycardia subjects at baseline, and inferred from this that parasympathetic control of heart rate was greatly impaired. Conversely with heart rate feedback, energy in the respiratory band increased over treatment, especially during in-session recordings. This is consistent with the view that the treatment effects observed were vagally mediated and that heart rate feedback was helpful to restore cardiovagal tone in these subjects. The finding of considerable and reliable intersubject differences in spectral respiratory energy, besides bearing clinical relevance, merits our attention if we are to use it as a statistic.

REFERENCES

Akselrod, S., Gordon, D., Ubel, F. A., Shannon, D. C., Barger, A. C., and Cohen, R. J., 1981, Power spectrum analysis of heart rate fluctuation: a quantitative probe of beat-to-beat cardiovascular control, Science, 213:220-222.

Anrep, G. V., Pascual, W., and Rossler, R., 1936, Respiratory variations of the heart rate. II - the central mechanism of the respiratory arrhythmia and the interrelations between the central and reflex mechanisms, Proc. Roy. Soc., 119:218-230.

Bauer, J. H., and Brooks, C. S., 1979, The long term effect of propranolol therapy on renal function, Am. J. Med., 66:405-410.

Blanchard, E. B., and Abel, G. G., 1976, An experimental case study of the biofeedback treatment of a rape-induced cardiovascular disorder, Behavior Therapy, 7:113-119.

Blanchard, E. B., and Epstein, L. H., 1978, A biofeedback primer, Addison-Wesley, Reading Ma.

De Boer, R. W., 1985, Beat-to-beat blood pressure fluctuations and heart rate variability in man, Thesis, Amsterdam University.

Campese, V. M., Romoff, M., De Quattro, V., and Massry, S. G., 1980, Relationship between plasma catecholamines, plasma renin activity, aldosterone and arterial pressure during postural stress in normal subjects, J. Lab. Clin. Med., 95:927-933.

Cheatle, M. D., and Weiss, T., 1982, Biofeedback in heart rate control and in the treatment of cardiac arrhythmias, in: "Clinical Biofeedback: efficacy and mechanisms", L. White and B. Turskey, eds., Guilford, New York.

Chess, G. F., Tam, R. M. K., and Calaresu, F. R., 1975, Influence of cardiac neural inputs on rhythmic variations of heart period in the cat, Am. J. Physiol., 228:775-780.

Davies, C. T. M., and Neilson, J. M. M., 1967, Sinus arrhythmia in man at rest, J. Appl. Physiol., 22:947-955.

Davies, H. E. F., 1975, Respiratory changes in heart rate, sinus arrhythmia in the elderly, Gerontologia Clinica, 17:96-100.

Eckberg, D. L., Drabinsky, M., and Braunwald, E., 1971, Defective cardiac parasympathetic control in patients with heart disease, New England J. Med., 285:877-883.

Eckholdt, K., Pfeiffer, B., and Schubert, E., 1980, Sympathetic and parasympathetic innervation at rest and work in man as judged by heart rate and sinus arrhythmia, in: "Interactions between Respiratory and Cardiovascular Control Systems", H. P. Koepchen, S. M. Hilton and A. Trzebski, eds., Springer, Berlin.

Eckholdt, K., Bodman, K. H., Camman, H., Pfeiffer, B., and Schubert, E., 1976, Sinus arrhythmia and heart rate in hypertonic disease, Advances in Cardiol., 16:366-369.

Engel, B. T., 1972, Operant conditioning of cardiac function: a status report, Psychophysiology, 9:161-177.

Engel, B. T., and Bleecker, E. R., 1974, Application of operant conditioning techniques to the control of cardiac arrhythmias, in: "Cardiovascular Psychophysiology", P. A. Obrist, A. H. Black, J. Brener and L. V. DiCara, eds., Aldine, Chicago.

Furedy, J. J., and Heslegrave, R. J., 1983, A consideration of recent criticisms of the T-wave amplitude index of myocardial sympathetic activity, Psychophysiology, 20:204-211.

Garnier, B., 1981, How to distinguish between "health" and "illness" in the psychosomatic cardiovascular field, in: "Psychosomatic cardiovascular disorders - when and how to treat?", P. Kielholz, W. Siegenthaler, P. Taggart and A. Zanchetti, eds., Huber, Bern.

Goldstein, R. E., Karsh, R. B., Smith, E. R., Orlando, M., Norman, D., Farnham, D., Redwood, D. R., and Epstein, S. E., 1973, The influence of atropine and vagally mediated bradycardia on the occurrence of ventricular arrhythmias following acute coronary occlusion in closed chest dogs, Circulation, 47:1180-1190.

Grassman, E. D., and Blomquist, R., 1977, Absence of sinus arrhythmia: a manifestation of sick sinus syndrome, Clin. Res., 25:4-8.

Grossman, P., and Wientjes, K., 1985, Respiratory-cardiac coordination as an index of cardiac functioning, in: "The Psychophysiology of Cardiovascular Control", J. F. Orlebeke, G. Mulder, and L. P. van Doornen, eds., Plenum Press, New York.

Grossman, P., and Wientjes, K., this volume, Respiration arrhythmia, vagal tone and respiration: some basic issues.

Grossman, P., 1983, Respiration, stress and cardiovascular function, Psychophysiology, 20:284-300.

Guyton, A. C., 1981, Medical Physiology, Saunders, Philadelphia Pa.

Hellman, J. B., and Stacy, R. W., 1976, Variation of respiratory sinus arrhythmia with age, J. Appl. Physiol., 41:738-743.

Hinkle, L. E., Carver, S. T., and Plakman, A., 1972, Slow heart rates and increased risk of cardiac death, Arch. Int. Med., 129:732-748.

Holmes, D. S., Solomon, S., Frost, R. O., and Morrow, E. F., 1980, Influences of respiratory patterns on the increases and decreases in heart rates in heart rate feedback training, J. Psychosomatic Res., 24:147-153.

Janssen, K. H. L., 1983, Treatment of sinus tachycardia with heart rate feedback, J. Behavioral Med., 6:109-114.

Janssen, K. H. L., and Berger, M. P. F., 1985, Heart rate feedback for sinus tachycardia: a group outcome study, Manuscript, Tilburg University.

Jennet, S., and McKillop, J. H., 1971, Observations on the incidence and mechanism of sinus arrhythmia in man at rest, J. Physiol., 213:58-59.

Johns, T. R., 1970, Heart rate control in humans under paced respiration and restricted movement: the effect of instructions and exteroceptive feedback, Unpublished doctoral dissertation, University of Maine.

Johnston, L. C., 1980, The abnormal heart rate response to a deep breath in borderline labile hypertension: a sign of autonomic nervous system dysfunction, Am. Heart J., 99:487-493.

Julius, S., 1977, Borderline hypertension: epidemiological and clinical implications, in: "Hypertension", A. Genest et al., eds., McGraw-Hill, New York.

Katona, P. G., and Jih, F., 1975, Respiratory sinus arrhythmia: noninvasive measure of parasympathetic cardiac control, J. Appl. Physiol., 39:801-805.

Levi, R. L., White, P. D., Stroud, W. D., and Hillman, C. C., 1945, Transient tachycardia: prognostic significance alone and in association with transient hypertension, J. Am. Ed. Assoc., 129:585-588.

Levy, M. N., 1971, Sympathetic-parasympathetic interactions in the heart, Circ. Res., 29:437-445.

Levy, M. N., DeGeest, H., and Zieske, H., 1966, Effects of respiratory center activity on the heart, Circ. Res., 18:67-78.

Levy, M. N., 1984, Cardiac sympathetic-parasympathetic interactions, Federation Proceedings, 43:2598-2602.

Liebhart, E. H., 1974, Attributionstherapie: Beeinflussung herzneurotischer Beschwerden durch Externalisierung kausaler Zuschreibungen, Zeitschr. f Klin. Psychol., 3:71-94.

Lopes, O. U., and Palmer, F. J., 1976, Proposed respiratory gating mechanisms for cardiac slowing, Nature, 264:454-456.

Lown, B., Verrier, R. L., and Rabinowitz, S., 1977, Neural and psychological mechanisms and the problem of sudden cardiac death, Am. J. Cardiol., 39:890-902.

Lumbers, E. R., McCloskey, D. I., and Potter, E. K., 1978, J. Physiol., 294:69.

McCabe, P. M., Porges, S. W., and Yongue, B. G., Spectral analysis of heart rate during depressor nerve stimulation: the validation of a non-invasive estimate of vagal tone, Soc. Neurosc.Abstr., 5:156.

McCanne, T. R., and Sandman, C. A., 1976, Proprioceptive awareness, information about response-reinforcement contingencies, and operant heart rate control, Physiol. Psychol., 4:369-375.

McCrady, J. D., Vallbona, C., and Hoff, H. E., 1966, Neural origin of the respiratory-heart rate response, Am. J. Physiol., 211:323-328.

Manuck, S. B., and Proietti, J. M., 1982, Parental hypertension and cardiovascular response to cognitive and isometric challenge, Psychophysiology, 19:481-489.

Manuck, S. B., Kaplan, J. R., and Clarkson, T. B., 1983, Behaviorally induced heart rate reactivity and atherosclerosis in cynomolgus monkeys, Psychosomatic Med., 45:95-107.

Matyas, T. A., and King, M. G., 1976, Stable T-wave effects during improvement of heart rate control with biofeedback, Physiol. & Behavior, 16:15-20.

Meyers, R. W., Pearlman, A. S., Hyman, R. M., Goldstein, R. A., Kent, K. M., Goldstein, R. E., and Epstein, S. E., 1974, Beneficial effects of vagal stimulation and bradycardia during experimental acute myocardial ischemia, Circulation, 49:943-947.

Miller, N. E., 1969, Learning of visceral and glandular responses, Science, 163:434-445.

Mulder, L. J. M., 1979, INSPAN, an algol computer program for the spectral analysis of the heart rate interval signal, a program description, Heymans Bull., 79-HB-439-RP.

Mulder, G., and Mulder, L. J. M., 1981, Information processing and cardiovascular control, Psychophysiology, 18:392-402.

Obrist, P. A., 1976, The cardiovascular-behavioral interaction as it appears today, Psychophysiology, 13:95-107.

Obrist, P. A., Galosy, R. A., Lawler, J. E., Gaebelein, C. H., Howard, J. L., and Shanks, E. M., 1975, Operant conditioning of heart rate: somatic correlates, Psychophysiology, 12:445-455.

Obrist, P. A., Wood, D. M., and Perez-Reyes, N., 1965, Heart rate during conditioning in humans: effects of UCS intensity, vagal blockade, and adrenergic block of vasomotor activity, J. Experim. Psychol., 70:32-42.

Paffenbarger, R. S., Thorne, M. C., and Wing, A. L., 1968, Chronic disease in former college students. VIII Characteristics in youth predisposing to hypertension in later years, Am. J. Epidemiol., 88:25-32.

Porges, S. W., McCabe, P. M., and Yongue, B. G., 1982, Respiratory-heart rate interactions: psychophysiological implications for pathophysiology and behavior, in: "Perspectives in cardiovascular psychophysiology", J. T., Cacioppo and R. E. Petty, eds., Guilford, New York.

Porges, S. W., this volume, Respiratory sinus arrhythmia: physiologic basis, quantitative methods, and clinical implications.

Roscoe, A. H., 1980, Heart rate changes in test pilots, in: "The Study of Heart Rate Variability", R. I. Kitney and O. Rompelman, eds., Clarendon, Oxford.

Sayers, B. M., 1973, Analysis of heart rate variability, Ergonomics, 16:17-32.

Scott, R. W., Blanchard, E. B., Edmundson, E. D., and Young, L. D., 1973, A shaping procedure for heart rate control in chronic tachycardia, Perceptual & Motor Skills, 37:327-338.

Sroufe, L. A., 1971, Effects of depth and rate of breathing on heart rate and heart rate variability, Psychophysiology, 8:648-655.

Steptoe, A., Melville, D., and Ross, A., 1984, Behavioral response demands, cardiovascular reactivity, and essential hypertension, Psychosomatic Med., 46:33-48.

Stoney, C. M., Langer, A. W., Sutterer, J. R., and Gelling, P. D., this
volume, Biofeedback assisted heart rate deceleration: specificity of
cardiovascular and metabolic effects in normal and high risk subjects.

Vaitl, D., 1975, Biofeedback-Einsatz in der Behandlung einer Patientin mit
Sinustachyardie, in: "Biofeedback Therapie", H. Legewie and L.
Nusselt, eds., Urban & Schwarzenberg, Munich.

Williamson, D. A., and Blanchard, E. B., 1979, Heart rate and blood
pressure feedback: a review of the recent experimental literature,
Biofeedback & Self-Regulation, 4:1-34.

Winkle, R. A., Glant, S. A., and Harrison, D. C., 1975, Pharmacologic
therapy of ventricular arrhythmias, Am. J. Cardiol., 36:629-635.

Yongue, B. G., McCabe, P. M., Kelley, S., Rivera, P., and Porges, S. W.,
1980, Changes in a respiratorily modulated component of heart period
variability as a result of pharmacological manipulations of vagal
tone in rats, Paper presented at the meeting of the Society for
Psychophysiological Research, Vancouver BC.

BIOFEEDBACK-ASSISTED CONTROL OF

HEART PERIOD VARIABILITY

D. Vaitl, W. Kuhmann and B. Ebert-Hampel

University of Giessen
Giessen
West Germany

In the last decade, we have conducted a series of experiments which were mainly focused at the modification of instantaneous variations of heart period (heart period variability, HPV). Historically speaking, this was suggested by casual observations in patients with sinus tachycardia who sometimes exhibited an exaggerated HPV during the prodromal phase of their attacks. Early experiments with normal subjects were aimed at the stabilization of instantaneous HPV by visual feedback techniques and the exploration of possible concomitant changes in cardiac-respiratory interaction. These findings are summarized in the first part of this chapter. Later in the chapter, we examine the clinical effectiveness of this approach with respect to changes in cardiac-respiratory interaction, control strategies used for HP stabilization, and symptoms of patients with heart-related disorders.

BACKGROUND

As previous chapters have demonstrated, HPV provides valuable information about the neural mechanisms involved in cardiac control. There are different types of variations (for classification see Luczak et al., 1980) ranging from long-term to short-term fluctuations in heart period (HP) (e.g. from $0-0.5 \times 10^{-4}$ Hz up to $0.5 \times 10^{-1}-0.5$ Hz). As illustrated in previous chapters, the relatively short-term variations of HP are closely related to respiratory, vasomotor, and thermoregulatory processes, which respond to both internal and external demands in a highly specific manner. Beyond these normal changes in HPV, the pathological aberrations of heart rhythms such as cardiac arrhythmias (e.g. sinus tachycardia, premature ventricular contraction, ventricular fibrillation) and excess HP variations are of paramount importance with respect to myocardial infarction and sudden cardiac arrest.

It has been demonstrated that the ventricular fibrillation threshold is lowered by psychological stress in dogs with ischemic coronary arteries (Lown, Verrier and Rabinowitz, 1977). Furthermore, the electric instability of the ischemic heart may be highly susceptible to imbalances of the neural input from higher brain structures. Skinner (Skinner and Reed, 1981) has demonstrated that the frontal cortex plays an important role in stressful situations when the excess dual autonomic tone, i.e. increases in both sympathetic and vagal discharges to the ischemic heart, is not inhibited by frontal cortex activities. Unusually large variations in HP could be observed by Yongue, Porges and McCabe (1979) in a small subgroup of stressed rats during periods of recovery from stress. These episodes were transient in nature and their offset and onset were sudden. Porges, McCabe and Yongue (1982) assume that the exaggerated respiratory sinus arrhythmia, as observed in this experiment, might be induced by state changes in the CNS which result in either an increase of vagal efferent discharge or an inhibition of sympathetic nervous system antagonism. In both cases, the onset and the offset of the large variations in HP are central in origin, although localized cardiac dysfunctions (ischemia, electrical instability, re-entry mechanism) cannot be excluded.

Because of the relevance of excess HPV for clinical issue, the ability to control such fluctuations becomes a potentially important concern. Therefore, despite the present uncertainty about the true origin and the underlying mechanisms of cardiac arrhythmias, especially of sudden increases of HPV, we raised the question initially of whether and to what extent normal subjects can learn to influence their HPV voluntarily. Such answered questions could suggest clinical implications and provide new perspectives for the management of cardiovascular disorders.

With these questions in mind, we have employed feedback techniques which provide subjects with information about heart rate (HR) and/or HPV and allow us to study the psychophysiological parameters involved in learned control of autonomic functions. Reviewing the literature on cardiac feedback studies, Williamson and Blanchard (1979) have concluded that compared to the host of studies on bidirectional HR control (speeding or slowing HR) the HPV feedback approach appears to be a relatively neglected area of biofeedback research. Early studies on HPV control have demonstrated the effectiveness of visual feedback in reducing instantaneous HP variations within a certain range (Hnatiow and Lang, 1965; Lang, Sroufe and Hastings, 1967; Sroufe, 1969; Harrison and Raskin, 1976).

These effects, however, are not solely brought about by feedback itself. As Harrison and Raskin (1976) pointed out, the short-term (single session) reductions in HPV are probably due to attending to a visual feedback display. While attempting to reduce HPV, transient decreases in HPV occur which are not dependent upon the information value of the feedback stimuli per se. This alternative interpretation is also in accord with the notion that HPV is reduced when mental load is increased through the number of stimuli (e.g. feedback signals) to be processed (Luczak et al., 1980). Thus, it may be possible that factors other than cardiac feedback are responsible for the positive results reported in the early studies on learned HPV control. Among these, respiratory activity appears to be one of the most critical variables as a mediator in cardiac feedback procedures, and has been proven to play an important role in both HR speeding and slowing tasks. In which way and to what extent, however, changes in cardiac-respiratory interactions are modified by HPV feedback procedures has not yet been examined explicitly. In order to investigate such processes underlying the feedback-assisted control of HPV, our group has conducted a series of experiments both in normals and patients with cardiac disorders such as cardiac arrhythmias and cardiophobic responses (Vaitl and Kenkmann, 1972; Vaitl, 1975b; Vaitl, Stegagno and Trombini, 1977; Vaitl, Kenkmann and Kuhmann, 1979; Ebert, Kuhmann and Vaitl, 1979; Ebert-Hampel, 1982; Kuhmann, 1984).

FEEDBACK METHODS USED

In almost all feedback experiments reported here the information given to the subjects consisted of a visual feedback of the cardiotachogram curve which was displayed on an oscilloscope in front of them (for details and explanation see left side of Figure 1 and Vaitl et al., 1979). All subjects were instructed to reduce the instantaneous fluctuations of their heart periods which would result, in turn, in a flattening of the amplitude of the ongoing cardiotachogram (i.e. stabilization of HPV). As also depicted in Figure 1 (right side), in several experiments another type of feedback has been employed which was characterized by a low-information feedback. Instead of the cardiotachogram curve as high-information feedback, a straight line was displayed on the oscilloscope which moved around the target according to momentary changes in heart periods. In order to smooth the up and down movement the position of this line was determined by a moving average of five heart periods. In order to determine if and how subjects learn to achieve control over their HPV, the information provided by the feedback display (high- and low-information) was systematically varied across different subject groups.

In the following section of this chapter, the main results of the single-session experiments will be summarized. They concern (a) the amount of HP stabilization achieved under different feedback conditions, and (b) the cardiac-respiratory interaction as modified by those experimental conditions.

STABILIZATION OF HEART PERIOD VARIATION (HPV)

All of these studies were designed in the same way. A baseline period of 5 minutes duration was followed by six training trials of 5 minutes each, during which different types of feedback were given. The feedback training trials were separated by pauses (1 minute) (Vaitl and Kenkmann, 1972; Vaitl et al., 1977). When standard deviations of HP are employed as variability measures, the following conclusions can be drawn from these studies:

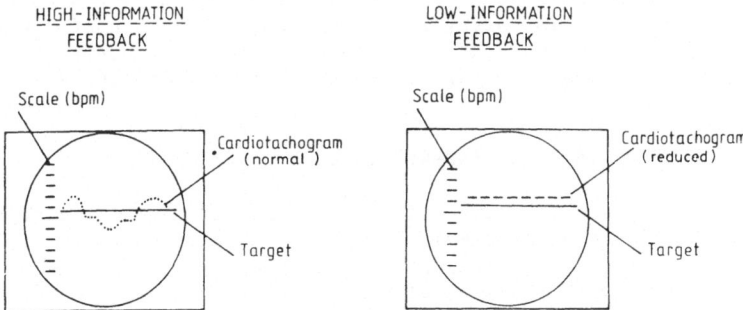

Fig. 1. Characteristics of high-information and low-information visual feedback. In high-information feedback, a cardiotachogram curve (50 beats) is displayed on an oscilloscope. This moves to rhythm of subjects' heart beats from right to left towards the scale (bpm). Subjects' task consisted in trying to get the single points of the cardiotachogram curve to approach the target (i.e. mean HR), continuously calculated by a moving average of 50 heart beats. In low-information feedback, subjects receive information only about momentary direction of change in the form of a straight line (reduced cardiotachogram). In addition, the amount of change is smoothed by a moving average of 5 heart periods. In both feedback, on the left side of the screen a bpm scale is displayed indicating 10 bpm steps (range 50–150 bpm).

Feedback is a necessary condition for HP stabilization. Without feedback, subjects were not able to reduce their HPV (Vaitl and Kenkmann, 1972; Vaitl, 1975a). This is true for subjects who never received feedback as well as for those subjects whose learned HP stabilization was tested during no feedback periods interspersed with feedback trials. Thus, transfer from feedback trials to non-feedback trials is minimal.

With respect to the contingency of feedback, the amount of information given (number of relevant parameters of the feedback signals displayed) appeared to be a critical variable in this kind of experiment. Subjects became more irritated and distracted and, as a consequence, their performance of voluntary HPV control was impaired, when many details of visual feedback had to be processed. On the other hand, too little information resulted in poorer motivation to control HPV or subjects falling asleep (Vaitl and Kenkmann, 1972; Vaitl, 1975a).

In studies of bidirectional HR control, it has been commonly accepted that noncontingent feedback represents an appropriate experimental control condition for effects induced by contingent feedback. This, however, does not hold for HPV feedback experiments. It could be shown that subjects were also able to stabilize their HR significantly under noncontingent feedback conditions (Vaitl, 1973). This effect is somewhat surprising, if one assumes that contingency does play the same role in HPV control tasks as in HR speeding/slowing tasks.

I has been postulated by several authors (for discussion see Cuthbert et al., 1981) that the performance of HR speeding is facilitated by contingent feedback compared to noncontingent feedback, whereas in HR slowing task reduced contingent information leads to better performance. In both cases, the contingency of feedback is a decisive parameter, which is positive for HR speeding and negative for HR slowing tasks. This, however, does not hold true for HPV stabilization. Both contingent and noncontingent feedback, when given continually on a beat-to-beat basis, reduce HPV to the same extent. This finding has been replicated several times (Vaitl, 1973; Cohors-Fresenborg et al., 1976; Kumann, 1984). Although the basic mechanism of this phenomenon is not yet fully understood, there is increasing evidence that the similarity of effects is mainly brought about by the comparable mental load induced by the same amount of feedback signals which are processed both under contingent and noncontingent feedback conditions.

STABILIZATION OF HPV AND CARDIAC-RESPIRATORY INTERACTION

It has been postulated that different types of visual feedback may induce different control strategies including specific respiratory maneuvers. Since changes in frequency and depth of breathing induced by HPV feedback are very small and inconsistent (Cohors-Fresenborg et al., 1976) compared to the pronounced respiratory manipulations as observed in HP speeding and slowing studies (Stegagno and Vaitl, 1979), a time-series approach has been chosen to study the cardiac-respiratory interactions under various feedback forms. This may lead to a better understanding of subjects' control strategies under those feedback conditions.

In a previous study (Vaitl et al., 1979) it could be demonstrated that the cross-correlation between the two time-series 'Heart Period' and 'Respiratory' (inspiration/expiration cycles) changed in a systematic fashion according to the feedback employed. The covariation between cardiac and respiratory activity was diminished when contingent feedback on a beat-to-beat basis was given. In contrast, noncontingent feedback displaying low HPV, or no feedback, led to closer covariations between these two time-series than continuous and contingent feedback.

In order to study these feedback-effects in more detail, the data of previous experiments have been reanalyzed by determining the weighted coherence measure (Porges et al., 1980). This measure, based upon cross-spectral analysis, provides a statistic that describes the proportion of variance shared by respiration and HP within the frequency band characteristic of respiration. It provides a quantitative estimate of the coupling between respiratory and cardiac activity. Little is known, however, about the physiological mediation underlying this estimate and its functional significance. Chapters by Porges, Grossman and Wientjes in this volume have addressed this issue in detail. Within the context of feedback-assisted HPV control, weighted coherence (C_W) measures are used for the moment solely as estimates of coupling. By comparing differences in C_W induced by different treatments (e.g. feedback versus no feedback), we have attempted to explore their functional significance, particularly their behavioral implications. Since all studies whose data were reanalyzed have been designed in the same way (baseline of 5 minutes, six training trials of six minutes duration each; for details of Vaitl and Kenkmann, 1972; Vaitl, Kenkmann and Kuhmann, 1979), multiple comparisons could be carried out.

For this purpose, three groups from earlier studies were selected as a first step (see Vaitl et al., 1979). Group 1 (n=16) was requested to control HPV by contingent (i.e. true) feedback; group 2 (n=15) and group 3 (n=15) were given noncontingent (i.e. false) feedback. These two later groups differed with respect to the amount of HPV feedback. Group 2 was provided with feedback displaying the normal range of HPV, whereas group 3 received very stable HPV feedback which reflected the almost ideal performance of HPV control. Both noncontingent data sets were continually generated by computer according to a predetermined algorithm.

As shown in Figure 2 the C_W values gradually diminished according to the type of feedback given. Compared to baseline levels, there was a significant increase in coherence measures under that noncontingent feedback condition which displayed low HPV; this type of feedback indicated that the task of HP stabilization was being successfully accomplished and did not require any improvement in performance. In contrast, a gradual decrease of the coherence measures occurred in the other noncontingent (normal HPV) feedback. When HP stabilization performance was determined by changes in standard deviation of HP, no differences between groups could be found.

These findings indicate that cardiac-respiratory coupling was mainly influenced by the extent to which subjects' counterregulatory processes were stimulated. Whenever the displayed apparent HPV was low, indicating that the training goals had been already achieved, no effort was made to reduce HPV further. However, counterregulatory maneuvers were needed whenever HPV feedback signalled larger instantaneous HP oscillations, as with contingent feedback or noncontingent feedback which occurred within the normal range of HPV.

In the next stage of analyses, similar changes in C_W were expected when, instead of noncontingency, the contingency of feedback was altered in a systematic manner. For this purpose, comparisons were made between low- and high-information feedback procedures, as illustrated in Figure 1 (data from Vaitl and Kenkmann study 1972, and Vaitl et al., study 1979). In order to determine the effect of feedback-information on C_W, another group (n=30) was added which did not receive and feedback (control group). On the basis of C_W values being influenced by counterregulatory processes, it was predicted that in the low-information feedback group (n=15), C_W values would be higher than in the high-information feedback group (n=15). The

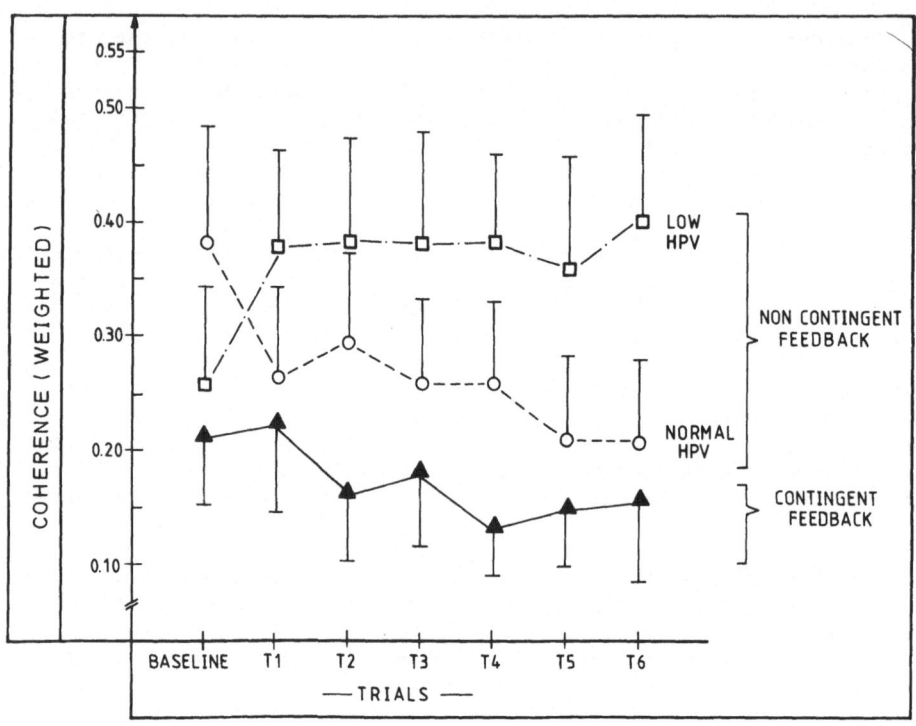

Fig. 2. Means and S.D. of weighted coherence during baseline and six
training trials (T1-T6) under contingent and noncontingent feedback conditions. Noncontingent feedback was given as cardiotachogram curve representing low HPV and normal HPV. This type of
feedback was taken from a data set stored in the computer and was
displayed on the screen point by point exactly to the rhythm of
subjects' heart beats.

highest C_W values ought to be obtained in the no-feedback group. As illustrated in Figure 3, sitting in a reclining chair and being instructed to
breath regularly, as the controls were to do, indeed resulted in greater C_W
values than in those groups who had to process the feedback information.
Significant differences between low- and high-information feedback groups
could be obtained only for the last three feedback trials. HP stabilization performance (determined in terms of standard deviation) was good in
the high-information, worse in the low-information and absent in the no-
feedback group.

In the last stage of reanalysis, an overall comparison was made which
included percent changes in C_W from baselines throughout different treatment trials (mean C_W across six trials for each group). This analysis
comprised three groups with no feedback ($n_1=14$, $n_2=15$, $n_3=15$), three groups
with high-information feedback ($n_1=10$, $n_2=14$, $n_3=15$), two groups with
low-information feedback ($n_1=15$, $n_2=15$), and two groups with noncontingent
feedback (low and normal HPV) which were the same as those depicted in
Figure 2.

Figure 4 illustrates very clearly that both high-information feedback
and noncontingent feedback with normal HPV reduced C_W values whereas no
feedback or noncontingent feedback of the low HPV type increased C_W values.
In low-information groups, the C_W values remain unaltered. This indicated
that changes in C_W were mainly brought about by manipulations of the cardiac
feedback. This appears very clearly when noncontingent feedback resulted

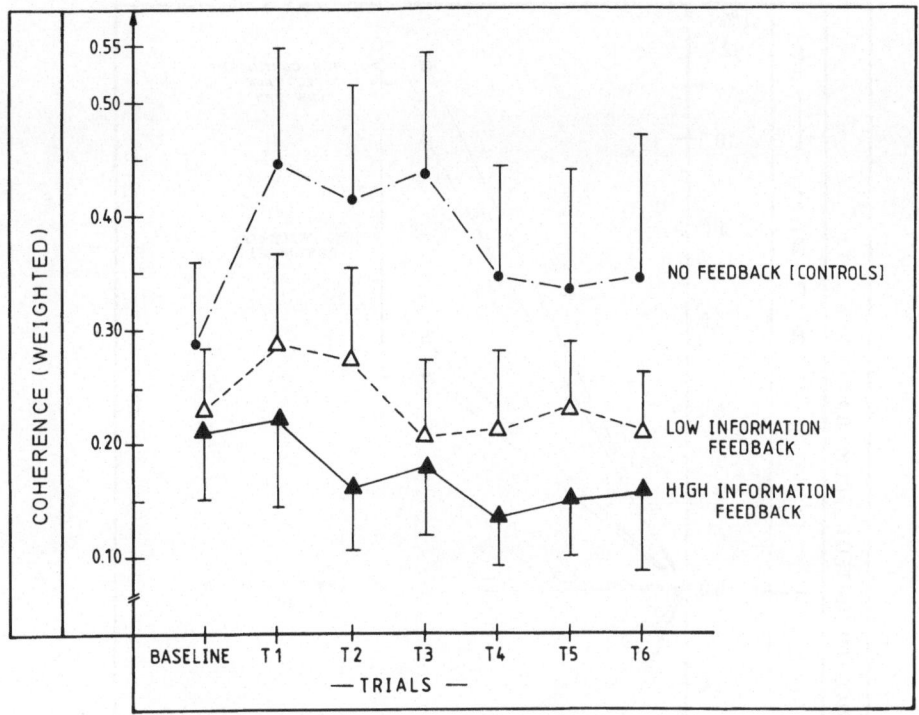

Fig. 3. Means and S.D. of weighted coherence during baseline and six
training trials (T1-T6) under low-information and high-information
feedback (cf. Figure 1) and under control condition (i.e. no
feedback).

in either low or normal HPV. Approximately 12% increase or decrease of Cw
could be produced when the HPV feedback was low or normal, respectively.
Accordingly, high-information feedback led to similar reductions in C_W as
the noncontingent, normal HPV feedback, whereas increases in C_W only
occurred when no feedback was given, i.e. when there was no need to exert
control over bodily function.

These systematic changes in C_W seem to reflect differences in subjects' behavioral strategies in various experimental conditions. HP
stabilization training with contingent visual feedback, which is given
continually on a beat-to-beat basis, may induce predominantly respiratory
control strategies: When the cardiotachogram curve displayed on the
oscilloscope goes up (i.e. HR increases), subjects might try to compensate
by exhaling or interrupting their inspiration cycle. The reverse may be
seen when HR tends to slow down: subjects start to inhale or to interrupt
their expiration cycle. In contingent and continually given feedback, the
slightest alteration of breathing (in frequency and/or depth) may induce
changes in HP which correspond to the instruction for HP stabilization.
However, these possible counterregulatory maneuvers must be very subtle, if
present, since no pronounced changes in respiration (either frequency or
depth; cf. Cohors-Fresenborg et al., 1976) could be detected, as mentioned
earlier.

In summary, the C_W measure apparently reflects the changes in cardiac-
respiratory interactions which occurred with different experimental manipulations. Such results revealed that one effect of feedback-assisted HP
stabilization is a partial reduction in cardiac-respiratory coupling. In
contrast, when no feedback signals are to be processed, cardiac-respiratory

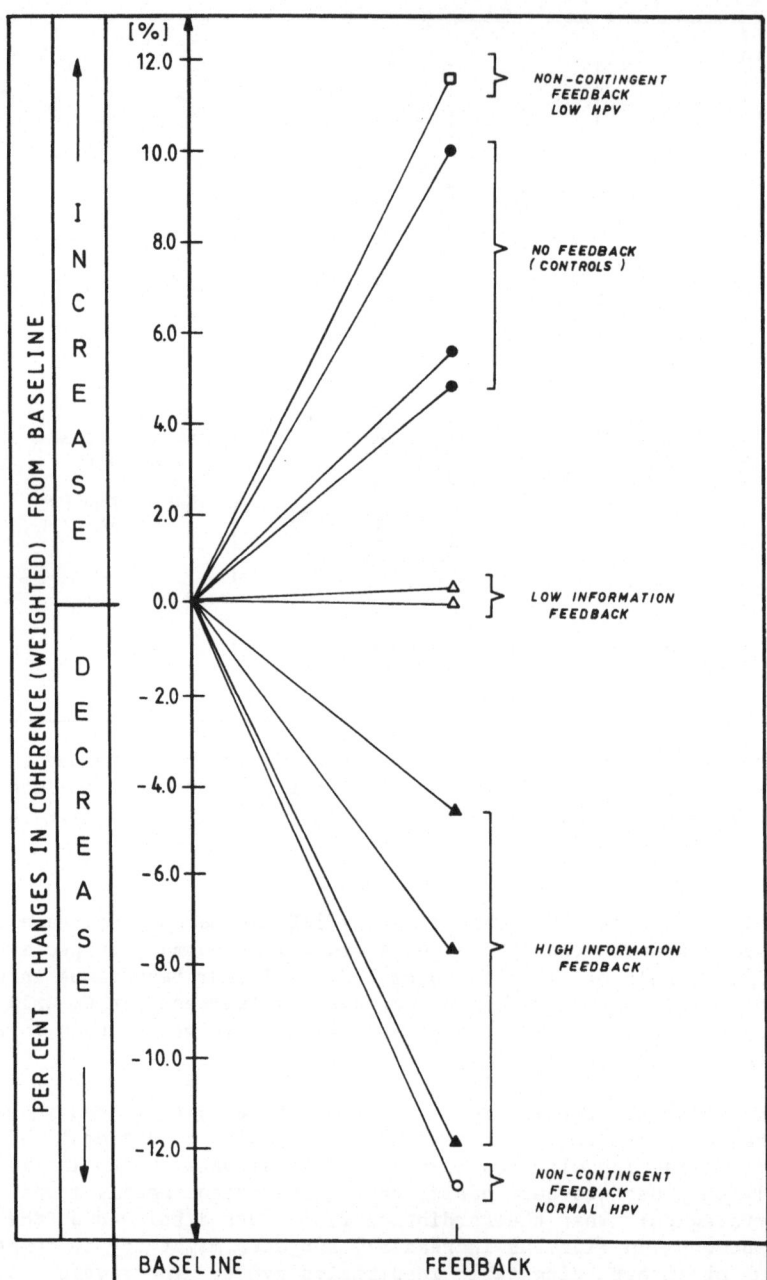

Fig. 4. Overall comparison of percent changes in weighted coherence measure from baseline to feedback trials for different groups which were provided by different information about how to reduce HPV. ——● No feedback (controls). ——△ Low information feedback (cf. Figure 1). ——▲ High information feedback (cf. Figure 1). ——□ Non-contingent feedback, low HPV. ——○ Non-contingent feedback, normal HPV.

coupling is augmented; this effect is probably due to adaptation to the experimental environment, as other influences on HPV (such as mental load) are reduced. This issue will be addressed further in the discussion section.

In the next section the long-term effects of HPV feedback training will be examined in a subgroup of patients with heart-related behavioral and emotional disorders.

CLINICAL OUTCOME STUDY

There are only a few studies which have examined the clinical use-fulness of cardiac feedback for the management of cardiovascular disorders, such as cardiac arrhythmias. A comprehensive and critical review has been presented by Cheatle and Weiss (1982). In this volume, Janssen and Beckering address the main clinical issues concerning HR feedback as an adjunct for medical treatment of patients with cardiac arrhythmias. In single case studies, it could be demonstrated that HR slowing feedback has been applied very successfully in clinical settings for reducing HR levels as well as for improving sinus tachycardia attacks (e.g. Scott et al., 1973; Engel and Bleecker, 1974; Vaitl, 1975b; Janssen, 1983). Recently, this was further established in a group outcome study by Janssen and Berger (1985). For other types of arrhythmias, however, feedback procedures have been proven clinically less effective compared to the reasonable cost-benefit ratio of pharmacological intervention (see Cheatle and Weiss, 1982).

In addition to these abnormalities, patients with such cardiac dis-orders can be characterized very reliably by a wide variety of behavioral and emotional disturbances, such as panic attacks, fear of sudden death, escape-avoidance behavior, social isolation, and drug abuse. Many of these patients are permanently seeking appropriate medical and/or psychological help, which is frequently ineffective for alleviating their various com-plaints. Therefore, we have attempted to improve and to stabilize such a group's still existing self-control activities by providing them with a cardiac feedback which is directly focused at the target organ, that is, the beating heart. This study was conducted in patients with cardiophobia or heart-related behavioral and emotional disorders (e.g. breathlessness, lump in the throat, dizziness, muscle tension, fear of sudden death, anxiety, depression, extreme escape-avoidance behavior (for detail see Ebert-Hampel, 1982)). The HPV feedback was chosen because of the fact that in the sample of patients studied, most of these psychological disturbances have been induced or preceded by perceived or real disturbances in cardiac functions (e.g. rapid heart beats, irregular heart beats, chest pain; data are based upon verbal reports and not upon continuous ECG monitoring). Therefore, a training aimed at cardiac stabilization was likely to be accepted by patients as a potentially successful aid for gaining cardiac self-control. In this context, a bidirectional heart-rate feedback training (HR speeding and/or slowing) would be contraindicated given the patients' previous experiences (e.g. tachycardia, fear of cardiac arrest) and heart-related complaints.

By using the HPV feedback approach, the study was designed to address both basic and clinical questions:

a. Are patients able to stabilize their HP under various feedback con-ditions and does this learned performance persist over time?
b. What roles do contingency (contingent vs. noncontingent) and con-tinuity (continuous vs. delayed, or cumulative) of feedback play during such training? Is there any superiority of contingent feed-back, as very frequently postulated in the literature on cardiac feedback, or is delayed feedback a more adequate procedure in order to avoid irritations emanating from continuous feedback?
c. Which individual control strategies for stabilizing HP are shaped by different kinds of feedback (contingent vs. noncontingent, cumulative vs. noncumulative?)

d. Is feedback training for HP stabilization effective at all in reducing somatic, behavioral, and emotional problems?

METHODS

Subjects

Out of a total of 242 patients who were referred to the Department of Clinical Psychology at the University of Muenster from different institutions (private practices, medical center) a sample of 33 patients was selected for the study. The criteria for selection were:

a. Reports of frequent and intense heart-related disturbances.
b. The heart-related problems were triggered by behaviorally defined situations (i.e. the behavioral analysis must reveal some relationship between heart-related disturbances and situations).
c. No cardiovascular disorder of organic origin (rejection rate: 29%).
d. No psychiatric disorder (rejection rate: 3%).

The histories of patients who were finally accepted for the study are presented in Figure 5.

Treatment Program

After two separate behavioral analyses and the completion of several questionnaires (see Ebert-Hampel, 1982), the training program of ten sessions (total duration approximately 45 minutes each) started. Each

PATIENTS

AGE AND SEX	
MALES: n = 17	AGE: 34,2 yrs (23 – 55 yrs)
FEMALES: n = 16	AGE: 32,8 yrs (21 – 43 yrs)

HISTORY OF SYMPTOMS	
MALES:	$\bar{X}$ = 5,4 yrs (0.8 – 20.0 yrs)
FEMALES:	$\bar{X}$ = 5.9 yrs (0.3 – 28.0 yrs)

FREQUENCY OF SYMPTOMS	
DAILY	53%
2 - 3 x / WEEK	36%
1 x / WEEK	9%
1 x / 2 WEEKS	2%

DURATION OF ATTACKS	
> 2 hrs	34 %
2 hrs	19 %
1 hr	44 %
< $\frac{1}{2}$ hr	3 %

Fig. 5. Patients' characteristics and history of their symptoms (for explanation see text).

288

session consisted of a baseline period (5 minutes) and six feedback trials (2 minutes each), each followed by transfer trials (2 minutes each) during which the patients were asked to perform HPV control without the aid of feedback signals.

Feedback Procedures

The feedback was given on an oscilloscope (see Figure 6). Two factors of feedback characteristics were systematically crossed: contingency (yes/ no) and continuity (yes/no). The resulting four experimental conditions were designed as follows: the continuous contingent/noncontingent feedback was given <u>during</u> each training trial, whereas the noncontinuous contingent/ noncontingent feedback was delayed and given cumulatively <u>after</u> each trial (for details see Figure 5 and cf. Ebert, Kuhmann and Vaitl, 1979).

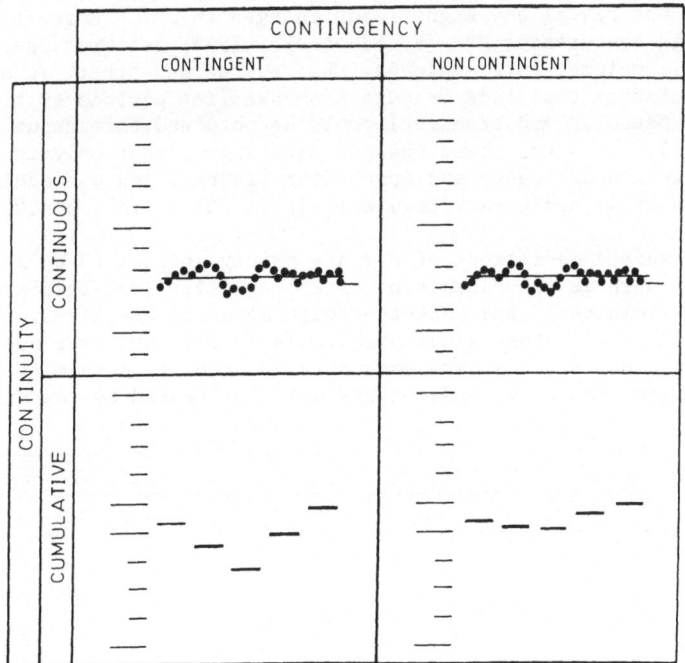

Fig. 6. Visual displays of the four feedback conditions: 1. Continuous-contingent feedback. 2. Continuous-noncontingent feedback. Feedback is displayed on the oscilloscope exactly as in contingent feedback. However, the variability of the cardiotachogram curve was manipulated systematically by computer routines according to a predetermined schedule (for details see Kuhmann, 1984). This implies that HPV is gradually reduced within sessions and across sessions. 3. Noncontinuous-contingent feedback. This feedback is given after each trials. Instead of a cardiotachogram curve, subjects receive feedback in form of five horizontal lines indicating HPV of the previous trial divided into five time segments of 30 seconds each. The scale on the left site represents 9 performance levels of HP stabilization indicating low (lower segments) and high HPV (upper segments). 4. Noncontinuous-noncontingent feedback. This feedback is also given after each trial. It is given in the same manner as in noncontinuous-contingent feedback. However, the same predetermined schedule as in continuous-noncontingent feedback is used here to manipulate the position of the five horizontal lines (according to the 9 performance levels represented by the scale on the left side).

RESULTS

Changes in Cardiac and Respiratory Activity

The first question concerns the changes in cardiac activity. In mean HR level, no significant changes occurred either within or across sessions. The mean HR of all four groups ranged from 68.9 to 75.1 bpm during baselines, from 67.7 to 71.9 bpm during training trials, and from 67.7 to 72.9 bpm during transfer trials.

The feedback-induced effects upon HPV appeared to be different depending upon the variability measure employed (see Kuhmann, 1984). When standard deviation of HP was employed, gradual decreases in HPV (i.e. stabilization) from baseline through feedback trials could only be observed in those groups which received continuous feedback. Irrespective of feedback contingency, in the cumulative feedback groups these variability measures did not reveal any significant changes in HPV. However, when peak-to-trough measures of HPV (Fouad et al., 1984; see Grossman and Wientjes, this volume) were employed, the reverse was true. In all groups, an increase of this amplitude measure from baseline periods to training phases (both feedback and transfer) could be obtained throughout training (see Figure 7). However, these changes were significant only in that group which received noncontingent and cumulative feedback and was additionally instructed to relax and breath regularly (F (1/10) = 7.45; p <.05).

Since standard deviations of HPV are mainly influenced by long-term trends in HPV such as unavoidable non-stationarities (one feedback/transfer trial lasted 2 minutes), and peak-to-trough measures are likely to be associated with respiratory sinus arrhythmia (RSA), autopower spectral analyses of the HPV signals were conducted in order to determine to what extent different frequency bands of HPV were influenced by the different

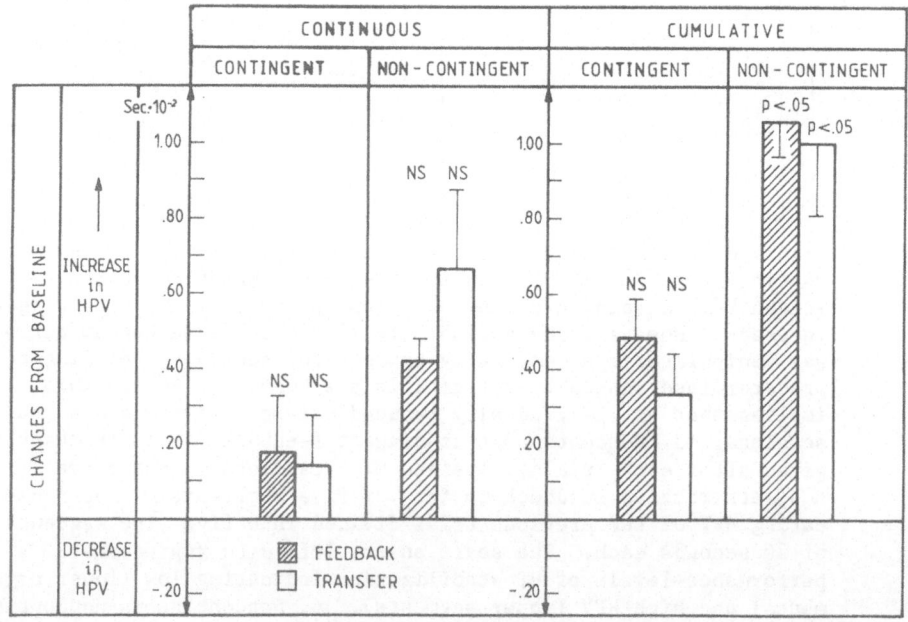

Fig. 7. Mean and S.D. of changes from baseline in peak-to-trough measures (sec × 10^{-2}) for HPV during training and transfer trials under continuous (contingent or noncontingent) and cumulative (contingent or noncontingent) feedback conditions.

290

feedback parameters employed. For this purpose, three major classes of HPV frequencies were selected and their changes from baseline were determined: one band of very low frequencies (VLF) from 0.001 up to 0.03 Hz, another band of low frequencies (LF) from 0.03 up to 0.15 Hz (band around 0.1 Hz), and a third one from 0.15 up to .35 Hz (high frequency, HF; cf. Baselli et al., 1985). During feedback trials, in all four groups the VLF were significantly suppressed. This indicates very clearly that the HP stabilization task per se is successful in regularizing the very slow trend in HPV (data are not shown here). Feedback-induced changes in LF and HF were determined separately for the four experimental conditions by calculating the mean differences between baseline values (10 for each experimental condition) and feedback trials (six trials per session, 10 sessions for each condition) for both frequency bands. Figure 8 represents the proportion of these changes in LF and HF. Similar changes from baseline could be observed for both LF and HF when feedback was continually given. Feedback contingency did not induce differences in LF and HF changes. The ratio of increases in both frequency bands (LF:HF) during feedback trials was approximately the same (1:2.2 for contingent feedback, 1:2.8 for noncontingent feedback). This implies that in both groups the HF band which is closely related to respiration has been enhanced at least twice as much as the LF band.

Compared to the continuous feedback conditions, cumulative feedback induced quite different changes in frequency bands under contingent as well as under noncontingent conditions. This mainly concerns the LF:HF ratio. As illustrated in Figure 8, the LF band is reduced by cumulative contingent feedback, but increased remarkably under the noncontingent feedback condition. In addition, changes in HF band also differed significantly. Only minimal increases in HF occurred when the cumulative feedback was noncontingent (LF:HF = 1:0.008). Under the contingent feedback condition, however, similar increases in the HF band could be observed as in the continuous feedback group. This implies that increases in the HF band did occur when contingent feedback information had continually or cumulatively to be processed, or when the information density was relatively high as in non-

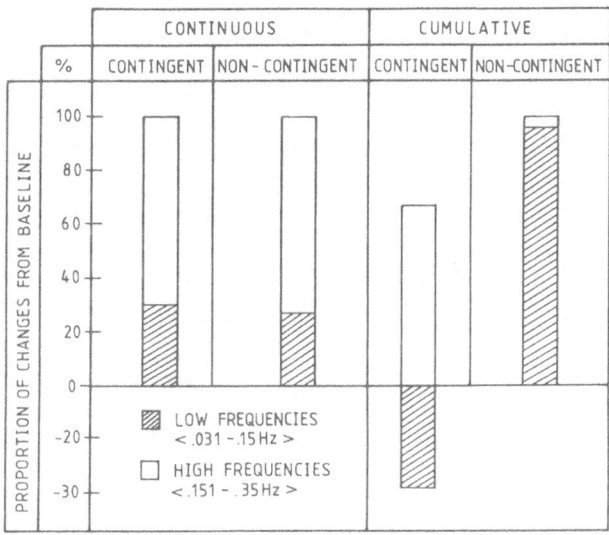

Fig. 8. Proportions (%) of mean changes in low and high frequency bands of HPV power spectrum from baselines to feedback trials across ten sessions for continuous (contingent/noncontingent) and cumulative (contingent/noncontingent) feedback conditions.

contingent continuous feedback. This increase, however, was remarkably smaller when the feedback information was noncontingent and delayed, but subjects were additionally encouraged to focus their attention on regular breathing and somatic relaxation. Only these circumstances favored increases in the LF band considerably. (Changes in cyclic fluctuations in the HF band were independent of the peak-to-trough measures, as observed in this particular group).

The next step of analysis concerns the cardiac-respiratory interaction. For this purpose, there again C_W measures were determined as we did for the single-session studies (see Figure 9). Under all feedback conditions, C_W measures increased significantly from baselines through feedback trials. Between groups, however, no significant differences could be obtained. When transfer trials were compared, however, the C_W values of the noncontingent, cumulative feedback group did differ quite substantially from the other three groups, which were not required to relax and to breath regularly. Interestingly, the C_W values for feedback trials were not reduced by contingent and continuous feedback as we have found in single-session studies. Here, in all groups, the coupling between respiratory and cardiac activity was enhanced during feedback trials compared to baseline levels. This is probably due to a general increase of regular breathing across the ten training sessions. This positive effect, however, did not appear until the third session, as Kuhmann (1984) has demonstrated by autocorrelational analysis of the respiration data. Less trial and error activity and greater familiarity with the feedback setting may have led to changes in respiration. Thus, it is understandable that feedback-induced reduction in C_W values, as seen particularly in contingent and continuous

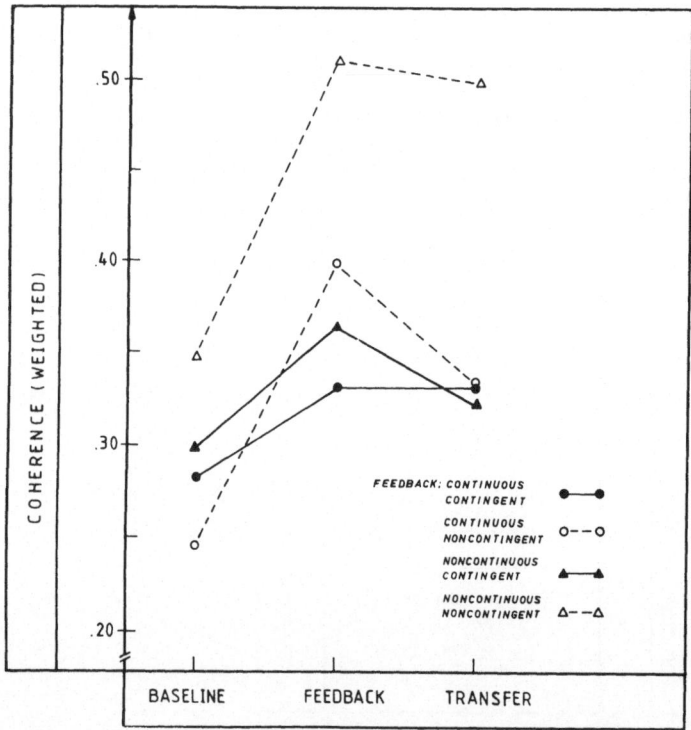

Fig. 9. Mean weighted coherence values during baseline, feedback, and transfer trials (6 per session, 10 sessions) for different feedback conditions: continuous-contingent; continuous-noncontingent; noncontinuous-contingent; noncontinuous-noncontingent.

feedback conditions in single-session studies, are certainly short-term
effects which fade out as soon as the feedback training lasts longer than
three sessions.

Behavioral Control Strategies

Behavioral control strategies concern all activities by which patients
attempt to produce changes in feedback signals toward the target response
requested by instruction. For this purpose, after each training session
patients were asked about the control strategies employed. Their verbal
reports were clustered (cf. Kuhmann, 1984) and categorized in four major
groups of statements (see Figure 10): a) Respiratory strategies (e.g.
regular breathing, shallow breathing), b) heart-related strategies (e.g.
attending to heart beats), c) relaxation and/or cognitive strategies (e.g.
reduction of muscle tension, thinking pleasant thoughts, thought stopping,
breath counting) and d) remainder, which comprised all those strategies
which are not included in the three previous ones.

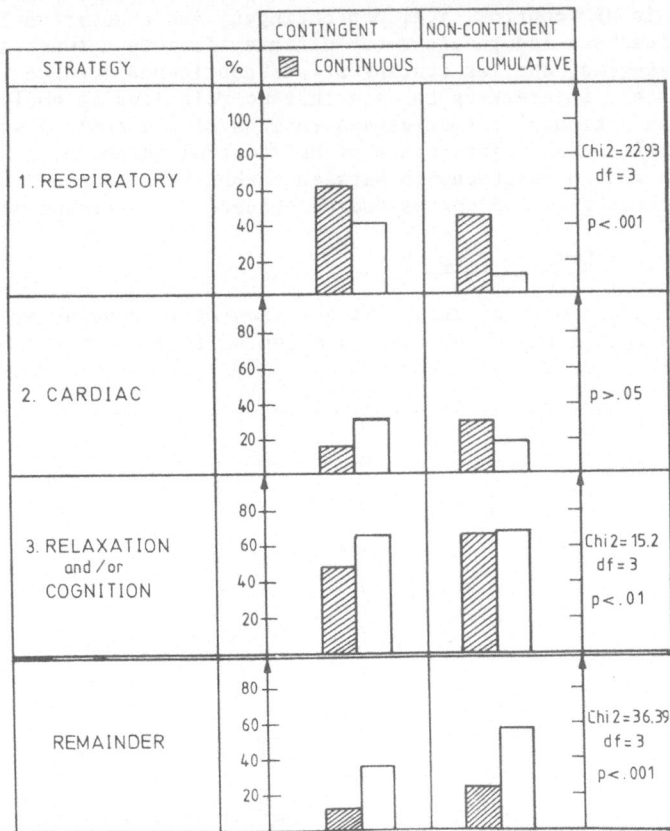

Fig. 10.   Percentage of strategies reported used by patients to control HPV
throughout the course of ten training sessions under contingent
(continuous or cumulative) and non-contingent (continuous or cumulative) feedback conditions. Chi-square statistics indicate statistical significance of the distribution of patients' statements with
regard to the categories of respiratory and cardiac control
strategies, bodily relaxation and/or cognitive strategies (e.g.
imagery, thought stopping, breath counting), and other strategies
not included in the previous ones (remainder).

From Figure 10, it becomes clear that respiratory maneuvers were mainly induced by continuous feedback, both under contingent and noncontingent conditions. In contrast, no significant differences could be found with respect to heart-related strategies. Relaxation and/or cognitive strategies, however, were very frequently reported, predominantly by those two groups who received cumulative feedback as well as by the noncontingent feedback group.

If one dichotomizes the strategies reported to be used into physiology-oriented strategies, such as respiratory or heart-related strategies, on the one hand (i.e. specific strategies) and cognition-oriented strategies, such as general relaxation or attentional processes, on the other hand (i.e. global strategies), the picture becomes more consistent. As illustrated in Figure 11, contingent as well as continuous feedback led patients to report global and specific strategies approximately to the same extent. Whenever the feedback was noncontingent or cumulative, patients tended to report more frequently global strategies than specific ones.

Thus, the differential feedback effects upon patients' verbal reports are mainly brought about by those forms of feedback that are assumed to be less effective in HPV control, i.e. noncontingent and cumulative feedback. Both types of feedback led to clear-cut differentiations between specific and global strategies, whereas contingent and continuous feedback forms did not. It is further interesting to note that no relationship could be observed between patients' effectiveness ratings of the control strategies utilized and their actual performance of HPV control (Kuhmann, 1984). Moreover, there was no relationship between verbal reports about respiratory control strategies and corresponding changes in breathing patterns.

Changes in Reported Symptom Frequency

From a clinical point of view, the question still remains as to whether, and to what extent, this manipulation of feedback information

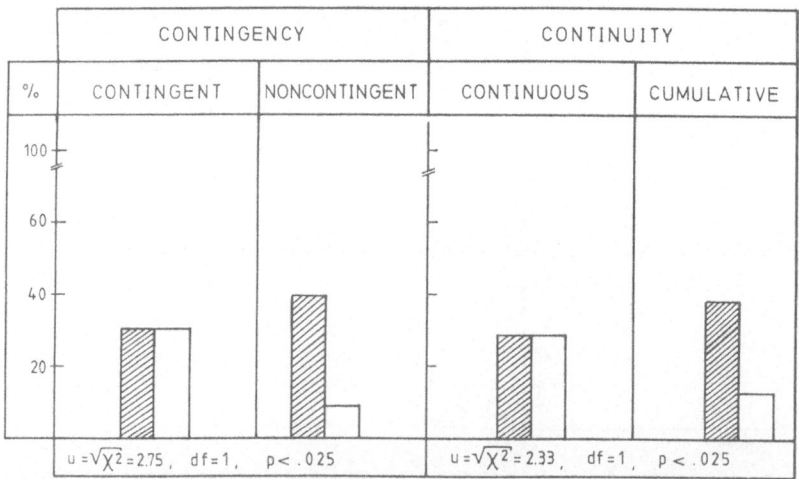

Fig. 11. Percentage of global and specific strategies used to control HPV across ten training sessions under contingent/noncontingent and continuous/cumulative feedback conditions. U-statistics indicate statistical significance of the distribution of patients' statements.

294

might be effective in reducing symptoms of patients with cardiophobic and heart-related disorders. In this context, we should focus our attention mainly on cardiac problems (for details and other psychological data collected cf. Ebert-Hampel, 1982, and Kuhmann, 1984). Changes in cardiac complaints were determined by a standardized questionnaire (Zenz, 1971). The dimension of cardiac complaints comprises heart-related disorders such as irregular heart beats, tachycardia, heart palpitations, acute chest pain or burning sensation in the heart region. As illustrated in Figure 12, for each feedback condition difference scores were calculated between pretreatment session (behavioral analysis sessions) and two follow-ups, 7 weeks and 6 months after the training was terminated. The results indicate very clearly that all groups did profit from biofeedback to a similar extent. However, only in those groups which received continuous feedback, either contingent or noncontingent, did the changes from pretreatment period yield statistical significance. In all groups, the most pronounced changes in heart-related disturbances occurred immediately after the last training

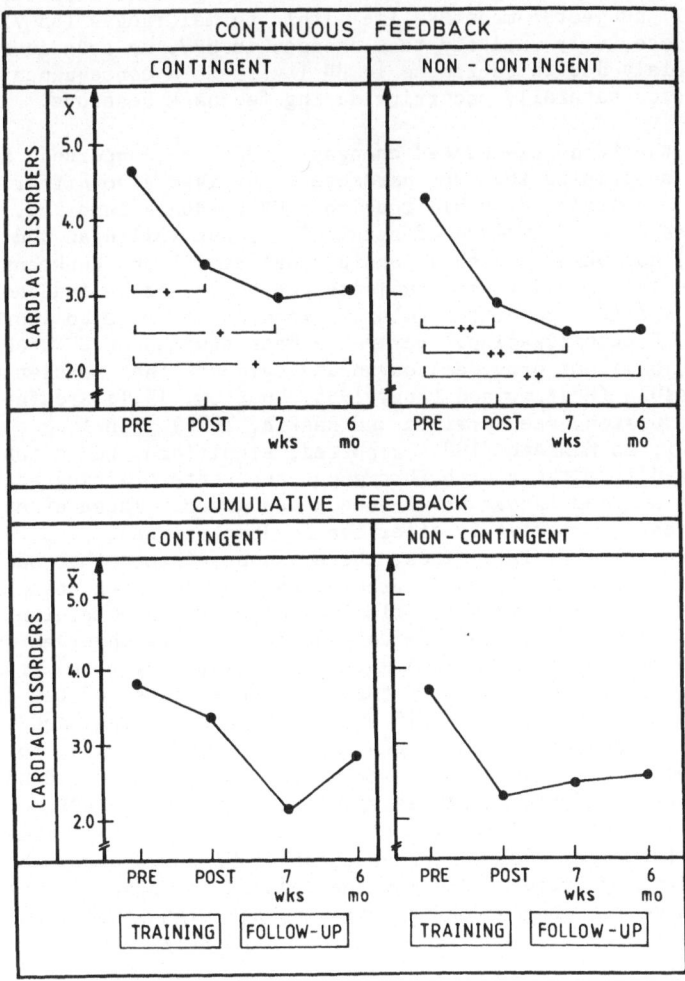

Fig. 12. Mean changes in test-scores (Zenz, 1971, Liste koerperlicher Symptome) for cardiac disorders under different feedback conditions (contingent-continuous, noncontingent-continuous, contingent-cumulative, noncontingent-cumulative) at pre-treatment (after 10 training sessions), 7 weeks and 6 months after training has been terminated (i.e. follow-ups). + = p<.05. ++ = p<.01.

session. This is not surprising if one assumes that the overall biofeed-back setting may exert a strong 'attention placebo' effect (patient-therapist relationship, instructions, explanations of cardiac functions etc.), which remained stable throughout half a year after the training period.

DISCUSSION

Summarizing the major findings of both the single-session studies and the clinical outcome study, the following conclusions can be drawn. These concern the changes in cardiac activity as well as the cardiac-respiratory interaction. Feedback studies on HPV control appear to represent an approach sui generis in the area of cardiac feedback because the changes in mean HR levels remain widely unaffected by the task of HP stabilization. One might have expected that HR slows down during such an easy task as HPV feedback. However, mean HR decreases from baselines to training trials in short-term as well as in long-term studies are not greater than 1-3 bpm. In addition, all subjects' mean HRs lie within normal ranges (65-75 bpm). It is, furthermore, very unlikely that changes in HPV, as seen in feedback studies, are solely due to decreases in HR levels as a consequence of general adaptation naturally occurring during feedback sessions.

As far as the feedback-induced changes in HPV are concerned, however, it is scarcely surprising that the parameters involved also differ from those examined and proposed by bidirectional HR feedback research. In HPV feedback studies, the 'knowledge of results' concept (Bilodeau and Bilodeau, 1969) has been favored as basic model (Vaitl and Kenkmann, 1972; Vaitl, 1975a). This implies that subjects can be taught by feedback information to act in a counter-regulatory fashion in order to improve performance of HP stabilization. Early feedback studies on HP stabiliz-ation, however, have not provided convincing evidence that persisting HPV control is possible (Hnatiow and Lang, 1965; Hnatiow, 1971; Sroufe, 1969, 1971; for a discussion, see Harrison and Raskin, 1976). In long-term studies, however, as Kuhmann (1984) reported, significant reduction in HPV could be obtained from the fourth throughout the tenth training session, when contingent and continuous HPV feedback was given. These effects, however, disappeared immediately after the feedback signals were turned off (i.e. during transfer trials). Thus, there is no evidence that subjects are able to transfer their learned performance from feedback to no feedback trials. This is in accord with the findings of the single-session studies. Moreover, increases in different HPV components could be observed when time-series reanalyses of those data were conducted. Power spectral analyses of HP signals revealed that throughout the course of ten feedback training sessions, both the .05 - .15 Hz (low frequency band) and .15 - .35 Hz (high frequency band) components increased from baseline to feedback trials. The low frequency rhythm was centered around 0.1 Hz (10-second-rhythm) which has been interpreted as spectral component of HPV reflecting changes in baroreceptor activity (Akselrod et al., 1981) or in diastolic blood pressure (De Boer, 1985). The spectrum of high frequency is associ-ated with respiratory cycles. The most pronounced increases in the 10-second rhythm occurred when no contingent feedback signal had to be pro-cessed and subjects were in addition instructed to relax and to breath regularly.

This experimental condition may serve as a point of reference from which the following interpretations can be delineated. First, let us assume that this task was less demanding than the other three were. In this case, no perturbation of ongoing HP fluctuations was experimentally induced; the cumulative, false feedback indicated increasing success and the relaxation instruction prevented subjects from making any further efforts to change their bodily functions. This led most likely to the observed predominance of low frequency components in HPV compared to the small portion left over for the respiration spectrum in this particular group. In addition, relaxation-induced reduction of peripheral vasomotor tone might also have facilitated the blood pressure-related rhythm to come into appearance so markedly. In contrast, none of the other experimental conditions produced increases of this oscillatory component to the same extent. Here, the component which has primarily been enhanced by those conditions was the respiration spectrum. This is probably due to the greater regularity of respiration (defined by autocorrelation coefficient) which was found to develop gradually throughout the course of the training (Kuhmann, 1984). Therefore, one may conclude that the respiratory component of HP fluctuations is increased rather than reduced by feedback.

The feedback-specific effects mainly concern the low frequency components of HPV. In both continuous feedback groups (contingent and non-contingent) the low frequency increased to a smaller degree than in the noncontinuous, noncontingent feedback groups and it was furthermore reduced under noncontinuous, contingent feedback conditions. This indicates that the high information density that had to be processed during continuous feedback as well as the low information of the cumulative, contingent feedback prevented the 10-second-rhythm from developing to as full an extent as was seen in the cumulative, noncontingent feedback group which was additionally instructed to relax and to breath regularly.

This fact, that the very low frequencies are generally reduced while the high frequencies, enhanced throughout the training, leads to some speculations which might have clinical relevance. In all four feedback groups, increases in the respiration-related frequency band occurred, which may reflect an increase in parasympathetic control of cardiac function. Although the feedback training was primarily aimed at reducing HPV, this component was not affected by subjects' voluntary maneuvers. In contrast, the short-term cyclic components of HPV did develop gradually throughout the training and could hardly be suppressed by any respiratory or cognitive strategy. With the exception of the cumulative, contingent feedback condition, as mentioned above, the same holds for the 10-second-rhythm. As Langhorst (this volume) demonstrated, this rhythmic component is closely related to a central rhythm which is basically inherent in common brain stem activities. Thus, if feedback of HPV has positive effects at all, they consist most likely in a general reduction of long-term fluctuations in HPV. Compared to this 'noise' variability, the inherent cyclic fluctuations and rhythmic components of HPV are facilitated and enhanced. This is probably due to general adaptation process which has been influenced by different HP stabilization tasks only to a very small extent.

The cardiac-respiratory interaction has also been influenced by the type of feedback given. As shown in single-session studies, contingent and noncontingent feedback when given on a beat-to-beat basis induced different cardiac-respiratory interactions as determined by weighted coherence (C_W) measures. Contingent feedback appeared to reduce the instantaneous co-variation of cardiac and respiratory cycle activity, whereas no feedback enhanced it. With regard to noncontingent feedback, however, two entirely different outcomes could be obtained. When noncontingent feedback displayed low HPV, indicating that the training goal had already been reached, C_W was increased; in contrast, under normal HPV conditions C_W was reduced to the same extent as under the contingent, high information feedback condition which confronted subjects with a higher amount of instantaneous HPV. These differential effects disappeared completely when more than one session of feedback was conducted.

In the clinical study, however, it could be shown that the cardiac-respiratory interaction was enhanced to a considerable amount, irrespective of the feedback contingency. Furthermore, the most markedly pronounced increases in the C_w measure did occur in that group which was cumulatively given a false feedback and was in addition requested to relax and to breath regularly. Thus, the differentiation between various feedback forms, as seen in single-session studies, can only be interpreted as short-term effects while general increases of cardiac-respiratory interaction during feedback trials across ten sessions indicate certainly long-term adaptation phenomena.

Prior to speculating about the C_w measure as index of vagal tone as proposed by several researchers (for discussion, see Porges' chapter in this volume), one should bear in mind that this measure can be influenced to a considerable amount by minimal changes in feedback information to be processed as well as by instructional control or a clinical setting. In this volume, Porges has demonstrated very clearly that C_w measures did not reflect decreases in vagal activity when pharmacologically induced by atropine. In contrast, a task-related phenomenon has been observed by Porges and Coles (1982) that might fit our findings. They reported significant reduction in C_w as the task (vigilance task, reaction time task) progressed, irrespective of high or low initial levels of C_w. This is in accord with the short-term effects of contingent, high information feedback, which resembles tasks with sustained attentional demands. Further research, however, is needed in order to elucidate the relationship between different attentional processes (phasic, sustained) and cardiac-respiratory coupling.

CONCLUSIONS

With respect to the scope of this volume the following major conclusions can be drawn:

1) Cardiac-respiratory interaction is mainly influenced by the amount of feedback-signals to be processed (i.e. short-term effects).
2) Cardiac-respiratory interaction is increased throughout feedback training across ten sessions, irrespective of the feedback form applied (i.e. long-term effects); this is probably due to a general adaptation.
3) Feedback-assisted heart period stabilization training suppresses the slow trends in heart period variability whereas the cyclic fluctuations (10-second rhythm and respiratory rhythm) are enhanced.
4) Under resting conditions, as within feedback settings, cardiac-respiratory interactions prove to be highly susceptible to external stimulus conditions. Changes in level of respiratory-cardiac interactions appear to be determined by a three-way interaction between 'mental load' (i.e. the amount of feedback signals to be processed), 'instruction' (or experimental setting) and time.

Acknowledgements

This research has been supported by a grant from the Deutsche Forschungsgemeinschaft (German Research Society) to the first author (VA 37, 1). I gratefully acknowledge the assistance of Diplome-Psychologist Harald Gruppe who carried out all the times-series analyses. I would also like to thank Dr Kees Janssen for his helpful advice during the preparation of the manuscript, and Dr Paul Grossman for suggesting the reanalysis of the data to explore whether HPV feedback enhanced endogenous cardiac rhythms (e.g. respiratory sinus arrhythmia) while at the same time reducing slow, nonstationary HP variations.

REFERENCES

Akselrod, S., Gordon, D., Ubel, F. A., Shannon, D. C., Barger, A. C., and
Cohen, R. J., 1981, Power spectrum analysis of heart rate fluctu-
ation: A quantitative probe of beat-to-beat cardiovascular control,
Science, 213:220–222.

Baselli, G., Cerutti, S., Civardi, S., Lombardi, F., Malliani, A., and
Pagani, M., 1985, Autoregressive modelling and spectral estimation
for the quantification of neural control mechanisms on heart rate
variability signals, in: "Melecon '85, Volume I: Bioengineering," A.
Luque, A. R. Figueiras, and J. M. R. Delgado, eds., Elsevier, North-
Holland, pp. 131–134.

Bilodeau, E. A., and Bilodeau, I. McD., 1969, "Principles of Skill Acquisition," Academic Press, New York.

Cheatle, M. D., and Weiss, T., 1982, Biofeedback in heart rate control and
the treatment of cardiac arrhythmias, in: "Clinical Biofeedback:
Efficacy and Mechanisms," Guilford Press, New York, pp. 164–194.

Cohors-Fresenborg, M., Czeschick, E., Hollen, W., Frhr. von, and Verstege,
R., 1976, "Biofeedback-Untersuchung zur Stabilisation der Herz-
frequenz unter verschiedenen Rueckmeldebedingungen," Master Thesis,
University of Muenster.

Cuthbert, B., Kristeller, J., Simons, R., Hodes, R., and Lang, P. J., 1981,
Strategies of arousal control: Biofeedback, meditation, and motivation, J. Exp. Psychol. Gen., 110:518–546.

DeBoer, R. W., 1985, "Beat-to-Beat Blood Pressure Fluctuations and Heart-
Rate Variability in Man: Physiological Relationships, Analysis
Techniques and Simple Model," Drukkerij Elinkwijk B.V., Utrecht.

Ebert, B., Kuhmann, W., and Vaitl, D., 1979, Effects of systematically
varied biofeedback training of heart rate on cardiophobic patients,
in: "Biofeedback and Self-Regulation," N. Birbaumer and H. D.
Kimmel, eds., Erlbaum, Hillsdale, N.J., pp. 425–436.

Ebert-Hampel, B., 1982, "Biofeedback und funktionelle Herzbeschwerden,"
Peter Lang, Verlag, Frankfurt/M.

Engel, B. T., and Bleecker, E. R., 1974, Application of operant con-
ditioning techniques to the control of cardiac arrhythmias, in:
"Cardiovascular Psychophysiology," P. A. Obrist, A. H. Black, J.
Brener, and L. V. DiCara, eds., Aldine, Chicago, pp. 456–476.

Fouad, F. M., Tarazi, R. C., Ferrario, C. M., Fighaly, S., and Alicandri,
C., 1984, Assessment of parasympathetic control of heart rate by a
noninvasive method, Am. J. Physiol., p. 246 (Heart, Circ. Physiol.),
15:H838–H842.

Harrison, R. S., and Raskin, D. C., 1976, The role of feedback in control
of heart rate variability, Psychophysiology, 13:135–139.

Hnatiow, M., and Lang, P. J., 1965, Learned stabilization of cardiac rate,
Psychophysiology, 1:330–336.

Hnatiow, M., 1971, Learned control of heart rate and blood pressure,
Perceptual and Motor Skills, 33:219–226.

Janssen, K. H. L., 1983, Treatment of sinus tachycardia with heart rate
feedback, J. Behav. Med., 6:109–114.

Janssen, K. H. L., and Berger, M. P. F., 1985, "Heart Rate Feedback for
Sinus Tachycardia: A Group Outcome Study," Manuscript, Tilburg
University.

Kuhmann, W., 1984, "Effekte und Mechanismen eines Langzeit-Biofeedback-
Trainings zur Kontrolle der Variabilitaet der Herztaetigkeit,"
Weiss, Dreieich.

Lang, P. J., Sroufe, L. A., and Hastings, J. E., 1967, Effects of feedback
instructional set on the control of cardiac-rate variability, J.
Exp. Psychol., 75:425–431.

Lown, B., Verrier, R. L., and Rabinowitz, S., 1977, Neural and psychological mechanisms and the problem of sudden cardiac death, Am. J.
Cardiol., 39:890–902.

Luczak, H., Philipp, U., and Rohmert, W., 1980, Decomposition of heart-rate variability under the ergonomic aspects of stressor analysis, in: "The Study of Heart-Rate Variability," R. I. Kitney and O. Rompelman, eds., Clarendon Press, Oxford.

Porges, S. W., Bohrer, R. E., Cheung, M. N., Deasgow, F., McCabe, P. M., and Keren, G., 1980, New time-series statistic for detecting rhythmic co-occurrence in the frequency domain: The weighted coherence and its application to psychophysiological research, Psychol. Bull., 88:580-587.

Porges, S. W., and Coles, M. G. H., 1982, Individual differences in respiratory-heart period coupling and heart period responses during two attention-demanding tasks, Physiological Psycholgy, 10:215-220.

Porges, S. W., McCabe, P. M., and Yongue, B. G., 1982, Respiratory-heart rate interactions: Psychophysiological implications for pathophysiology and behavior, in: "Perspective in Cardiovascular Psychophysiology," J. Cacioppo and R. Petty, eds., Guilford Press, New York.

Scott, R. W., Blanchard, E. B., Edmundson, E. D., and Young, L. D., 1973, A shaping procedure for heart rate control in chronic tachycardia, Perceptual and Motor Skills, 37:327-338.

Skinner, J. E., and Reed, J. C., 1981, Blockade of the frontocortical-brainstem pathway prevents ventricular fibrillation of the ischemic heart in pigs, Am. J. Physiol., 240:H156-H163.

Sroufe, L. A., 1969, Learned stabilization of cardiac rate with respiration experimentally controlled, J. Exper. Psychol., 71:391-393.

Sroufe, L. A., 1971, Effects of depth and rate of breathing on heart rate and heart rate variability, Psychophysiology, 8:648-655.

Stegagno, L., and Vaitl, D., 1979, Voluntary heart rate acceleration under conditions of binary feedback and social competition, in: Biofeedback and Self-Regulation," N. Birbaumer and H. D. Kimmel, eds., Erlbaum, Hillsdale, N.J., pp. 197-204.

Vaitl, D., and Kenkmann, H. -J., 1972, Stabilisation der pulsfrequenz durch visuelle rueckmeldung, Zeit. Klin. Psychol., 1:251-271.

Vaitl, D., 1973, Heart rate control under false feedback conditions, in: "Biofeedback and Self-Control," D. Shapiro, T. C. Barber, L. V. DiCara, J. Kamiya, N. E. Miller, and J. Stoyva, eds., Aldine, Chicago, p. 502.

Vaitl, D., 1975a, Zur problematik des biofeedback, dargestellt am beispiel der herzfrequenzkontrolle, Psychol. Rundschau, 26:191-211.

Vaitl, D., 1975b, Biofeedback-einsatz in der behandlung einer patientin mit sinus-tachykardie, in: "Biofeedback-Therapie. Lernmethoden in der Psychosomatik, Neurologie und Rehabilitation," H. Legewie and L. Nusselt, eds., Urban and Schwarzenberg, München.

Vaitl, D., Kenkmann, H. -J., and Kuhmann, W., 1979, Heart-rate stabilization feedback and concomitant physiological changes, in: "Biofeedback and Self-Regulation," N. Birbaumer and H. D. Kimmel, eds., Erlbaum, Hillsdale, N.J.

Vaitl, D., Stegagno, L., and Trombini, G., 1977, Stabilizzatione della frequenza cardiaca mediante feedback visivo in condizioni di rilassamento farmacologicamente indotto, Arch. Psicol. Neurol. Psich., 38:204-222.

White, L., and Tursky, B., 1982, "Clinical Biofeedback: Efficacy and Mechanisms," Guilford, New York.

Williamson, D. A., and Blanchard, E. B., 1979, Heart rate and blood pressure biofeedback. II. A review and integration of recent theoretical models, Biofeedback and Self-Regulation, 4:35-50.

Yongue, B. G., Porges, S. W., and McCabe, P. M., 1979, "Changes in Vagal Control of the Heart Following Signaled and Unsignaled Shock," Paper presented at the Meeting of the Society for Psychophysiological Research, Cincinnati.

Zenz, H., 1971, Empirische befunde über die giessener fassung einer beschwerdeliste, Zeit. Psychothera. med. Psychol., 21:7-13.

CLINICAL APPLICATIONS

HYPERVENTILATION AS DIAGNOSTIC STRESS TEST FOR VARIANT ANGINA
AND CARDIOMYOPATHY: Cardiovascular Responses, Likely Triggering
Mechanisms and Psychophysiological Implications

S. A. Mortensen, H. Nielsen and Paul Grossman*

Rigshospitalet, Copenhagen
*Institute for Stress Research
and Free University, Amsterdam

INTRODUCTION

The recognition that coronary artery spasm (CAS) is an important
pathogenic factor in evolving myocardial ischemia has generated new
possibilities for selective and effective antianginal treatment (Maseri
et al., 1978; Severi et al., 1980; Fischer, Hansen and Sandoe, 1978).
Prinzmetal's variant angina (PVA) (Prinzmetal et al., 1959) is characterized by attacks of chest pain at rest, often in the early morning hours,
and most typically associated with electrocardiographic (ECG) signs of
transmural myocardial ischemia. The CAS in PVA develops upon a wide
spectrum of coronary artery lesions from normal or nearly normal arteries
to severe coronary artery disease with involvement of two to three of the
main vessels (Severi et al., 1980; Bertrand et al., 1979). However, the
clinical picture may be atypical, with manifestations of arrhythmias or
syncopes obscuring and delaying the diagnosis of CAS in those subjects with
only moderate chest discomfort.

Several provocative measures have been employed (Table 1) as diagnostic tests performed to reproduce attacks of CAS. These procedures may
be separated into the following categories: (1) pharmacological interventions using ergot alkaloids (ergonovine; Heupler et al., 1978), alkal-
ization (tris-buffer; Yasue et al., 1978), cholinergic drugs (metha-
choline), adrenergic drugs (epinephrine), posterior pituitary hormones
(vasopression; Chahine, 1980); and (2) physiological stimuli including the
cold pressor test (Raizner et al., 1980), exercise test (Yasue, 1978) and
hyperventilation (Groves et al., 1975; Yasue et al., 1981; Girotti et al.,
1982; Weber et al., 1981; Pujadas et al., 1981; Mortensen, Vilhelmsen and
Sandoe, 1981). Mechanically induced CAS by coronary catheters is well-
known but without clinical value. Evidence of emotionally induced spasm
has been recently indicated in patients with angina pectoris who performed
a psychologically stressful quiz (Schiffer et al., 1980).

The present report deals with cardiovascular-respiratory relations in
patients evidencing increased coronary vascular reactivity. One purpose of
this Chapter is to review our experiences using hyperventilation as a
diagnostic test for patients with PVA or chest pain related to other types
of heart disease. Another primary goal of this paper, however, is to
extrapolate our findings to issues of potential importance for the psychophysiology of specific cardiovascular disorders. With regard to the latter

Table 1.

PROVOCATIVE TESTS	CORONARY ARTERY SPASM
PHARMACOLOGICAL INTERVENTIONS:	ERGOT ALKALOIDS
	ALKALIZATION
NON-PHARMACOLOGICAL TESTS:	COLD PRESSOR TEST
	EXERCISE LOAD
	HYPERVENTILATION
	PSYCHOLOGIC STIMULI
COMBINED PROCEDURES	

aim, our orientation is upon relations between psychological stress, hyperventilation and cardiovascular responses with specific reference to our high-risk patient population. A brief justification for such a focus would seem at this point to be merited.

HYPERVENTILATION, PSYCHOPHYSIOLOGY AND CARDIOVASCULAR RISK

Hyperventilation, defined as ventilation in excess of carbon dioxide production, is a normal response to different forms of psychological stress (e.g., demanding mental tasks, physical pain and anticipation of aversive stimulation; Grossman, 1983; Wientjes and Grossman, 1985). One study, for example, found that 40% of aviation cadets learning to fly hyperventilated during their training flights (Balke, Elles and Wells, 1958), whereas another investigation reported that over 90% of its subjects hyperventilated in anticipation of a painful electric shock (Suess et al., 1980). Taken as a whole, such studies also suggest that the degree of hyperventilation (defined as reduction in alveolar CO_2 level) may be directly proportional to the perceived intensity of psychological stressor (Grossman, 1983; Wientjes and Grossman, 1985). Other evidence, furthermore, indicates that there are large individual differences in the propensity to hyperventilate in specific situations, often related to psychological characteristics (Stoney, Langer, Sutterer and Gelling, this volume; Suess et al., 1980). In a recent study, Wientjes and Grossman (1985) found both consistent individual differences in hyperventilatory responses across several conditions and an enhanced tendency toward hyperventilation across individuals as increased mental effort was required during a monetary-incentive reaction-time task; more severe hyperventilators tended also to be more dispositionally situationally anxious. Of particular relevance to cardiovascular risk, another experiment reported that Type-A subjects showed greater reductions in CO_2 levels than B's during an aversive mental task (Stoney et al., this volume). Hence, psychological stress seems often to produce hyperventilatory reactions, although the degree of CO_2 reduction apparently depends upon individual-specific factors, as well as the type and intensity of the stress stimulus.

There is also an abundance of evidence pointing toward cardiovascular effects of hyperventilation that could spell particular risk for heart and circulatory system patients: hyperventilation among both, normals and patients, produces complaints of chest pain, tachycardia, atypical ECG responses, myocardial vasoconstriction and impaired myocardial oxygen supply (see Grossman, 1983; Grossman and Wientjes, in press, for reviews). As we shall soon see, voluntary hyperventilation among PVA patients consistently elicits the coronary vasospasm, ECG abnormalities and chest pain which characterize a PVA episode. Given that such attacks are very serious, jeopardizing events when taking place without medical supervision, this evidence powerfully suggests that spontaneous stress-induced hyperventilation could seriously compromise the health of PVA, and perhaps other cardiovascular patients.

It is rather well established that hyperventilation is implicated in the development and prolongation of stress-related, functional cardiovascular disorders in which there is no evidence of organic pathology (e.g., Syndrome X; see Grossman and Wientjes, 1985). Chronic anxiety has been frequently related to this type of dysfunction. It is also clear that such disorders may often coexist with organic heart disease (Bass et al., 1983; Friedman, 1947; Yu, Yim and Stanfield, 1959). The present report underlines the seriousness of risk that may occur when these two kinds of disturbance interact in the same individual. By clinically observing the cardiac effects of hyperventilation upon several different patient groups and normals, our findings may help to indicate just which organic heart disorders are most dangerous in combination with psychosomatic hyperventilation-related disturbances.

SUBJECTS INVESTIGATED

During the last three years prolonged hyperventilation has been used in our clinic (the Department of Medicine B, Rigshospitalet University Hospital, Copenhagen) as a means of provocation for all consecutive patients suspected of having PVA and for selected cases with chest pain of obscure origin. The diagnosis of variant angina was made on the basis of the following criteria: (a) typical and repeated attacks of anginal pain at rest during a period of more than one month; (b) significant and transient ST-segment elevations in several leads (at least 2 mm) not present in the baseline ECG; (c) relief of symptoms by nitrates; and (d) no rise in myocardial enzymes in relation to the attacks.

Fourteen of our 23 patients were clinically diagnosed from spontaneous attacks; in the remaining nine patients where there were longer symptom-free intervals or atypical manifestations of spasm, the diagnosis of PVA was made using the hyperventilation test in seven of nine, whereas two of nine subjects were classified as Syndrome X (SYX) (Kubler and Opherk, 1983).

We furthermore studied fifteen selected patients with dilated cardiomyopathy (i.e., a primary disease of the heart muscle characterized by impaired systolic ventricular functioning). The patients were classified clinically, noninvasively (echocardiography) and invasively (routine heart catheterization supported by endomyocardial biopsy). These patients were all suffering from chest discomfort or pain. A "control series" of 24 patients with other cardiac and non-cardiac diseases (Table 2), plus seven normal subjects, were studied parallel to the PVA patients.

Table 2.

HYPERVENTILATION AND CORONARY ARTERY SPASM
CONTROL-GROUP (N=24)

OESOPHAGEAL DYSFUNCTION & GASTROINTESTINAL DISEASE (10)
MUSCULOSKELETAL DISORDERS (5)
CORONARY ARTERY DISEASE (4)
VARIOUS HEART DISEASES (4)
PHEOCHROMOCYTOMA (1)

HYPERVENTILATION TEST - METHODS

Prolonged strenuous hyperventilation (HVT) with a frequency of about 35 respirations per minute (min) was performed during a period of 6 min. A twelve-leads ECG was obtained continuously with a paper speed of 10 mm/sec for a period of 20 min. Baseline ECG, and ECG every second minute was obtained during the test at a paper speed of 25 mm/sec. Blood pressure (arm-cuff) was determined every second minute, and arterial blood samples were taken immediately before and after the period of forced breathing to ensure that a sufficient level of hypocapnia had been reached. A venous cannula was placed in the cubital fossa for intravenous medications or blood-drawing during the HVT.

The tests were usually performed at "the critical time" of the day during which symptoms had occurred in the past (usually in the early morning), and control-tests were performed at successive days usually in the afternoon. Multiple tests were performed during the 24-hour cycle in selected cases to study the circadian variation in sensitivity to the HVT, just as serial tests were carried out before and after treatment with two calcium channel blockers, Verapamil (isoptin[R]) and nifedipine (adalat[R]). In addition to the HVT, all patients underwent bicycle exercise tests and had standard echocardiograms obtained. Coronary arteriography was performed in 20 of 23 patients with PVA and SYX and in the majority of the controls.

The HVT was considered positive if: (1) chest pain + ST-deviation (> 2 mm) was provoked or (2) ST-elevation (> 2 mm) ensued. The time of appearance and the duration of pain and ECG events were registered in minutes calculated from the start of overbreathing.

HYPERVENTILATION TEST - PRECAUTIONS

All tests were performed either in the coronary care unit, the stress-testing laboratory or the catheterization laboratory, with optimal facilities for resuscitation including DC-defibrillator. Informed consent to participate in the HVT was obtained.

The HVT was stopped immediately if there were signs of ST-segment elevation or chest pain. The following medications were ready for i.v. use (in loaded syringes): (1) nitroglycerin; (2) isoptin[R]; and (3) atropine. Further, nitroglycerin for sublingual use and adalat[R] capsules were avail-

Table 3.

PATIENT DIAGNOSIS	HVT PERFORMED	POSITIVE HVT	NEGATIVE HVT	INCONCLUSIVE HVT
VASOSPASTIC ANGINA (21)	7/21	6	0	1
SYNDROME X (2)	2/2	2	0	0
DILATED CARDIOMYOPATHY (15)	15/15	0	13	2
VARIOUS TYPES OF HEART DISEASE AND EXTRACARDIAC PAIN (24)	24/24	0	23	1
NORMAL SUBJECTS (7)	7/7	0	7	0

able. As inability to stop hyperventilation was seen in a few cases, we had a plastic bag at hand for CO_2 rebreathing.

Patients with clinical and/or exercise-ECG evidence of severe coronary artery disease were excluded from the test because of the potentially great risk of complications from provoked CAS or vasoconstriction. Serial ECG's and myocardial enzyme determinations preceded the HVT, and cases of unstable angina and threatening myocardial infarction were excluded.

OBSERVATIONS AND ILLUSTRATE CASE REPORTS

1. Variant Angina

The series of patients with PVA collected from 1976 to 1983 consisted of 13 males and 8 females with a mean age of 53.6 years (range 36-76 years). The "controls", 18 males and 6 females had a mean age of 48.7 years (range 19-77 years). Coronary arteriography performed in 18 to 21 patients with PVA showed single-vessel disease in ten, two-vessel disease in one and normal coronary arteries in seven cases. Table 3 shows the outcome of the HVT in the different patient categories in "the diagnostic situation" (without antianginal treatment), i.e., when the patients were admitted for evaluation of their symptoms with chest pain.

Fourteen out of 21 suspected PVA patients had had spontaneous attacks of chest pain and ST-segment elevation so that the diagnosis of CAS could be established without any provocative test. In the remaining seven, the attacks were either infrequent and/or atypical with arrhythmias and fainting spells, and in this group six responded positively to HVT with ST-segment elevation (2-10 mm), and concomitant chest pain in five. In one case the HVT was inconclusive because of reduced ventilatory capacity (obstructive lung disease); however, this patient had on a previous occasion presented spontaneous attacks of pain and ST-elevation.

Symptoms (pain and ECG-changes) subsided within a few minutes (1-3 minutes) whether nitroglycerin was given or not. Two patients experienced arrhythmias after the test, one patient had ventricular ectopic beats and one patient suffered serious arrhythmias and conduction disturbances as the HVT provoked spasms in both the left and right coronary artery (Mortensen et al., 1981).

The changes in acid-base balance and pCO_2 were expected to exceed the following limits to ensure sufficient hyperventilation: pH > 7.60 and pCO_2 < 3.00 kPa (1 kPa = approximately 7.5 mmHg). The HVT's were positive when scheduled at the same time of day as when spontaneous attacks had previously occurred (usually in the morning); the control-tests scattered throughout the rest of the day were negative.

Different therapeutics may modulate the disease activity of PVA and the response to HVT. Nine of 11 patients treated with different beta-blockers experienced more frequent and severe attacks during the treatment periods and none of the patients improved with this treatment (Sandoe, Vilhemsen and Mortensen, 1982). Treatment with calcium channel blockers prevented the positive response to all HVT's performed on successive days in the PVA patients, even in the early morning.

CASE STUDIES

Case 1. A typical result of the HVT is shown in Figure 1 (right panel) with ST-elevation in the inferior leads (II, III and aVF) from a

307

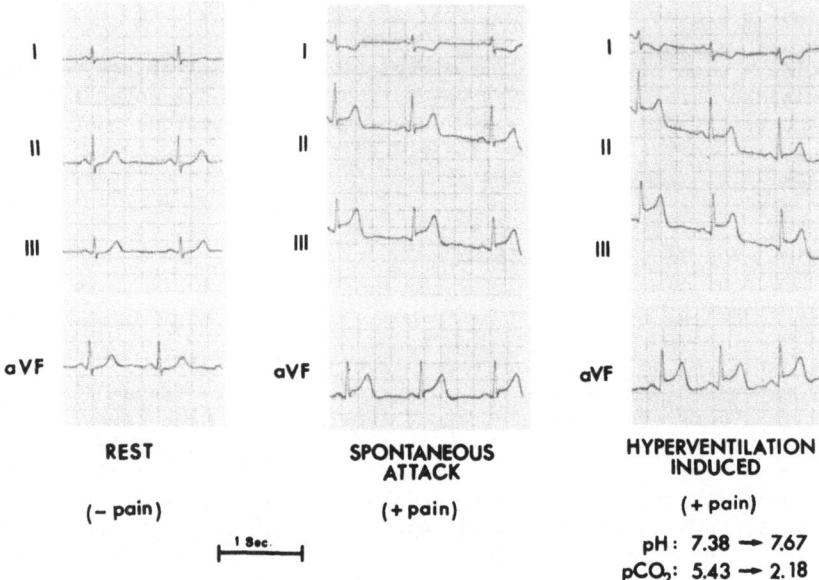

I

II

III

aVF

REST

(− pain)

I

II

III

aVF

SPONTANEOUS
ATTACK

(+ pain)

1 Sec.

I

II

III

aVF

HYPERVENTILATION
INDUCED

(+ pain)

pH: 7.38 → 7.67
pCO₂: 5.43 → 2.18

Fig. 1. ECG obtained from a 37-year-old male during spontaneous attack of chest pain suggesting transmural ischemia of the inferior myocardial wall. The same pattern was induced by hyperventilation (right panel).

37-year-old male who had a 75% stenosis of the right coronary artery. A spontaneous attack (middle panel) demonstrates the same pattern elicited just prior to a scheduled HVT, suggesting that the psychological stress from the planned investigation was a sufficient stimulus to elicit CAS in this patient, who was in the waxing phase of symptoms. This patient responded positively to the test during the hyperventilatory breathing itself, unlike most of the patients who showed delayed CAS response during the recovery from HV (approximately 5-6 minutes after stopping the HVT).

Case 2. In another patient from the series, a 57-year-old male who had experienced attacks with chest pain and arrhythmias in the early morning (Figure 2), simultaneous recording of cross-sectional echocardiography and ECG was performed during HVT. While the ECG showed ST-elevation in leads II, III and aVF, and the patient experienced chest pain, the posterior and inferior wall of the left ventricle and the inferior part of the septum gradually developed akinesia. Spontaneous relief of pain and ECG changes were accompanied by hyperkinesia of the previous akinetic myocardial segments on the echocardiogram which lasted a few minutes (Egeblad, Vilhelmsen and Mortensen, 1982).

2. Syndrome X

Two patients from the series, one male and one female, showed ST-depression both during exercise and HVT (Figure 3). Both had absolutely normal coronary arteries. In the male patient a biphasic response from the HVT was registered. Initially chest pain and marked ST-depression was provoked in several leads after approximately four to five minutes of hyperventilating. These events faded away during the next one to two minutes; however, after a symptom-free interval of two minutes, the ECG-response recurred accompanied by a significant decline in mean blood pressure (from 120 to 80 mmHg) with shivering and general discomfort. Pretreatment with a calcium channel blocker (adalat[R]) plus isosorbid-

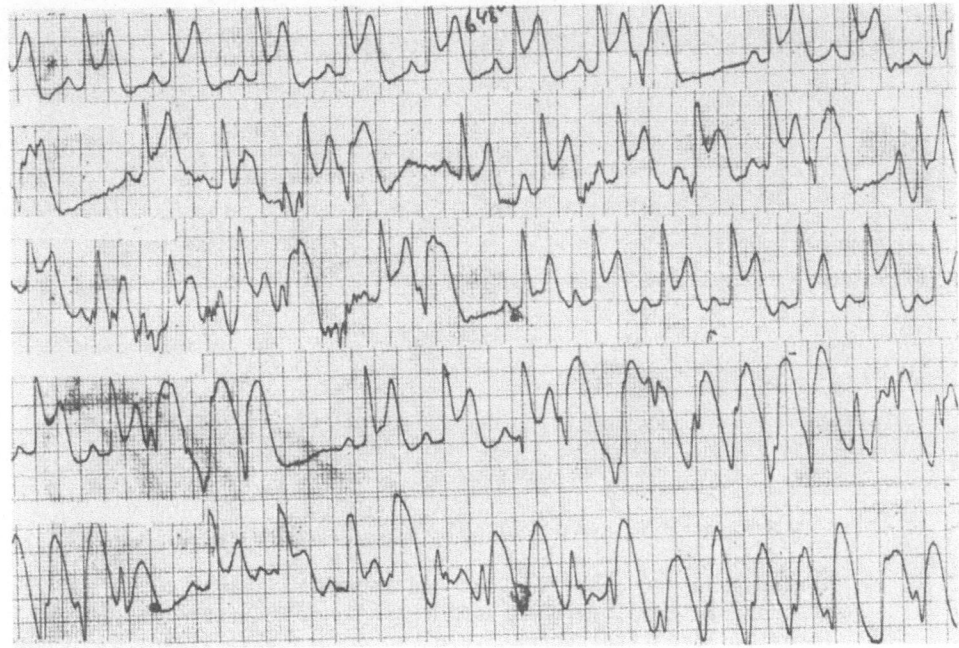

Fig. 2. ECG monitoring showing sinus rhythm and ST elevation, followed by
multiform ventricular tachycardia. Slight chest discomfort was
present. The attack subsided after a few minutes in this patient
with variant angina.

diuitrate (cardopax[R]) prevented the positive response from the HVT in this
patient. An undefined metabolic abnormality (Richardson, 1974) may be
responsible for these findings, and the SYX cases, perhaps, could be
included in the poorly defined entity of "latent cardiomyopathy".

3. Cardiomyopathy

A microspasm theory has been proposed from animal studies in dilated
(congestive) cardiomyopathy (Factor and Sonnenblick, 1982) and the use of
verapamil in these experiments proved effective in preventing the development of the disease. These observations might be applied to humans, as
spasm tendency may be involved in the early stage of cardiomyopathy
favoring the prophylactic use of calcium channel blockers instead of beta-
blockers as proposed by others (Swedberg et al., 1979).

None of our fifteen patients with dilated cardiomyopathy responded to
the HVT with chest pain and significant ST-segment changes. However, most
of the patients showed increased frequency of premature ventricular beats,
and five patients experienced some chest discomfort. This may be totally
non-specific, but local tissue ischemia from vasoconstriction might be
possible. Two of the patients were unable to complete the HVT efficiently.

The HVT may prove useful for research purposes in these patients as a
stress test, e.g., during cardiac catheterization when studies of myocardial metabolism are carried out.

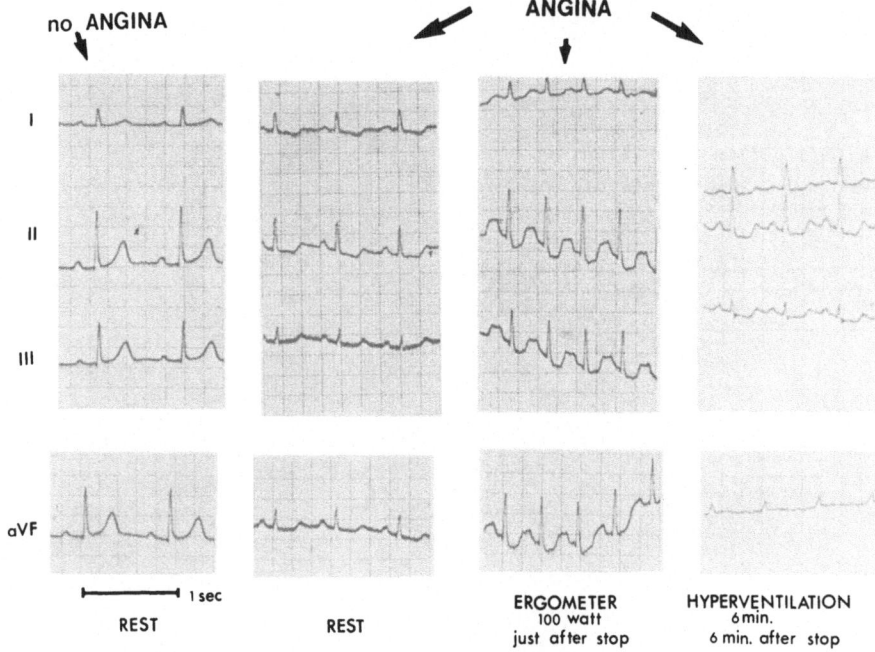

no ANGINA   ANGINA

I

II

III

aVF

| | 1 sec

REST   REST   ERGOMETER   HYPERVENTILATION
                                  100 watt   6 min.
                              just after stop   6 min. after stop

Fig. 3. The response to exercise test and hyperventilation of a
46-year-old female with Syndrome-X. The ST-depressions in the
inferior leads are suggestive of subendocardial ischemia. Chest
pain and ECG changes appeared 6 minutes after stopping the hyperventilation (i.e. in the recovery phase).

4. Controls

None of the seven normal subjects or the 24 "control patients" with a
range of cardiac diseases, oesophageal dysfunction, skeletal and muscular
disorders, were positive responders to the HVT. One patient with ischemic
heart disease showed 1 to 2 mm ST-depression during HVT without pain.

5. Follow-up Studies

Twenty-three patients with PVA and SYX were followed from eight to 81
months (mean, 42 months). At the follow-up study nineteen were still
alive; four had died (two sudden deaths and two non-cardiac deaths). One
patient had suffered acute myocardial infarction, and eight had developed
hypertension. Further, one of the hypertensive patients had suffered a
cerebrovascular attack.

Thirteen of the nineteen survivors had been treated on a long-term
basis with calcium channel blocker, and nine were free of chest pain while
four had pain at exercise. Control-HVT's were all negative in this group
(Table 4). Six patients were not on treatment, either because they had
discontinued the treatment themselves because of disappearance of symptoms
or because of complaints from side-effects. Four of the latter group had
negative HVT's suggesting spontaneous remission of the vasospastic disease
(Waters et al., 1981). In two cases there were a positive HVT so that the
calcium channel blocker treatment was started again.

Thus, symptoms at rest were prevented in all patients treated by
calcium antagonists; however, one-third still had some complaints during
physical activity. Nearly one-fourth of 19 patients were in remission at
the long-term follow-up investigation.

Table 4.

HYPERVENTILATION AND CORONARY ARTERY SPASM
FOLLOW-UP 19 PATIENTS WITH PVA AND SYX

	HVT PERFORMED	HVT OUTCOME	
		POS.	NEG.
13 PATIENTS ON TREATMENT [x)]	10		
A. NO SYMPTOMS (N=9)		0	6
B. PAIN AT EXERCISE (N=4)		0	4
6 PATIENTS WITHOUT TREATMENT	6		
C. NO SYMPTOMS (N=5)		1	4
D. PAIN AT EXERCISE + REST (N=1)		1	-

x) CALCIUM CHANNEL BLOCKERS

ADVERSE EFFECTS AND LIMITATIONS OF THE HYPERVENTILATION TEST

The severe arrhythmias after HVT in one of our patients caused no sequelae (Mortensen et al., 1981); however, these events should keep the investigator in mind that a potentially life-threatening state may be provoked (although it is a non-pharmacological test), stressing the importance of optimal facilities for resuscitation. Apart from the case just mentioned, no complications have occurred in the present series. A few patients have had a marked psychological reaction during the HVT with anxiety and prolonged ventilatory recovery (necessitating the use of CO_2-rebreathing in a plastic bag).

Inconclusive tests may be produced in patients with obstructive lung disease and decreased ventilatory capacity. The HVT stimulus may, furthermore, not be strong enough in patients who are already chronically hyperventilating. Additionally, borderline or negative tests may be due to reduced sensitivity at the time of the test (Maseri and Chierchia, 1982).

RESPONSES TO HYPERVENTILATION AND DISCUSSION OF TRIGGERING STIMULI

Hyperventilation induces a number of effects, especially upon the cardiovascular system (Grossman, 1983). ECG changes are frequently registered during sudden and forceful hyperventilation with a duration of about one-half to one minute, i.e., acute hyperventilation. Apart from increases in heart rate, flattening or inversion of T-waves may be seen (Wasserburger and Alt, 1961; Joy and Trump, 1981; Thompson, 1943). The mechanisms by which acute hyperventilation produces ECG changes are unknown although various explanations have been reported, e.g., shortening of the repolarization with asynchrony in the ventricles, fluctuations in plasma potassium and increased sympathetic activity. It is noteworthy that the changes may persist through the period of hyperventilation and that the abnormalities disappear when recovery from acute/chronic overbreathing takes place. Simple explanation and physiotherapy have been able to restore the normal breathing in chronic cases, together with disappearance of the chest pain complaints (Evans and Lum, 1977). However, in cardiac patients, especially subjects with latent or manifest arteriosclerotic disease, acute hyperventilation may be potentially detrimental (Grossman, 1983). A fall in the arterial pCO_2 and subsequent increased coronary vascular tone, together with sympathetic dominance, may compromise the myocardial oxygen supply, theoretically leading to ischemic attacks. Conversely, a predominant vagal tone seems to exert a protective function in animal experiments in the setting of myocardial infarction (Goldstein et al., 1973), and presumably this is a propitious mechanism in humans as well.

Hence, changes in the respiratory pattern may interact with cardio-vascular risk factors (Grossman, 1983), triggering a pathophysiological sequence with increased levels of catecholamines, vasomotor changes and subsequent myocardial infarction, arrhythmias or sudden death. This hypothesis with regard to ischemic heart disease is currently being tested (see Freeman, this volume).

Some interesting observations have been made by Nowlin et al. (1965) and Murao et al. (1972). They registered significant ECG changes (ST-depression and ST-elevations plus ventricular arrhythmias), especially at night, during episodes of REM-sleep in a series of patients with nocturnal angina. A tachypneic condition was proposed as a trigger mechanism for these attacks. These ECG patterns were comparable with the result of prolonged hyperventilation observed in patients suspected of CAS (Groves et al., 1975; Yasue et al., 1981; Girotti et al., 1982; Weber et al., 1981; Pujadas et al., 1981; Mortensen et al., 1981). Our results point to a high specificity of the HVT in PVA, used without additional stimuli as a non-pharmacological provocative test. We have been reluctant to use injections of vasoactive drugs (e.g., ergonovine), as there have been reports of deaths from sustained CAS with this approach (Buxton et al., 1980).

Sensitivity to the HVT showed circadian variations (Mortensen et al., 1981) rendering this test a clinically useful maneuver for monitoring the effectiveness of drug therapy. It is probable that attacks of CAS may be provoked solely during acute/subacute phases of the disease. But this may make the HVT especially relevant in the clinical situation, and possibly more specific than the ergonovine test, which can provoke oesophageal spasm as well (Dart et al., 1980).

The mechanisms by which the HVT provokes CAS are probably multifactor-ial, and the most significant triggering factors remain to be clarified:

The state of activity of the vasospastic disease seems crucial, as it was not possible in our study to provoke spasm when the patient was in a "cool phase" of the disease (i.e., spontaneous remission). Subjects in a waxing phase responded to the test in the recovery period after discontin-uation of the hyperventilation, and one patient in a "hot phase" responded during the overbreathing with chest pain and ECG changes compatible with transmural myocardial ischemia.

The cyclic character of variant angina may modulate the intensity of the HVT stimulus, as the frequency of anginal pain is most pronounced in the early morning hours. The finding that the HVT was invariably positive at the time of the day when spontaneous attacks had occurred in the past and negative during the rest of the 24-hour cycle (Mortensen et al., 1981) may reflect involvement of circadian variations in certain hormones, e.g., prolactine or melatonine level.

The intensity of hyperventilation measured as changes in pH and pCO_2 seems important. Tests performed during sensitive periods of the day where blood-gases were only moderately affected were invariably accompanied by a slight or negative response.

It is still unknown whether it is the alkalosis or the hypocapnia that predominates in the pathogenesis of CAS; however, presumably it is the latter. A sudden drop in arterial pCO_2 level causes the symptomatology of cerebral vasoconstriction (Grossman and Swart, 1984), and the low pCO_2

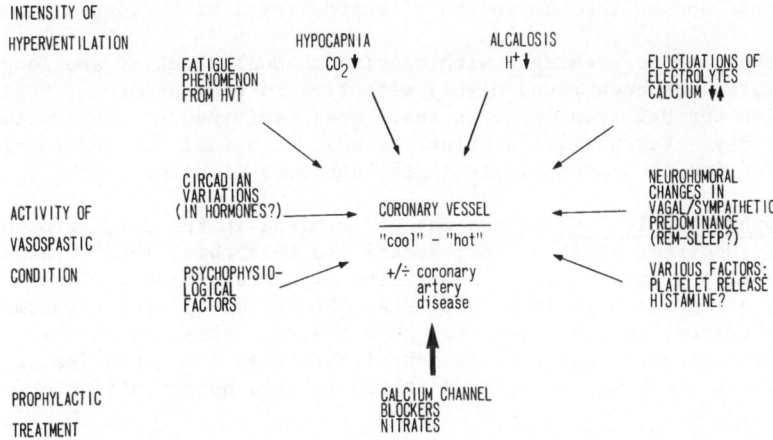

Fig. 4. Hyperventilation and coronary artery spasm – trigger mechanisms.

level may induce vasoconstriction in the myocardial resistance vessels and/or conductance vessels as well, especially when the vessel wall is hypersensitive (Maseri and Chierchia, 1982). According to experiments by Fleckstein and co-workers (1976), a decrease in hydrogen ion concentration may be responsible for the vasoconstriction since hydrogen ions exert a calcium-antagonistic action in relation to active calcium transport, so that a high pH might dispose to vasoconstriction. Previous reports have pointed to increased coronary vascular tone during hyperventilation, both in normal subjects and in coronary artery disease (Neill and Hattenhauer, 1975; Rowe, Castillo and Crumptom, 1962) with impaired oxygen release in the myocardium (as the affinity of oxygen to hemoglobin is increased due to the Bohr effect).

Changes in plasma calcium might influence the vasomotor tone crit- ically in the recovery phase after the HVT when calcium again rises, bringing about vasoconstriction.

The sequence of events leading to CAS may have been subject to a fatigue effect, as spasm provocation was not possible when a positive response with the HVT had occurred a short time before. This is in accordance with findings of others (Girotti et al., 1982).

Various neuro-humoral involvements may also play a role. The bene- ficial effect of plexectomy on the severity of symptoms of PVA (Bertrand, Lablanche and Tilmant, 1981) points to an influence of the autonomic nervous system, but the relative significance of vagal/sympathetic pre- dominance is unclear. One can speculate that the change from high vagal tone during the night towards increased sympathetic influence in the early morning may be involved in the attacks of pain and arrhythmias in PVA. Conversely, humoral factors alone may be responsible, as CAS was provoked by ergonovine in a patient whose heart was totally denervated (i.e., auto- transplanted; Angell, 1981).

Naturally occurring substances, such as histamine, may be involved in the pathophysiology of CAS provoked by HVT (excess release from the mast cells), as histamine injected in humans has elicited spasm (Bristow, Ginsbur and Harrison, 1982).

313

An additional plausible hypothesis is that local <u>endothelial factors</u> (prostacycline) and <u>platelet factors</u> (factor 4 and thromboxane A_2) may perpetuate and worsen the CAS in the affected vessel with reduced flow.

The <u>prophylactic treatment</u> with calcium channel blockers and long-acting nitrates has been found highly effective in preventing the positive response from the HVT even when the tests were performed at the critical time of the day. Verapamil (isoptinR) as well as nifedipine (adalat) were equally effective as a prophylaxis in the subjects studied.

<u>Psychophysiological disorders</u> may be involved in the trigger mechanisms of CAS (Schiffer et al., 1980; Maseri and Chierchia, 1982; Grossman, 1983). Maseri's group has found a striking high prevalence of Type A personality among their patients with PVA. Stoney et al. (this volume) has found, furthermore, that A-types tend more towards hyperventilatory response under stress. Hence it is conceivable that some episodes of CAS among PVA individuals may arise from stress-related hyperventilation.

CONCLUSIONS

The pathophysiological sequences leading to coronary artery spasm remain obscure, but new horizons for research might appear from studying the respiratory influences upon the coronary circulation. Stress-related spontaneous hyperventilation and subsequent vasoconstriction may compromise the myocardial oxygen supply in coronary artery disease, resulting in some the acute manifestations of this disease (i.e., arrhythmias and sudden death). Therefore patients with clinical suspicion of severe coronary pathology should not be subjected to the possible detrimental consequences of hyperventilation. Conversely, as a diagnostic test, prolonged hyperventilation has been found clinically useful in patients with suspected Prinzmetal's variant angina. In our patient sample the test was rather specific, and it was valuable in assessing disease activity and drug treatment. However, the method may be used as a stress-test in other clinical groups (in parallel or as alternative to ergometry). Although responses to hyperventilation are significant and the mechanisms are of utmost interest, they remain to be clarified.

REFERENCES

Angell, W., 1981, Autotransplantation and aorta-coronary bypass. Paper presented at: International symposium on pathophysiology of angina pectoris and coronary artery spasm. Therapeutic implication; 25-26 September, Sevilla, Spain.

Balke, B., Ellis, J. P., and Wells, J. G., 1959, Adaptive responses to hyperventilation, <u>J. Appl. Physiol.</u>, 12:269.

Bass, C., Cawley, R., Wade, C., Ryan, K. C., Gardner, W. N., Hutchinson, D. C. S., and Jackson, G., 1983, Unexplained breathlessness and psychiatric morbidity in patients with normal and abnormal coronary arteries, <u>Lancet</u>, 1:605.

Bertrand, M. E., and Cherrier, F., 1979, L'angine de poitrine de Prinzmetal: 20 ans après, <u>Archives Mal Coeur</u>, 72:939.

Bertrand, M. E., Lablanche, J. M., and Tilmant, P., 1981, Treatment of Prinzmetal's variant angina. Role of medical treatment with nifedipine and surgical coronary revascularization combined with plexectomy, <u>Am. J. Cardiol.</u>, 47:174.

Bristow, M. R., Ginsburg, R., and Harrison, D. C., 1982, Histamine and the human heart: the other receptor system, <u>Am. J. Cardiol.</u>, 49:249.

Brunelli, C., Lazzari, M., Simonetti, I., L'Abbata, A., and Maseri, A., 1981, Variable threshold of exertional angina: a clue to a vasospastic component, <u>European Heart J.</u>, 2:155.

Buxton, A., Goldberg, S., Hirshfeld, J. W., Wilson, J., Mann, T., Williams, D. O., Overlie, P., and Oliva, P., 1980, Refractory ergonovine-induced coronary vasospasm: importance of intracoronary nitro-glycerin, Am. J. Cardiol., 46:329.

Chahine, R. A., 1980, The provocation of coronary artery spasm, Catheterization & Cardiovascular Diagnosis, 6:1.

Dart, A. M., Davies, H. A., Lowndes, R. H., Dalai, J., Ruttley, M., and Henderson, A. H., 1980, Oesophagal spasm and angina: diagnostic value of ergometrine (ergonovine) provocation, European Heart J., 1:91.

Egeblad, H., Vilhelmsen, R., Mortensen, S. A., Richardson, P. J., and Livesley, B., 1974, Angina pectoris with normal coronary arteries, Lancet, 1:677.

Evans, D. W., and Lum, L. C., 1977, Hyperventilation: an important cause of pseudoangina, Lancet, 1:155.

Factor, S. M., and Sonneblick, E. H., 1982, Hypothesis: is congestive cardiomyopathy caused by a hyperreactive myocardial microcirculation (microvascular spasm)?, Am. J. Cardiol., 50:1149.

Fleckstein, A., Nakayama, K., Fleckstein-Grùn, B., and Byon, Y. K., 1976, Interactions of H-ions, Ca-antagonistic drugs and cardiac glycosides with excitation contractions coupling of vascular smooth muscle, in: "Ionic Action on Vascular Smooth Muscle", E. Betz, ed., Springer-Verlag, Berlin-Heidelberg-New York.

Friedman, M., 1947, Studies concerning the etiology and pathogenesis of neurocirculatory asthenia. V: the introduction of a new test for the diagnosis and assessment of the syndrome, Psychosomatic Med., 9:233.

Gaash, W. H., Lufshanoski, R., Leachman, R. D., and Alexander, J. K., 1974, Surgical management of Prinzmetal's variant angina, Chest, 66:614.

Girotti, L. A., Crosatto, R., Messuti, H., Kaski, J. C., Dyszel, E., Rivas, C. A., Araujo, L. I., Vetulli, H. D., and Rosenbaum, M. B., 1982, The hyperventilation test as a method for developing a successful therapy in Prinzmetal's angina, Am. J. Cardiol., 49:834.

Goldstein, R. E., Karsh, R. B., Smith, E. R., Orlando, M., Norman, D., Farnham, G., Redwood, D. R., and Eptstein, S. E., 1973, The influence of atropine and vagally mediated bradycardia on the occurrence of ventricular arrhythmias following acute coronary occlusion in closed-chest dogs, Circulation, 47:1180.

Grondin, C. M., 1981, Sympathetic denervation and aorto-coronary by-pass. Paper presented at: International symposium on pathophysiology of angina pectoris and coronary artery spasm. Therapeutical implications, 25-26 September, Sevilla, Spain.

Grossman, P., 1983, Respiration, stress and cardiovascular function, Psychophysiology, 20:284.

Grossman, P., and Swart, J. C. G., 1984, Diagnosis of hyperventilation syndrome on the basis of reported complaints, J. Psychosomatic Res., 28:97.

Grossman, P., and Wientjes, K., 1985, Respiratory-cardiac coordination as an index of cardiac functioning, in: "Psychophysiology of Cardio-vascular Control," J. F. Orlebeke, G. Mulder, and L. J. van Doornen, eds., Plenum, New York.

Groves, M. B., Marcus, F. I., Ewy, G. A., and Phibbs, B. P., 1975, Coronary arterial spasm in variant angina produced by hyperventilation and valsalve - documented by coronary arteriography, in: "Coronary Artery Medicine and Surgery Section V, Variant Angina and Surgical Treatment", J. C. Norman, ed., Appleton-Century-Crofts, New York.

Hansen, J. Fischer, and Sandoe, E., 1978, Treatment of Prinzmetal's angina due to coronary artery spasm using verapamil, European J. Cardiol., 7:327.

Heupler, F. A., Proudfit, W. L., Razavi, M., Shirey, E. K., Greenstreet,

R., and Sheldon, W. C., 1978, Ergonovine maleate provocative test
for coronary arterial spasm, Am. J. Cardiol., 41:631.

Joy, M., and Trump, D. W., 1981, Significance of minor ST segment and T
wave changes in the resting electrocardiogram of asymptomatic
subjects, Br. Heart J., 45:48.

Kübler, W., and Opherk, D., 1983, Unusual causes of angina pectoris: the
syndrome X, in: "What is angina?", Proceedings of a symposium held
in The Hague, 15-16 October, D. G. Julian, K. I. Lie, L. Wilhelmsen,
and A. B. Hässle, eds., Mölndal, Sweden.

Maseri, A., Severi, S., Nes, M. de, L'Abbate, A., Chierchia, S., Marzilli,
M., Ballestra, M., Parodi, O., Biagina, A., and Distante, A., 1978,
Am. J. Cardiol., 42:1019.

Maseri, A., and Chierchia, S., 1982, Coronary artery spasm: demonstration,
definition diagnosis, and consequences, Prog. Cardiov. Diseases,
25:169.

Mortensen, S. A., Vilhelmsen, R., and Sandoe, E., 1981, Non-pharmacological
provocation of coronary vasospasm. Experience with prolonged
hyperventilation in the coronary care unit, European Heart J.,
4:391.

Murao, S., Harumi, K., Katayama, S., Mashima, S., Shimomura, K., Murayama,
M., Matsuo, H., Yamamoto, H., Kato, R., and Chen, C., 1972, All-
night polygraphic studies of nocturnal angina pectoris, Japanese
Heart J., 13:295.

Neill, W. A., and Hattenhauer, M., 1975, Impairment of myocardial O_2 supply
due to hyperventilation, Circulation, 52:854.

Nowlin, J. B., Troyer, W. G., Collins, W. S., Silverman, G., Nichols, C.
R., McIntosh, D., and Estes, E. H., 1965, The association of
nocturnal angina pectoris with dreaming, Annals Internal Med.,
63:1040.

Prinzmetal, M., Kennamer, R., Merliss, R., Wada, T., and Bor, N., 1959,
Angina pectoris, I: a variant form of angina pectoris, Am. J. Med.,
27:375.

Pujadas, G., Tamashiro, A., Ruades, J., and Aldasoro, J., 1981, Coronary
vasospasm provoked by the hyperventilation test, Am. J. Cardiol.,
47:450.

Raizner, A. E., Chahine, R. A., Ishimori, T., Verani, M. S., Zacca, N., and
Jamai, N., 1980, Provocation of coronary artery spasm by the cold
pressor test, Circulation, 62:925.

Rowe, G. C., Castillo, C. A., and Crumpton, C. W., 1962, Effects of hyperventilation on systemic and coronary hemodynamics, Am. Heart J.,
63:67.

Sandoe, E., Vilhelmsen, R., and Mortensen, S. A., 1982, Arrhythmias in
Prinzmetal's variant angina and their management by calcium antagonists, Revista Portugesa de Cardiologia, 1:23.

Schiffer, F., Hartley, L. H., Schulman, C. L., and Abelmann, W. H., 1980,
Evidence of emotionally-induced coronary arterial spasm in patients
with angina pectoris, Br. Heart J., 44:62.

Severi, S., Davies, G., Maseri, A., Marzullo, P., and L'Abbate, A., 1980,
Long-term prognosis of "Variant" angina with medical treatment, Am.
J. Cardiol., 46:226.

Suess, W. M., Alexander, A. B., Smith, D. D., Sweeney, H. W., and Marion,
R. J., 1980, The effects of psychological stress on respiration: a
preliminary study of anxiety and hyperventilation, Psychophysiology,
17:535.

Swedberg, K., Hjalmarson, A., Waagstein, F., and Wallentin, I., 1979,
Prolongation of survival in congestive cardiomyopathy by beta-
receptor blockade, Lancet, 1:1374.

Thompson, W. P., 1943, The electrocardiogram in the hyperventilation
syndrome, Am. Heart J., 25:372.

Wasserburger, R. H., and Alt, W. J., 1969, The normal RS-T segment
elevation variant, Am. J. Cardiol., 8:184.

Waters, D. D., Szlachcic, J., Théroux, P., Dauwe, F., and Mizgala, H. F., 1981, Ergonovine testing to detect spontaneous remissions of variant angina during long-term treatment with calcium antagonistic drugs, Am. J. Cardiol., 47:179.

Weber, S., Pasquier, G., Guiomard, A., Lancelin, B., Maurice, P., Gourgon, R., and Degeorges, M., 1981, Application clinique du test de provocation par l'alcalose dus spasme artèriel coronaire, Archives Mal Coeur, 74:1389.

Wientjes, K., and Grossman, P., 1985, The respiratory response and respiration-related risk factors in stress, Report Institute for Perception-TNO Soesterberg, The Netherlands.

Yasue, H., 1978, Beta-adrenergic blockade and coronary arterial spasm, in: "Management of Ventricular and Tachycardia - Role of Mexiletine", Proceedings of a symposium held in Copenhagen 25-27 May, E. Sandoe, D. G. Julian and J. W. Bell, eds., Excerpta Medica, Amsterdam.

Yasue, H., Nagao, M., Omote, S., Takizawa, A., Miwa, K., and Tanaka, S., 1978, Coronary arterial spasm and Prinzmetal's variant form of angina induced by hyperventilation and tris buffer infusion, Circulation, 58:56.

Yasue, H., Omote, S., Takizawa, N., Masao, N., Hyon, H., Nishida, S., and Minoru, H., 1981, Comparison of coronary arteriographic findings during angina pectoris associated with S-T elevation or depression, Am. J. Cardiol., 47:539.

Yu, P. N., Yim, B. J., and Stanfield, C. A., 1959, Hyperventilation syndrome, Arch. Int. Med., 103:902.

HYPERVENTILATION AND ISCHAEMIC HEART DISEASE

Leisa J. Freeman

Department Cardiology
Charing Cross Hospital, Fulham Palace Road
London W6 8RF

It is increasingly obvious that the paradigms that hold sway over cardiology at present are not providing adequate solutions. Risk factor management has been disappointing [1] and coronary artery bypass grafting is not the simple answer to angina pectoris, usually considered to be due solely to the rigid coronary atheromatous narrowings demonstrated at angiography [2].

Hyperventilation has long been known to be associated with marked cardiovascular instability [3], yet many working with coronary disease have lost sight of this fact, recognizing it as merely a bothersome psychiatric disorder. However, it has been identified in the type A behavior pattern [4], coronary artery spasm [5], arrhythmias [6], and as an important disqualifier in cardiac rehabilitation [7]. The biobehavioral antecedents of symptomatic coronary artery disease make it clear that there are powerful dynamic factors that intervene to thrust a person from health into a cardiac catastrophe, be it myocardial infarction, angina pectoris, tachydysrhythmia, or even sudden cardiac death, and that these events seldom, if ever, come out of the blue. It is then on this background of disordered homeostasis that we postulate hyperventilation may exert its most devastating cardiovascular effect (see Figure 1).

BIOBEHAVIORAL ANTECEDENTS

There is a slow and grudging realization that the extent and degree of coronary narrowings seen at arteriography do not hold a simple and linear relationship to the severity of the symptoms experienced by a patient. For example, recordings of thousands of arteriograms have shown that two people might have the same degree of coronary stenoses, and yet one might have severe and life-threatening symptoms, and the other may be troubled occasionally by a fleeting pain or no symptoms at all [8]. Moreover, the coronary appearances at a time when a patient is experiencing many attacks of severe angina each day, and his conditions is called "unstable" or "pre-infarction" and later when he has minimal symptoms, are remarkably unchanged [9].

Clearly the problem is not solely structural and the best correlates appear to be biobehavioral. For example, sleep disturbances (waking fatigued, poor quality sleep and long sleep latency) show a very high

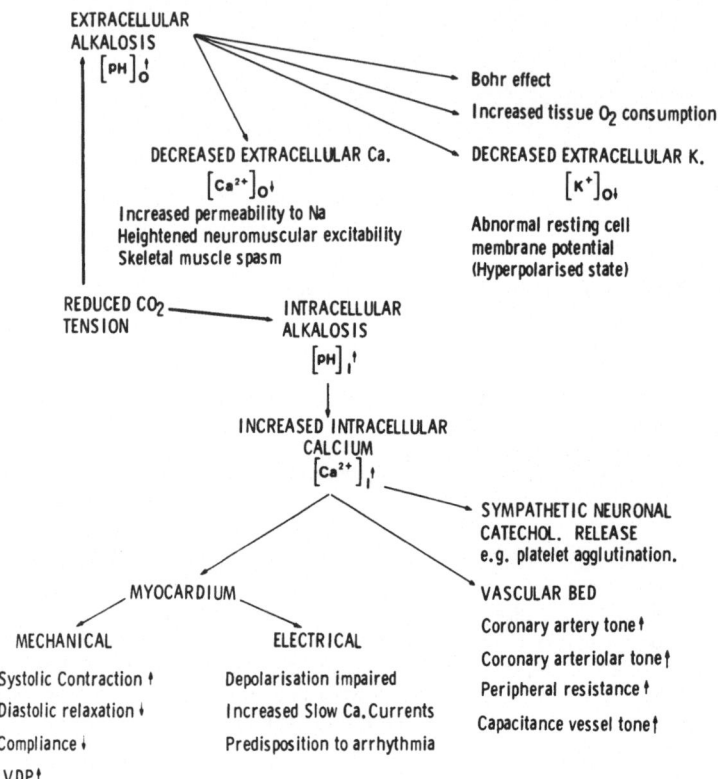

Fig. 1. The mechanisms by which hyperventilation, causing a fluctuating reduction of the blood CO_2 tension, induces vasomotor instability and disturbances of function. (Courtesy of Abdul Hamid-Al-Abbasi, 1982). [ ]$_O$ = extracellular concentration, e.g., $[K^+]_O\downarrow$ decreased concentration of extracellular ionized potassium. [ ]$_I$ = intracellular concentration, e.g., $[Ca^{2+}]_I\uparrow$ increased intracellular concentration of ionized calcium. LVDP = Left ventricular end-diastolic pressure.

correlation with the symptoms of angina occurring with emotion, exertion or after meals, yet the coronary artery appearance holds no similar predictive value [10]. This pattern of exhaustion has been well described [11,12], each task to be performed seemingly taking more effort than had formerly been the case, and longer hours are worked but less achieved. Sleep becomes inadequate, increasing the exhaustion and promoting another vicious circle of deterioration. There are cycles of rage and frustration, despair and hopelessness.

The struggle to achieve former levels of performance is reflected by increased sympatho-adrenal-medullary and pituitary-adrenal-cortical arousal [13]. It is of interest to note again that denial of helplessness and general life dissatisfaction (both of which are associated with markedly elevated levels of cortisol) were the strongest correlates of rest and nocturnal angina in a recent study of symptoms, behavior and angiographic findings [10].

Although mild hyperventilation is a normal response to many situations, both real and imagined [39], we believe that the respiratory response to such everyday stimuli frequently becomes disproportionate when an individual is thus compromised by exhaustion and extreme arousal. It is interesting that Da Costa's original link between chest pain and hyperventilation pointed out the marked exhustion and struggle required to keep up with colleagues, which seemed a prerequisite for an abnormal breathing pattern to exert its potent effect [14].

ROLE OF HYPERVENTILATION IN THE PRODUCTION OF ANGINAL SYNDROMES

Firstly, the symptoms of fatigue, breathlessness, palpitations and chest pain, closely mimic those of organic heart disease, to the extent that invites much unnecessary coronary arteriography. Bass et al. [15] have shown that this is a very common problem, marked hypocapnia being present in 67% of patients who had normal or near-normal coronary arteriograms when they were investigated with a view to surgical treatment for angina-like pain. Further, patients who by virtue of their age have marked coronary artery disease, may require less medication or avoid surgery altogether, if recognition and removal of the hyperventilation abolishes the majority of their symptoms.

Secondly, cardiac arrhythmias generated by hyperventilation can lead to the prescription of drugs which depress myocardial function and increase the risk of sudden death. We have documented cases of hyperventilation inducing atrial fibrillation, atrial flutter and paroxysmal atrial tachycardia [16], and elegant electrophysiological studies have demonstrated how hyperventilation switches on the alternate bundle in some cases of Wolff-Parkinson-White syndrome [17]. We have identified a particular type of right ventricular ectopic which we use as a marker of hyperventilation [18] (Figure 2). We are uncertain of its etiology, but consider it may be due to altered right ventricular dynamics associated with increased venous return. Its incidence decreases as the hyperventilation is treated, and its identification can save further drug intervention. No less important is the marked cardiovascular hyper-reactivity documented in these patients who hyperventilate to simple activity [19]. In a recent study of hyperventilation in cardiac rehabilitation, we frequently noticed gross heart rate and blood pressure responses to small amounts of effort when we performed exercise testing [7]. This clearly produces myocardial ischemia earlier than might otherwise have been expected. Hyperventilation may also confuse the issue on some occasions by producing pseudoischemic electrocardiographic changes. These include T-wave flattening, and QT prolongation (as a result of the respiratory alkalosis) and ST-segment depression/T-wave inversion, probably as a result of asynchronous myocardial repolarization due to sympathetic dominance [20].

Thirdly, hyperventilation can reduce coronary blood flow by a combination of coronary vasospasm and a Bohr shift to the left, which decreases the amount of oxygen available to the tissues [21]. Maseri et al. [22] have demonstrated the overriding importance of spasm in patients with variant (Prinzmetal) angina which characteristically occurs not with effort, but at night or at rest. Moreover, there is increasing evidence that spasm is a major factor in unstable or cresendo angina and angina occurring early after coronary artery bypass grafting [23] and infarction. There is also evidence that it may produce frank infarction [24]. Hyperventilation appears to produce this effect through fluctuating hypocarbia inducing alkalosis and large fluxes of ionized calcium. Smooth muscle contraction is a biphasic response and both stages are pH dependent. The alkalosis associated with hyperventilation, allows the release of the tightly bound intracellular ionized-calcium-initiating contraction. This phase accounts for 70% of the overall smooth muscle tension generated. A slower tonic phase then follows, when freely exchangeable extracellular calcium ions enter the smooth muscle cell through the slow calcium channels located in the cell membrane. It is only this second phase that can be inhibited by calcium blocking agents, such as nifedipine and verapamil [25].

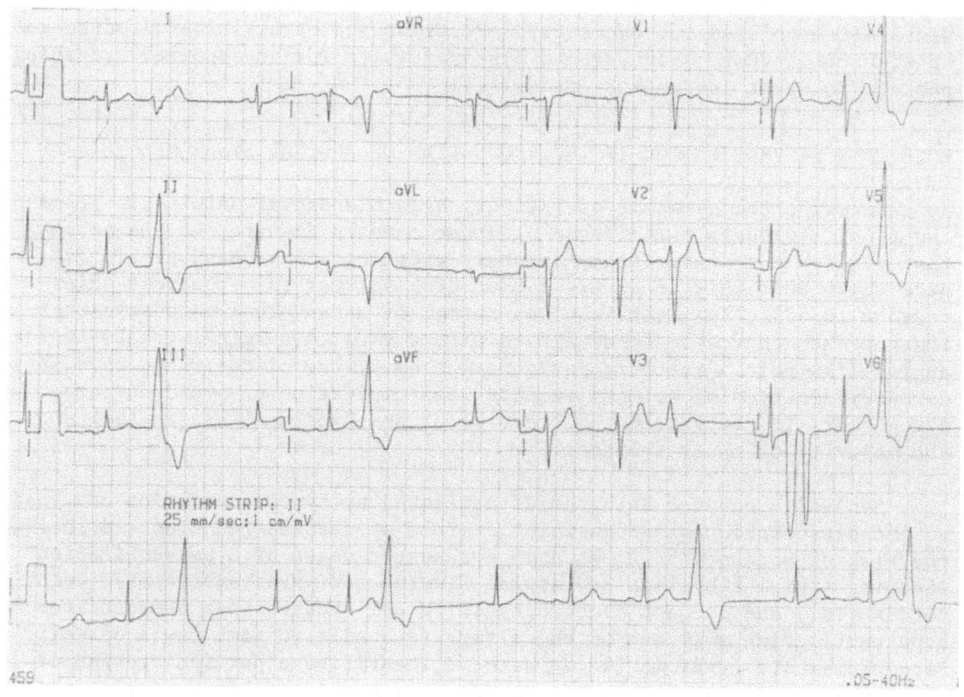

Fig. 2. An electrocardiogram showing frequent right ventricular ectopy. A history consistent with a diagnosis of hyperventilation was subsequently obtained and provocation testing was positive. The characteristics of the ectopic beat to note are the following: 1. LBBB pattern in the chest leads and a QRS interval of at least 0.12 seconds. The LBBB pattern in the chest leads can be distinguished from the typical LBBB electrocardiographic pattern by the fact that the initial forces are directed anteriorly and are very slowly inscribed. 2. The main QRS force is directed inferiorly and to the right. 3. The R wave from V1 to V3 is relatively tall and wide. 4. The horizontal vectorcardiogram rotates counterclockwise.

Fourthly, it is possible that hyperventilation may also lead to increased left ventricular stiffness. This may be an indirect effect. Adrenaline excretion has been measured up to three times normal in patients who hyperventilate and this may be sufficient to produce subendocardial ischemia, necrosis and subsequent scarring [27]. The mechanical dysfunction can often be detected clinically by an audible and palpable atrial gallop, which waxes and wanes with the patient's observed neuroendocrine arousal [28]. This catecholamine myocytolysis has also been implicated in sudden cardiac death [29]. Further excessive catecholamine surges may flood the intracellular compartment of the myocardial cells with ionized calcium, which may not only augment contraction but impair diastolic relaxation and increase myocardial stiffness [30].

INCIDENCE OF THE HYPERVENTILATION SYNDROME IN IHD

The true incidence of hyperventilation is extremely hard to assess, for many omit to even look for it once they have demonstrated organic disease. Brashear [31] assessed the incidence of the hyperventilation syndrome in cardiology outpatients as between six and eleven percent, a figure, which in our experience, is extremely conservative. In a recent study we did of patients undergoing cardiac rehabilitation, 66% of patients were considered to hyperventilate. This diagnosis was made on the basis of four or more clinical criteria. Thirty-nine percent were found to hyperventilate with activity, 44% with emotive topics and 17% as an ingrained habit [7].

In another study performed at this institution, the incidence of hyperventilation was assessed in patients undergoing diagnostic coronary arteriography for chest pain with exertional angina pectoris (> 1 mm ST-segment depression with exercise) and good left ventricular function (LVEDP < 15 mm Hg). 16.6% (5/30) were found to have resting hypocapnia (< 30 mm Hg) and 56.6% (17/30) had a positive test for hyperventilation. Moreover, 39% recognized that this manoeuver provoked symptoms similar to those experienced in daily life, including typical chest pain in nine patients. ST-segment depression was produced in four patients and ST-elevation in one (6 standard leads monitored) [32].

In patients with coronary artery spasm (Prinzmetal angina), a recent study has demonstrated the dominant role of hyperventilation in the production of ST-segment elevation in 11 of 14 patients (78%) with variant angina [33]. Girotti et al. [34] demonstrated vasospasm produced by hyperventilation at angiography and found that it had a 70% sensitivity and a 100% specificity. Although the potent effect of hypocapnia is realized, few at present seem to link a laboratory manoeuver with the possibility of spontaneous hyperventilation producing the symptoms in the patient's daily life [35,39].

ETIOLOGY OF THE HYPERVENTILATION IN ISCHEMIC HEART DISEASE

Once organic and physiological causes of hyperventilation have been eliminated, the likely origin of the disordered breathing has been considered to be either a response to an emotional trigger or an ingrained habit. Common emotional stimuli have been considered to be the threat of death, real or imagined, in the patient or a close relative or friend, or witnessing a traumatic and unpleasant event, the nature of which is subsequently suppressed; or severe, and often unexpressed, grief, anger or hostility [31]. Most patients with a coronary illness spend some days in a Coronary Care Unit where they experience fear of their own death, witness a death, or watch the drama of resuscitation by the 'crash' team. It is hardly surprising that an upper thoracic mode of breathing is then frequently observed [36]. Such emotional triggers are more likely to produce an attack at night or at rest (characteristic times for vasospasm to be a dominant mechanism in producing myocardial ischemia), or during discussions about their illness and its effect on life style and business.

Hyperventilation may start as a habit, perhaps in the army, or following abdominal operations, or as expressions of comeliness or virility, and only begin to exert significant effects when the homeostasis has been violated by struggle, defeat and exhaustion. Studies of patients with the coronary-prone behavior pattern (Type A) have identified a particular type of vocal stylistics, with frequent sighs, an explosive pattern of speech and upper chest breathing [5]. Many patients with angina of effort develop pain at a set distance or after a particular activity and it is possible that hyperventilation diminishes the painful sensation [37].

It is then reasonable to assume that in some instances hyperventilation may become part of the preparatory response to exertion [39]. Since alkalosis has been shown to reduce the angina threshold [38], it is possible to visualize a vicious circle developing and the hyperventilation becoming a dominant and persistent habit.

CONCLUSION AND TREATMENT

Hyperventilation can clearly produce profound physiological effects and the patient with the ischemic heart disease seems exquisitely susceptible. Moreover, its recognition and effective treatment may save the patient from costly, invasive and expensive investigations and heavy drug regimes designed to treat symptoms, but not the cause. It appears inappropriate to treat the hyperventilation alone without as much attention being paid to the restoration of adequate sleep and arousal levels, which had so ably provided such a sensitive substrate. In our unit we have employed an acronym, S.A.B.R.E.S., to remind each trainer of the therapeutic goals: to achieve adequate sleep (S) (with sedation if necessary), modification of arousal (A) by counselling; breathing control (B) to produce a relaxed and abdominal mode of breathing that avoids inappropriate hyperventilation in response to effort, emotion or other activities of daily life; a sensible balance of rest and effort (R.E.) that avoids isometric effort and approaches performance realisitically, and finally reestablishment of the patient's self-esteem (S), a process we see achieved by the patient's realization that he has considerable power to improve his own symptoms.

Acknowledgements

It would not have been possible to write this Chapter without the help, advice and encouragement of Dr. P. G. F. Nixon. Leisa J. Freeman is supported by a Charing Cross Governors Research Fellowship.

REFERENCES

1. M C. Petch, The progression of coronary artery disease, Brit. Med J., 283:1073 (1981).
2. J. Pidgeon, N. Brooks, P. Magee, J. R. Pepper, M. F. Sturridge, and J. E. C., Wright, Reoperation after previous aortocoronary bypass surgery, Br. Heart J., 53:269 (1985).
3. T. Lewis, The soldiers heart and effort syndrome, Shaw, London (1918).
4. C. D. Jenkins, The coronary prone personality, in: "Psychological Aspects of Myocardial Infarction and Coronary Care", W. E. Gentry and R. B. Williams, eds., The CV Mosby Co., Saint Louis, (1975).
5. K. Rasmussen, J. P. Bagger, J. Bottzaun, and P. Henringsen, Cold pressor test and hyperventilation as provocation of coronary artery spasm, Eur. Heart J., 5:354 (1985).
6. K. Wildenthal, D. S. Fuller, and W. Shapiro, Paroxysmal atrial fibrillation induced by hyperventilation, Am. J. Cardiol., 21:436 (1968).
7. P. G. F. Nixon, H. Al-Abassi, J. King, and L. J. Freeman, Hyperventilation in cardiac rehabilitation, Holistic Medicine, 1:5 (1986).
8. E. Sowton, The treatment of angina pectoris, Practitioner, 223:471 (1979).
9. N. E. Neil, T. Wherton, J. Fluri-Lumdeen, and I. Cohen, Acute coronary insufficiency. Coronary occlusion after intermittent ischemic attacks, N. Engl. J. Med., 302:1157 (1980).
10. C. D. Jenkins, B. E. Stanton, M. D. Klein, J. A. Savageau, and D. E. Harken, Correlates of angina pectoris among men awaiting coronary artery bypass surgery, Psychosomatic Med., 45(2):141 (1983).
11. A. Appels, The year before myocardial infarction, in: "Biobehavioral Bases of Coronary Heart Disease", T. M. Dembroski, T. H. Schmidt and G. Blumchen, eds., Karger, Basel (1983).
12. P. G. F. Nixon, The human function curve, The Practitioner, 217:265-770 and 935-944 (1976).

13. J. P. Henry, and J. P. Meehan, Psychosocial stimuli, physiological specificity and cardiovascular disease, in: "Brain Behavior and Bodily Disease", H. Weiner, M. A. Hofer and A. J. Stunkard, eds., Raven Press New York (1981).

14. J. M. Da Costa, On 'Irritable heart', Am. J. Med. Services, 61:17 (1871).

15. C. Bass, C. Wade, W. N. Gardener et al., Unexplained breathlessness and psychiatric morbidity in patients with normal and abnormal coronary arteries, Lancet, 1:605 (1983).

16. L. J. Freeman, A. Conway, and P. G. F. Nixon, Heart rate, emotion and hyperventilation, J. Psychosom. Res., (1986) (In press).

17. G. S. Butrous, G. C. Kaye, A. W. Nathan et al., Respiratory modulation of A-V pathway conduction, Abstracts of the 57th scientific session of the Am. Heart Assoc. Monograph No. 107, Circulation II, 70(4):217 (1984).

18. L. J. Freeman, and P. G. F. Nixon, Chest pain and the hyperventilation syndrome - some etiological considerations, Postgrad. Med. J., 61, 957 (1985).

19. L. C. Lum, The syndrome of habitual chronic hyperventilation, in: "Modern Trends in Psychosomatic Medicine - III", O. Hill, ed., Butterworths, London (1981).

20. D. Lary, and W. Goldschlarger, Electrocardiographic changes during hyperventilation in patients with normal coronary arteriograms, Am. Heart J., 87:383 (1974).

21. W. A. Neil, and M. Hattenhauer, Impairment of myocardial oxygen supply due to hyperventilation, Circulation, 52:854 (1975).

22. A. Maseri, and S. Chiercha, Coronary artery spasm, definition, diagnosis and consequences, Progr. Cardiovas. Dis., 25(3):169 (1982).

23. B. Zingone, A. Salvi, and B. Branchini, Perioperative coronary artery spasm leading to myocardial ischemia after venin graft surgery, Br. Heart J., 288:1073 (1981).

24. P. B. Oliva, and J. C. Breckinridge, Arteriographic evidence of coronary artery spasm in acute myocardial infarction, Circulation, 56:366 (1977).

25. R. Ginsberg, M. Bristow, J. Schroeder, D. Harrison, and E. Stimson, Potential pharmacologic mechanisms involved in coronary artery spasm, in: "Drug-induced Heart Disease", M. R. Bristow, ed., Biomedical Press, Elsevier, North Holland (1980).

26. H. Folgering, and A. Cox, Betablockade with metoprolol in the hyperventilation syndrome, Respiration, 41:33 (1981).

27. L. J. Freeman, and P. G. F. Nixon, Dynamic causes of angina pectoris, Am. Heart J., 110(5):1087 (1985).

28. P. G. F. Nixon, Non-invasive techniques in angina pectoris, in: "Angina Pectoris", O. Paul, ed., Medicom Press, New York (1974).

29. R. B. Eliot, and J. C. Buel, Role of the central nervous system in sudden cardiac death, in: "Biobehavioral Bases of Coronary ARtery Disease", T. M. Dembroski, T. H. Schmidt and G. Blumchen, eds., Karger, Basel (1983).

30. W. G. Nagler, The ionic basis of contractility, relaxation and heart failure, in: "Modern Trends in Cardiology", M. F. Oliver, ed., Butterworths, London (1975).

31. R. A. Brashear, Hyperventilation syndrome, Chest, 161:257 (1983).

32. L. J. Freeman, and P. G. F. Nixon, Hyperventilation and ischemic heart disease, Biol. Psychol., (1986) (In press) (Abstr).

33. F. Crea, G. Davies, F. Romeo et al., Myocardial ischemia during ergonovine testing: different susceptibility to coronary vasoconstriction in patients with exertional and variant angina, Circulation, 69(4):690 (1984).

34. L. A. Girotti, J. R. Crossato, H. Messuti et al., The hyperventilation test as a method for developing successful therapy in Prinzmetal angina, Am. J. Cardiol., 49:834 (1982).
35. L. J. Freeman, and P. G. F. Nixon, Are progressive heart damage and coronary artery spasm linked with the hyperventilation syndrome?, Br. Med. J., 291:851 (1985).
36. S. Hymes, and P. Neurberger, Breathing pattern found in heart attack patients, Res. Bull., 2:10 (1980).
37. C. J. Glynn, J. W. Lloyd, and Folkhards, Ventilatory response to intractable pain, Pain, 201 (1981).
38. W. A. Neill, G. A. Pantley, and V. Makornchai, Respiratory alkemia during exercise reduces angina threshold, Chest, 80(2):149 (1981).
39. P. Grossman, Respiration, stress and cardiovascular function, Psychophysiology, 20:284 (1983).

VASOVAGAL SYNCOPE:

ANTECEDENT PSYCHOSOCIAL FACTORS AND PATHOPHYSIOLOGY

William H. Sledge and Kees H.L. Janssen*

Yale University Department of Psychiatry
*Tilburg University Department of Psychology

INTRODUCTION

This paper is a summary of reports on the psychosocial antecedent factors in syncope and a review of some of the pathophysiological findings of other investigators. We attempt an integration of findings in our consideration of these two aspects of syncope. Our main concern will be with vasovagal syncope, but we will also examine micturition syncope by way of comparison.

Syncope, most commonly in the form of vasovagal (vasodepressor) syncope, is a relatively common occurrence. When syncope is not associated with, or the result of, systemic or neurological disease, it is usually a benign condition. It achieves importance in occupational (e.g., aerospace) or social contexts where sudden loss of consciousness is dangerous or not tolerated. Occasionally syncope may be a repeated and crippling manifestation of psychopathology and uncontrolled anxiety in which case it assumes importance for the debilitating consequences of repeated loss of consciousness. So while there are clinical reasons to understand syncope, it is not a major public health problem. No one dies of syncope itself, although some (Engel, 1978) believe some forms of sudden death have a similar pathophysiology.

Nevertheless, syncope merits serious and intensive study. A full understanding of the pathophysiology of syncope, particularly vasovagal syncope, can take us towards a more complete understanding of functions in the cardiovascular system, particularly of the mechanisms that maintain homeostatic regulation of blood pressure and vascular tone. For vasovagal syncope is par excellence an example of homeostatic breakdown, and a very interesting one, for it is not a disease in the usual sense. There is no tissue change (as far as we know) and no alteration of function (except in the acute instance). It seems that we all have the capacity for vasovagal syncope given the right circumstances of emotional arousal.

The literature (Engel, 1962) on the pathophysiology gives us a good, if incomplete, understanding of the basic physiological events. The circulatory collapse that results from this emotional fainting is not caused by vasomotor failure but instead by strong emotional excitation of parasympathetic nerves (Guyton, 1981). Early manifestations of this fainting usually include sweating, pallor, rapid pulse, mild hypertension

and hyperventilation. These symptoms seem to occur when the person sees
himself endangered by imminent threat. In his report of this stage, the
fainter will often mention nausea, yawning, sighing and weakness. Fainting
itself usually occurs a few minutes later, often after the emotional triggering event has changed. The immediate precursor of the faint is a sudden
fall in peripheral vascular resistance, producing a systemic vascular
hypotension and bradycardia, and further irregularity of respiration.
The latter cardiovascular changes result in a cerebral ischemia of which
fainting is the direct result (Guyton, 1981; Engel, 1961).

Engel and Romano (1947) proposed that this fainting arises when the
subject facing danger prepares for running or other activity, but muscular
activity is not carried out. Tracing their interpretation back to Cannon's
classical studies, they propose that the body is trapped by its own wisdom.
Essentially, vasovagal syncope starts as a purposeful reaction to a situation of real, threatened, or fantasized danger. This reaction turns
detrimental only when subsequent behavior aimed at solving the crisis is
physically or socially inhibited. This interpretation is based, in part,
on the earlier demonstration by several authors (Barcroft and Swan, 1953;
Blair et al., 1953) that vasodilator effects are induced in skeletal
muscles of humans subjected to emotional stress. Normally muscle contractions then help to push blood in the valved veins toward the heart. In
Engel's (1961) view such contractions do not occur in syncope, so that
blood pools in the enlarged vascular bed.

Graham (1961) differs from this view of Engel and others by postu-
lating that fainting occurs after a threat has either been carried out or
can be seen to have safely passed. In Graham's view, vasovagal syncope
constitutes a diphasic autonomic response. The manifestations in the early
hyperdynamic phase of syncope can be attributed to anxiety. The second,
hypodynamic phase is attributed to a relief from anxiety when the person
sees himself as no longer threatened, either because danger has safely
passed, or because the threat has actually been carried out. This is
accompanied by a sudden cessation of the physiological processes elicited
by the hyperdynamic first phase. These processes invariably are
accompanied by opposing vagal reflex mechanisms, to prevent excessive rise
of heart rate and blood pressure. If the hyperdynamic processes cease
abruptly, the massive vagal influences will be unopposed, and fainting may
occur.

According to Guyton (1981), vasovagal fainting probably results from
powerful stimulation of the anterior hypothalamic vasodilator center.
Stimulation of this center (medial preoptic area) is known to induce
several effects: bladder contraction, and decreased heart rate and blood
pressure. This is concordant with Schmidt's (1975) view in which the
triggering emotion and fear are thought to have their impact on the
effector organs through the limbic system. A crucial role is attributed to
the cingulate gyrus "depressor area", stimulation of which results in
sudden inhibition of sympathetic peripheral vascular tone, with a fall in
blood pressure and pulse (Löfving, 1961). This reflex is transmitted from
the cingulum to the hypothalamic sympatho-inhibitory area, and from there
to the vasodepressor center of the medulla oblongata (Folkow et al., 1964).
This model helps us understand why in syncope it often is so difficult to
establish whether hypotension occurs first or bradycardia; the rapidity of
the chain of events strongly favors the simultaneous activation of a
vasodepressor and a cardio-inhibitory reflex (Stevens, 1966).

An alternative explanation for the events in Graham's diphasic model
has been advanced more recently (Engel, 1978; Vingerhoets, 1984): fainting
occurs when there is a sudden shift from a fight-flight reaction to a
conservation-withdrawal reaction (Henry and Stephens, 1977; Henry, 1976).

The former reaction is regulated by orbital frontal cortex, amygdala, and sympathetic nervous system, resulting in behavioral arousal, display and aggression. Concomitant with this reaction, increased levels of catecholamines, testosterone, fatty acids and glycogenolysis will be observed. The conservation-withdrawal reaction conversely involves activation of the pituitary-adrenal axis with increased ACTH and cortisol levels, and vagal activation. Inhibition of ongoing behavior, restricted mobility and low sex and maternal drives are features of this reaction in animals. Generally biochemical and cardiovascular changes in syncope seem to fit quite well predictions following from Henry and Stephens' model (Vingerhoets, 1984). However, given the sudden and precipitous character by which these cardiovascular changes and fainting usually occur in vasovagal syncope, neural rather than humoral factors must be taken as the primary basis for its etiology (Weissler and Warren, 1959; Goldstein et al., 1982).

As stated before, vasovagal fainting is commonly accompanied by irregularity of breathing. Several authors have noted the association of onset of syncope with hyperventilation, a common symptom of emotional stress. As a result of this there is a fall in arterial carbon dioxide content. The effects of this hypocapnea in lowering cerebral blood flow, arterial pressure and in increasing muscle blood flow are well-known, and may accentuate the circulatory embarrassment in syncope. Indeed, hyperventilation and other breathing maneuvers have been found to facilitate the induction of syncope in several experimental studies (Stevens, 1966; Dermskian and Lamb, 1958; Lamb et al., 1958). Also in clinical studies, hyperventilation has been found to play a prominent role in the onset of syncope (Curtis and Thyer, 1983; Ruetz et al., 1967; McHenry et al., 1961; Graham et al., 1961). It has been advanced that cardiac arrhythmias and resulting decrease in cardiac output would explain this association of hyperventilation to syncope (Lamb et al., 1958). However, these changes in cardiac function are not a common observation under syncope, and it would appear that bradycardia plays at the most only a contributing role in syncope (Weissler and Warren, 1959). Besides by way of trigger, respiratory changes in syncope can also be observed to parallel the cardiovascular changes. In this view the above-mentioned cingulate gyrus depressor area can be conceived as not exclusively engaging the autonomic nervous system, but in addition when intensely activated, exerting a generalized inhibitory influence on respiration and somatomotor control (Löfving, 1961).

EMOTIONAL FACTORS IN SYNCOPE

In any case, there is a consensus that the fainting in vasovagal syncope is not caused by vasomotor failure but instead by strong emotional excitation of the parasympathetic nerves to the heart, and of the vasodilator nerves to the skeletal muscles, thereby slowing the heart and reducing the arterial pressure. This makes it pertinent to identify the qualities of the emotional affect that would predispose for syncope. We have conducted several studies with aircrew to pursue this question (Sledge, 1978; Sledge and Boydstun, 1979; 1982). Here we will summarize the findings in these reports in order to discuss possible models by which emotions may relate to vasovagal syncope as well as just how vasovagal syncope may be distinguished from other types of fainting, e.g., micturition syncope. To make the multifaceted concept of emotion more amenable to our purposes, we will attend to several distinct aspects: psychoenvironmental; cognitive; affective; and physiological.

In brief, our method was as follows: over an eight-and-one-half month period, we studied every fainting aviator (N = 34) referred to a central aeromedical evaluation-consultation facility at the United States Air Force

School of Aerospace Medicine (USAFSAM). The Air Force rules require every fainting aviator to be referred to this setting for an evaluation before being considered for return to flying status. Fainting automatically disqualifies an aviator from further flying duties, and a waiver is necessary to return to flying. We believe we had a cross-sectional, random sample of the population of people who are aviators and fainters. Each subject remained at our facility for several days. All of them had a routine USAFSAM clinical evaluation which, for syncope, included a complete history and physical examination with specialty examinations in otolaryngology, ophthalmology, neurology and others as indicated, and a variety of laboratory examinations which usually included an EEG, skull x-rays, brain scan, tilt-table test, and routine blood and urine tests. In addition, for our study the patients were given psychological tests, a hyperventilation challenge, and extended interviews with a research psychiatrist that delved into more detail about the syncopal episode. For comparison purposes we studied a randomly selected control group of aviators referred to USAFSAM who had never fainted. There were 26 control patients.

Our diagnostic findings for syncope revealed 24 patients (70%) with vasovagal syncope; four patients (12%) with micturition syncope and six patients (18%) with a variety of causes of syncope that we called the miscellaneous group. This last group included a student pilot who had an inflight episode of loss of consciousness secondary to G forces, one who had subacute bacterial endocarditis, two with hyperventilation syndrome and two with syncope of unknown etiology. These last two were probably variants of vasovagal syncope.

None of these 34 patients had syncope secondary to other medical or neurological disorders. The criteria for the diagnosis of vasovagal syncope included pertinent negatives, such as the absence of severe pain, blood loss, infection, high fever, mind-altering drug abuse, excessive alcohol use, or other possible etiologies of a physiological nature immediately prior to the episode of fainting. Vasovagal syncope was differentiated from neurotic syncope reactions (including hysterical fainting) by the history of the fainting episode and the findings of the USAFSAM psychiatric interview. Vasovagal syncope patients, in general, have a gradual onset of "pre-syncopal" symptoms and gain consciousness rapidly upon assuming a recumbent position; hysterical loss of consciousness is sudden, usually without premonitory signs and not necessarily related to posture. All patients in our study were unconscious.

Four patients were diagnosed as having micturition syncope. The criteria for this diagnosis included absence of stigmata of systemic, cardiovascular, and central nervous system disease as possible etiological factors and the close association of micturition in time with the onset of loss of consciousness - within one minute of completing the act of micturition.

The control group consisted of 26 randomly chosen patients who had been referred to USAF for a potentially aeromedical significant problem; however, neurological and psychiatric problems were excluded as well as were patients who had a history of previous episodes of fainting symptoms. The controls had the same research assessment as the syncopal group. On basic demographic characteristics, the controls and the fainters were quite similar.

For the purposes of this report we will only statistically compare the vasovagal and control groups because of the relatively small sample sizes of the other two syncopal groups. However, we will present and summarize the findings from the vasovagal, micturition and control groups.

RESULTS

Biomedical

In Table 1 we see the biomedical findings for the syncopal subjects. There are a few mildly abnormal findings scattered throughout the group but only one (subacute bacterial endocarditis) had a condition that could account for the episode of fainting. One should note there were four patients (12%) who spontaneously noted that they re-experienced their same presyncopal symptoms with the hyperventilation challenge (two vasovagal, two miscellaneous syncope). However, another 16 patients (47%) indicated their hyperventilation experience was very similar to but not quite the same as their presyncopal symptoms. These latter subject responses were always in reply to being questioned about the similarities or differences between the two activities.

Psychological Tests

There were minor statistical differences between the vasovagal syncopal patients and the non-syncopal controls (Sledge and Boydstun, 1982). These differences do not appear to be clinically significant. There were no apparent differences between the vasovagal, micturition and miscellaneous syncopal groups on the psychological tests (16PF, Cornell Medical Index, and Fear Inventory).

Onset Conditions of Syncope

We divided onset conditions into broad psychosocial factors occurring within the three months prior to fainting and immediate psychosocial factors that occurred at the time of fainting. In terms of broad onset factors (Table 2), the vasovagal syncopal patients differed from the controls along several dimensions of job related feelings. The vasovagal group was more frustrated and fearful, less satisfied and more desirous of a change. The micturition syncope group resembled the vasovagal group and the miscellaneous group had the highest proportion of all who had negative feelings about work (Table 2).

Of note is the number (three or 75%) of micturition syncope patients who had an antecedent physical illness (all of a trivial nature) such as upper respiratory tract infections or colds. The miscellaneous group had an 83% incidence of people who reported they were ill before they fainted. The vasovagal patients do not differ from the controls in the incidence of antecedent illnesses; however, the incidence seems large for all groups (42% to 83%).

As stated before there is a consensus that syncope is triggered by an emotional reaction to some aspect of the immediate antecedent situation. Little is known, however, as to what specific aspect in the triggering situation would contribute most to eliciting the syncope. Therefore in our assessment of immediate antecedent factors, we considered not only the social dimensions of the situation, but also the level of affect arousal, as well as cognitions and fantasies immediately before the faint.

In terms of affect arousal at the time of fainting, we noted that vasovagal and miscellaneous group subjects seemed to differ from the micturition and control subjects. (When we questioned the asymptomatic controls, we used for the reference time the time when they learned they had to be referred to the USAFSAM.) Affects were rated on a scale of 0 to 4, with 0 = no arousal, and 4 = very strong - almost out of control. The mean scores of these affects are presented in Table 3. The vasovagal group was statistically significantly higher than the controls on depression and

Table 1. Clinical Findings of Vasovagal Syncope Patients

Patient	Laboratory findings during the SAM Evaluation				Previous episodes		Miscellaneous comments
	Brain scan	Skull x-ray	EEG	Tilt table	Presyncope	Loss of consciousness	
1	Neg	None	Neg	Neg	Yes	1	Incontinence of urine, diagnosed as hyperventilation syndrome
2	None	Neg	Neg	Neg	Yes	14	Prior alcohol use
3	Neg	Neg	Grade I	Neg	Yes	None	Diagnosed as hyperventilation syndrome
4	Neg	Neg	Neg	None	Yes	4	
5	Neg	Neg	Neg	Neg	No	None	Prior alcohol use
6	None	Neg	Neg	Neg	Yes	1	
7	Neg	Neg	Neg	Neg	No	None	
8	Neg	Neg	Grade II	Neg	No	None	
9	Neg	Neg	Neg	Neg	No	None	
10	Neg	Neg	Neg	Neg	No	None	Prior alcohol use
11	Neg	Neg	Neg	Neg	Yes	3	Trauma on falling; urinary incontinence
12	None	Neg	Neg	Neg	No	None	
13	Neg	Neg	Neg	Neg	Yes	None	Prior alcohol use
14	Neg	Neg	Grade III	Neg	Yes	2	Prior alcohol use
15	Pos	Pos	Neg	None	No	None	Significant trauma on falling (skull fracture)
16	Neg	Neg	Neg	Neg	Yes	1	

No.							Comments
17	Neg	None	Neg	Neg	Yes	None	Trauma on falling
18	Neg	Neg	Neg	Neg	No	None	
19	None	Neg	Neg	Neg	Yes	2	
20	Neg	Neg	Neg	Pos	Yes	None	Negative CAT scan during SAM evaluation
21	Neg	Neg	Neg	Neg	Yes	1	Trauma on falling
22	Neg	Neg	Grade I	Neg	Yes	2	
23	None	Neg	Neg	Pos	Yes	2	
24	None	Neg	Neg	Neg	Yes	None	
MICTURITION SYNCOPE							
25	Neg	Neg	Neg	Neg	No	None	Probable hyperventilation as antecedent
26	None	Neg	Neg	Pos	No	1	Inflight episodes
27	Neg	Neg	Neg	Pos	Yes	None	Had viral illness
28	None	Neg	Neg	Neg	No	1	
MISCELLANEOUS							
29	None	Pos	Neg	Neg	No	None	Had viral-type illness; inflight episode; no diagnosis made
30	Neg	Neg	Neg	Neg	Yes	None	Inflight episode related to improper anti-G straining maneuver
31	None	Neg	Grade I	Neg	No	None	Hyperventilation syndrome
32	None	Neg	Grade I	Neg	No	None	
33	None	None	Neg	None	No	None	Lost consciousness apparently secondary to SBE
34	Neg	Neg	Neg	Pos	Yes	1	Normal CAT Scan. Probably hyperventilation syndrome

Reprinted with permission from: W. H. Sledge and J. A. Boydstun, Syncope in Aircrew, Aviation, Space, and Environmental Medicine, 53:258-265 (1982).

Table 2. Onset Conditions for Syncope and Control Groups

Condition	Micturition syncope (N = 4)	Vasovagal syncope (N = 24)	Control (N = 26)	Miscellaneous (N = 6)	Vasovagal vs. control probability (level x²)
Actual object loss	1 25.0%	5 20.8%	8 30.8%	1 16.7%	N.S.*
Threatened object loss	1 25.0%	11 45.8%	8 30.8%	4 66.7%	N.S.
Separation	1 25.0%	8 33.3%	5 19.2%	2 33.3%	N.S.
Anniversary	0	2 8.3%	2 8.0%	0	N.S.
Extramarital affair	0	2 8.3%	0	0	N.S.
Self-esteem diminished	1 25.0%	12 50.0%	10 38.5%	6 50.0%	N.S.

Feelings about job:				
Resentful	0	7 29.2%	3 11.5%	2 33.3%	N.S.
Fearful	1 25.0%	6 25.0%	1 3.9%	3 50.0%	.03
Satisfied	3 75.0%	15 62.5%	24 92.3%	3 50.5%	.003
Neutral	0	3 12.5%	7 26.9%	1 16.7%	N.S.
Frustrated	1 25.0%	11 45.8%	4 15.4%	3 50.0%	.02
Desired change	1 25.0%	9 39.1%	2 7.7%	2 33.3%	.009
Significant job stress	0	7 29.2%	4 15.4%	4 66.7%	N.S.
Antecedent physical illness	3 75.0%	11 45.8%	11 42.3%	5 83.3%	N.S.

*N.S. no significant

Reprinted with permission from: W. H. Sledge and J. A. Boydstun, Syncope in Aircrew, Aviation, Space, and Environmental Medicine, 53:258-265 (1982).

Table 3. Affect Arousal at Reference Time (Mean Scores)

Affect	Micturition syncope (4)	Vasovagal syncope (24)	Misc. (6)	Control (26)
Anger	.25	.71	1	.50
Resentment	.25	.79	1	.50
Depression	0	.42	.5	.31
Fear	.67	1.17	1.33	.58
Helplessness	.25	1.75	1.5	.81
Anxiety	.75	1.58	1.5	.92
Elation	0	.08	0	.46
Frustration	.50	1.29	1.17	.77
Worry	.50	1.33	1.5	1.04

Reprinted with permission from: W. H. Sledge and J. A. Boydstun, Syncope in Aircrew, _Aviation, Space, and Environmental Medicine_, 53:258-265 (1982).

helplessness and were almost statistically significantly different on the affects of fear and elation (Sledge and Boydstun, 1978). The micturition syncope scores are below the controls in all categories except fear, and here there is only a slight difference. In interpreting these findings one must note that three of the micturition syncope patients had been recumbent (two were asleep) immediately before their faint.

We dichotomized the patients into those with a high affect arousal immediately before fainting and those who did not have a high affect arousal based on the number and degree of aroused affects noted. To be in the high affect group, a patient must have had three of the nine affects at the moderately intense level - a rating of two or higher. There was no micturition syncope patient in the high affect group, but twelve (50%) vasovagal subjects, four (67%) miscellaneous subjects, and four (15%) controls were in the high affect group. For the vasovagal versus control comparison, frequencies were significant at $p < 0.01$ (chi square = 6.87, df = 1); for the miscellaneous group versus control comparison, the frequencies were significant at $p < 0.03$ (Fisher's Exact Test); the micturition syncope group versus the controls was not statistically significantly different (Fisher's Exact Test).

On other immediate antecedent factors the vasovagal syncope group stands out on this measure as well (Table 4). More often than not (75% or 18 subjects), the vasovagal group members found themselves in situations that were threatening in real and/or symbolic terms, and they were unable to counter the threat. This was not true for the other syncopal groups.

This finding bears further exploration. We inquired in detail what our fainters were thinking about just before they fainted. Eighteen vasovagal syncopal patients gave a clear account of their immediate situation as well as their presyncopal thoughts. None of the micturition syncope patients remembered their presyncope thoughts, and one of the miscellaneous syncope patients (with the diagnosis of syncope of unknown etiology) had memory of presyncopal thoughts. All 18 of the vasovagal subjects reported a social situation that manifested some fantasized threat to their well being. Eleven were involved in a medical procedure (9 venipunctures or injections, 1 ECHO cardiogram, 1 suture removal); three were not actively involved in a medical procedure but were worried about their health; four were in social situations where there was no bodily threat but a clear threat to self-esteem. Their fantasies were almost always over-reactions to the reality of the social situation and were all characterized by a

Table 4. Immediate Events Prior to the Onset of Syncope

Event	Micturition	Vasovagal	Miscellaneous
Medical procedure	1(25%)	12(50%)	0
Pain	0	6(25%)	0
Sight of blood	0	6(25%)	0
Fantasy of harm	0	11(45%)	0
Perceived inability to act	0	18(75%)	1(16.7%)

Reprinted with permission from: W. H. Sledge and J. A. Boydstun, Syncope in Aircrew, Aviation, Space, and Environmental Medicine, 53:258-265 (1982).

perceived threat and an inability to counter the threat. These findings are summarized in Table 5. Despite a great variety of actual situations, a variety of different personalities and personal circumstances, the basic emotional structure of the fantasy (threat to self and inability to act) was the same in all circumstances.

To summarize our findings to this point:

1. All syncopal groups resemble one another on broad onset conditions in that they differ from a control group along the dimensions of job distress and dissatisfaction.
2. Micturition syncope patients had a higher incidence of antecedent physical illness and were frequently recumbent immediately before fainting.
3. Vasovagal and miscellaneous syncope patients differed from the micturition syncope patients in that immediately before fainting they tended to be in a state of emotional arousal, characterized by a feeling of helplessness, fear, and "depression".
4. Hyperventilation was clearly an important component of at least four (12%) of our patients. We believe, however, hyperventilation was a component of another 16 (47%) patients.
5. The vasovagal syncope patient had a high incidence of an antecedent fantasy that was remarkably similar among all patients and was not found in the micturition syncope patients and most of the miscellaneous patients.

CONCLUSION

The way to syncope is a complex one, and there are perhaps multiple pathways to the specific cardiovascular-respiratory dynamics that eventuate in diminished cerebral profusion and loss of consciousness. From the clinical perspective, the role of psychosocial factors seems to be both specific and non-specific. All groups seem to have some particular stressors in their lives. All syncope groups report some form of distress about work which is different from the control group.

The micturition patients tended to have had a physical illness and to have been recumbent prior to fainting but were not in a state of relative emotional arousal. For these micturition patients it may be that the usual regulatory mechanisms maintaining orthostatic homeostasis were less responsive or stable, and the act of micturition further led to a relative parasympathetic discharge with subsequent increased peripheral vaso-dilatation and reduced cardiac output so that syncope eventuated. In this instance psychosocial variables seem to play a background or non-specific role, if any role at all. Indeed, the mechanism in micturition syncope may

Table 5. Pre-Symptom Thoughts of Syncopal Patients

*Case	Social situation	Participants		Fantasy	
		Subject	Object	Action	Outcome
1	Routine dental visit	Dentist	Self	Dentist to administer local anesthesia	Vague sense of harm to mouth
2	Patient has just had echocardiogram performed for purpose of aeromedical examination	Medical technician	Self	Technician made an exclamatory remark	Patient believed examination indicated he had a severe, fatal disorder
3	Indoctrination experience to a military academy	Upper-classman	Self	Patient was singled out for abuse	Public ridicule of patient
4	Patient is waiting for intramuscular injection of allergy medication	Self	Nurse	Resentment towards nurse for having to wait	Unable to express resentment
		Nurse	Self	Believed nurse to be incompetent as she approached him for injection	Believed he would be harmed in some fashion by her
5	Annual aeromedical examination	Medical technician	Self	Technician had trouble getting blood; patient felt he could not object	Patient believed he would be harmed by an air embolus
6	Important briefing before prestigious audience	Audience	Self	Patient made hostile slip of the tongue and perceived audience laughter as ridicule	Public mortification

7	Annual aeromedical examination	Medical technician	Self	Believed technician was taking "too many tubes"	Vague sense of being harmed through excessive blood taking
8	Sutures removed in a strange hospital	Medical technician	Self	Patient believed technician was inexperienced and believed sutures were being removed "too early"	Wound would open
9	Patient was being tested on the ground phase of a surprise check ride	Flight commander	Self	As he was being tested patient believed he was missing some of the questions	Believed he may not pass the test and would be grounded
10	Patient was visiting family on a holiday and had eaten excessively	Self	Self	Became ill and experienced uncontrolled vomiting	Believed he would suffocate
11	Patient was about to embark on an undesired assignment; believed he had a pneumothorax but his flight surgeon had dismissed it	Flight surgeon	Self	Believed flight surgeon did not take him seriously	Believed he may die from his condition
12	Routine annual aeromedical examination	Medical technician	Self	Routine uneventful venipuncture	Believed a nerve in his arm would be damaged
13	Routine flu shot	Medical technician	Self	Patient believed he would get the flu and that he would faint when he got the injection	Believed he would be embarrassed

Table 5. Continued

		Fantasy			
		Participants			
*Case	Social situation	Subject	Object	Action	Outcome
14	Patient was about to receive intramuscular injection for an orthopedic condition	Foreign M.D.	Self	Patient did not trust M.D. who was about to administer injection	Vague fear of being harmed
15	Routine aeromedical examination	Medical technician	Self	Patient was about to undergo routine venipuncture	Feared he would faint and be embarrassed
16	Patient was eating with mother who was telling a story about his cousin	Cousin	--	Cousin was in an accident; patient fainted when he heard the outcome of the accident	Cousin's face was mutilated
17	Routine aeromedical examination	Medical technician	Self	Technician was having difficulty obtaining blood; patient felt constrained from complaining	Venipuncture was especially painful
18	Night duty assignment	Air force	Self	Felt he could not complain about unpleasant night duty assignment	Believed he was being taken advantage of

*Case number here do not correspond to case numbers in Table 1.
Reprinted by permission of Elsevier Science Publishing from Antecedent Psychological Factors in the Onset of Vasovagal Syncope, by W. H. Sledge, Psychosomatic Medicine, 40:568-579. Copyright 1978 by the American Psychosomatic Soc., Inc.

be purely physiological (Lyle et al., 1961). Proudfit and Forteza (1959) have emphasized the importance of the circulatory changes associated with the Valsalva maneuver performed during micturition. In the presence of circulatory pressor tone already compromised by assuming the upright position after recumbency, even minimal increases in intracranial and intrathoracic pressures can profoundly disturb the cardiovascular equilibrium. Gastaut and Fischer-Williams (1957) suggested that in addition to reduced vasomotor tone and sudden rise to erect posture, increased parasympathetic activity associated with micturition may be an important factor in the onset of this form of syncope.

In vasovagal syncope the psychosocial factors may have both a non-specific as well as a specific influence. The vasovagal patients also have the background factors of the job distress (i.e., the non-specific influence). Added to that non-specific influence is the extraordinarily specific nature of the immediate situation with the high affect arousal and the specific feelings of helplessness, fear and the fantasy of a threat and an inability to respond to the threat. Engel (1962 and 1978) has made similar observations and put forth the idea of the emotional components of the diphasic response of syncope. He noted that vasovagal syncope occurs in the face of submission to a threatening situation which must be denied. Furthermore, the data suggest an extension of Engel's formulation of threat to the body as the provoking thought to include psychosocial threats such as humiliation, mortification, and job failure. It is quite remarkable that the basic predication of these patients' presymptom cognition (i.e., "There is a threat X and I must submit to threat X") was quite the same across a variety of social contexts and defensive operations of individual patients. Although the specific nature of the threat varied from patient to patient, it was present in each case in which presyncope thoughts were recalled. In all instances except one case, there was a perceived threat emanating from a real figure in the patient's immediate social context. Interestingly, usually these figures occupied or represented a position of authority in relation to the patient. Perhaps this perception of a threat from a greater authority often constrained these, for the most part, aggressive and outspoken people from taking action.

Affectively, there was a sense of resignation and helplessness in challenging the threat; there was the feeling of "giving in". In Case 10 (Table 5), although there was no higher authority, the patient nevertheless felt helpless and believed there was nothing to stop him from suffocation from his repeated vomiting. The importance of the affects of helplessness and hopelessness (giving up - given up response) for the onset of various psychophysiological disorders has been noted (Luborsky et al., 1973; Adamson and Schmale, 1965).

Another feature of some note is that even though the presymptom fantasies were derived from the immediate social context, the fantasized outcome was clearly exaggerated and realistically unwarranted except (perhaps) in the cases of perception of social embarrassment or public ridicule.

The data suggest some support for the "two-condition hypothesis" of symptom onset suggested by Luborsky and Auerback (1969) in which the broad context and the specific, immediate psychological context are both necessary, but neither is a sufficient, independent condition for the onset of symptoms. In the instance of our vasovagal aviators, the broad context may be the condition of being dissatisfied with work. The "background" state or broad context may then set the stage for psychological over-reaction to situations usually adaptively managed by the patient. This psychological over-reaction may be accompanied by the physiological correlate of autonomic hyperreactivity. When confronted with the narrow immediate context, which, for vasovagal fainters, seems to be the relatively specific stress of anticipation of bodily or social harm, the patient over-reacts maladaptively. With adaptive breakdown, there occurs a psychophysiological arousal state. In our vasovagal patients, this state may be autonomic nervous system instability in the form of a sympathetic hyperresponse to the idea or perception of threat followed by a para-sympathetic hyperresponse (with vasodilatation and reduced cardiac output) to the state of "giving up" to the threat which then leads to reduced blood pressure, cerebral hypoperfusion, and syncope.

Our experience gives support then for the idea of a switch in the adaptive-defensive function of the vasovagal fainter from a fight-flight mode with its associated sympathetic arousal to the conservation-withdrawal mode with its vagal activation. The submission to threat activates the conservation-withdrawal system. We are left with a model for the onset of vasovagal syncope as depicted in Figure 1. Micturition syncope could be understood in an analogous model as suggested in Figure 2.

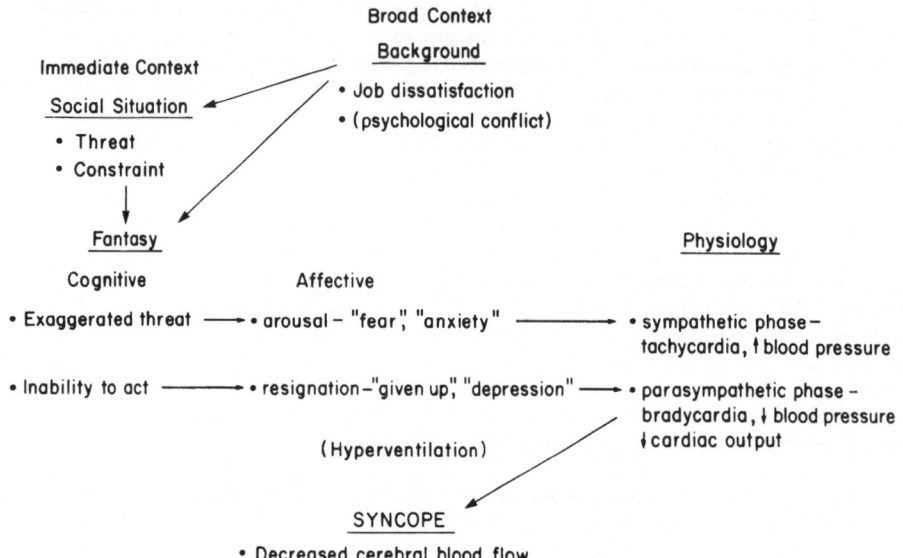

Fig. 1. Model for onset of vasovagal syncope.

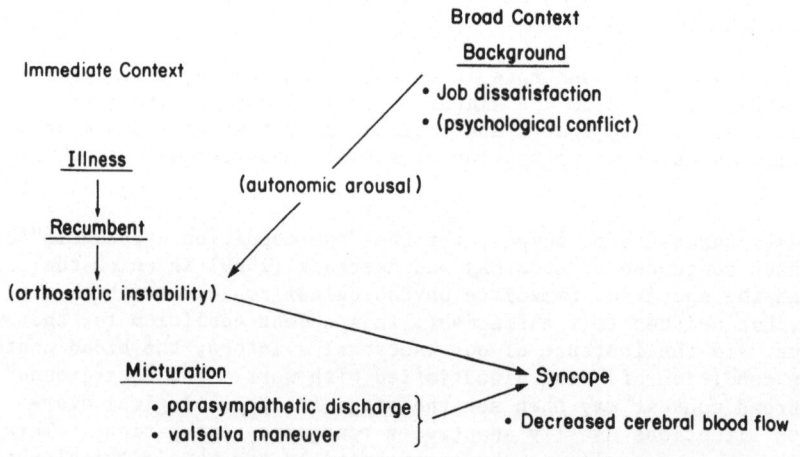

Fig. 2. Model for onset of micturition syncope.

An intriguing question is why there is the seeming specificity of the form and content of the presymptom cognition in our vasovagal syncope patients. It is difficult to imagine that only fainters have these thoughts; surely many have such thoughts but do not faint. But here, all the fainters who could remember what they were thinking before their loss of consciousness report an extraordinarily similar presymptom fantasy. Could it be there is some similar personality constellation that is relatively specific for vasovagal fainters or this occupational group? Could it be that this particular fantasy (consciously or unconsciously) is a necessary but not sufficient condition for the onset of vasovagal syncope? There is some epidemiological evidence that in our culture, vasovagal syncope occurs more commonly among men than women (Engel, 1978; Simons et al., 1977). This can be related to the need for males in our culture to exaggerate bravery and to inhibit the overt expression of fear. Shame for failure to live up to such standards constitutes the classic psychodynamic precondition for syncope (Engel, 1978). This holds _par excellence_ for aircrew, given their occupational requirements and the highly discriminating selection process they go through.

The percentage of subjects in our sample succumbing to syncope after hyperventilation may seem limited, but we cannot be sure in how many of the other subjects changes in prefaint breathing pattern occurred that remained unnoticed. In our examination of the subjects, the hyperventilation challenge was cautiously imposed and certainly did not aim at having the subject actually faint. Interestingly, about 12% of the vasovagal syncope subjects spontaneously admitted that bodily sensations they experienced during the provocation had a striking resemblance to those in a real presyncope period and another 16 (47%) admitted such a resemblance on questioning. This observation is in line with the existing clinical evidence (Curtis and Thyer, 1983; Ruetz et al., 1967; Graham et al., 1961; McHenry et al., 1961) for a close association of respiratory changes and vasovagal syncope. Further investigation of this relationship seems warranted and may bear relevance for the preventive management of identified vasovagal syncope.

Although we do not have answers for the questions above, surely the study of this psychophysiological disorder in the context of a highly selected and homogeneous group has much promise as a model for the investigation of mind-body interface issues.

Acknowledgements

The authors wish to acknowledge the central role of Col. James Boydstun, USAF, MC, who collaborated in the conduct of the studies summarized here and the support of these studies by the United States Air Force, Systems Command, School of Aerospace Medicine.

REFERENCES

Adamson, D. J., and Schmale, A. H., 1965, Object loss, giving up, and the onset of psychiatric disease, Psychosom. Med., 27:557-576.

Barcroft, H., and Swan, H. J. C., 1953, "Sympathetic Control of Human Blood Vessels", Arnold, London.

Blair, D. A., Glover, W. E., Greenfield, A. D., and Roddie, I. D., 1959, Excitation of cholinergic vasodilator nerves to human skeletal muscle during emotional stress, J. Physiol., 148:633-639.

Curtis, G. C., and Thyer, B., 1983, Fainting on exposure to phobic stimuli, Am. J. Psychiatr., 140:771-774.

Dermskian, G., and Lamb, L. E., 1958, Cardiac arrhythmias in experimental syncope, J. Am. Med. Assoc., 168:1623-1630.

343

Engel, G. L., 1962, "Fainting 2nd Ed.", Charles C. Thomas, Springfield, IL.

Engel, G. L., 1978, Psychologic stress, vasodepressor (vasovagal) syncope, and sudden death, <u>Ann. Internal Med.</u>, 89:403-412.

Engel, G. L., and Romano, J., 1947, Studies of syncope: IV, biologic interpretation of vasodepressor syncope, <u>Psychosom. Med.</u>, 9:288-294.

Folkow, B., Langston, J., Oberg, B., and Prerovsky, I., 1964, Reactions of the different series coupled vascular sections upon stimulation of the hypothalamic sympatho-inhibitory area, <u>Acta Physiol. Scand.</u>, 61:476-483.

Gastaut, H., and Fischer-Williams, M., 1957, Electroencephalographic study of syncope; its differentiation from epilepsy, <u>Lancet</u>, 2:1018-1025.

Goldstein, D. S., Spanarkel, M., Pitterman, A., Toltzis, R., Gratz, E., Epstein, S., and Keiser, H. R., 1982, Circulatory control mechanisms in vasodepressor syncope, <u>Am. Heart J.</u>, 104:1071-1075

Graham, D. T., 1961, Prediction of fainting in blood donors, <u>Circulation</u>, 23:901-906.

Guyton, A. C., 1981, "Medical Physiology", Saunders, Philadelphia.

Henry, J. P., 1976, Understanding the early pathophysiology of essential hypertension, <u>Geriatrics</u>, 31:59-72.

Lamb, L. E., Dermskian, G., and Sarnoff, C. A., 1958, Significant cardiac arrhythmias induced by common respiratory maneuvers, <u>Am. J. Cardiology</u>, 2:563-571.

Löfving, B., 1961, Cardiovascular adjustments induced from the rostral cingulate gyrus, <u>Acta Physiol. Scand.</u>, 53, supplement 184.

Luborsky, L., and Auerback, A. H., 1969, The symptom-context method, <u>J. Am. Psa. Assoc.</u>, 17:68-99.

Luborsky, L., Docherty, J. P., and Penick, S., 1973, Onset conditions for psychosomatic symptoms: a comparative of immediate observation with retrospective research, <u>Psychosom. Med.</u>, 35:187-204.

Lyle, C. B., Monroe, J. T., Blinn, D. E., and Lamb, L. E., 1961, Micturition syncope, <u>NEJM.</u>, 265:982-986.

McHenry, L. C., Fazekas, J. F., and Sullivan, J. F., 1961, Cerebral hemo-dynamics of syncope, <u>Am. J. Med. Sci.</u>, 241:173-178.

Proudfit, W. L., and Forteza, M. E., 1959, Micturition syncope, <u>NEJM.</u>, 260:328-330.

Ruetz, P. O., Johnson, S. A., Callahan, R., Meade, R. C., and Smith, J. J., 1967, Fainting: a review of its mechanisms and a study in blood donors, <u>Med.</u>, 46:363-384.

Schmidt, R. T., 1975, Personality and fainting, <u>J. Psychosom. Res.</u>, 19:21-25.

Seligman, M. E. P., 1975, "Helplessness: on depression, development, and death", Freeman, San Francisco.

Simons, C., Schultheis, K. H., and Kihle, K., 1979, Synkopen <u>in</u>: "Lehrbuch der psychosomatischen Medizin", Von Uexkull Th. et al., eds., Urban & Schwarzenberg, Munich.

Sledge, W. H., 1978, Antecedent psychological factors in the onset of vasovagal syncope, <u>Psychosom. Med.</u>, 40:568-579.

Sledge, W. H., and Boydstun, J. A., 1979, Vasovagal syncope in aircrew, <u>J. Nerv. Ment. Dis.</u>, 167:114-124.

Sledge, W. H., and Boydstun, J. A., 1982, Syncope in aircrew, <u>Aviation, Space, Environmental Med.</u>, 53:258-265.

Stevens, P. M., 1966, Cardiovascular dynamics during orthostasis and the influence of intravascular instrumentation, <u>Am. J. Cardiol.</u>, 17:211-218.

Vingerhoets, A. J. J. M., 1984, Biochemical changes in two subjects succumbing to syncope, <u>Psychosom. Med.</u>, 46:95-103.

Weissler, A. M., and Warren, J. V., 1959, Vasodepresssor syncope, <u>Am. Heart J.</u>, 57:786-794.

HEART RATE VARIABILITY IN AUTONOMIC

NEUROPATHS AND NEWBORN BABIES

R. I. Kitney

Engineering in Medicine Laboratory
Department of Electrical Engineering
Imperial College, London, United Kingdom

INTRODUCTION

This Chapter will discuss two areas where the application of HRV analysis is likely to be of clinical significance. First the application to HRV is neuropaths and second to HRV in the newborn. In both case the discussion will draw on the information presented in the previous Chapter which relates to normal adult HRV.

APPLICATION OF HEART RATE VARIABILITY ANALYSIS TO NEUROPATHY

The results presented in my earlier Chapter concern normal physiology. In recent years heart-rate variability monitoring has led to the discovery that in diabetic neuropathy the autonomic efferents to the heart can be partially or wholly affected (Wheeler and Watkins, 1973; Weiling et al., 1982). In neuropathic diabetics vagal denervation is almost certainly the cause of the loss of heart rate variability (HRV) (Lloyd-Motsyn and Watkins, 1976). These findings are consistent with our own results from normal subjects which indicate that the parasympathetic efferent to the SA node is of primary importance in HRV. In addition to the various statistical measures employed in the assessment of HRV (Sayers, 1973; 1980), some attempts have been made to describe the phenomenon in control theory terms (Kitney, 1980; Hyndman, 1980). The analysis described in this study was applied to the results of Watkins and Mackay (1980).

Figure 1 illustrates the results of these authors. Figure 1a shows the results of five representative normal subjects from which it can be seen that peak HRV occurs at 0.1 Hz. This is consistent with our results (Figure 12 earlier Chapter). Figure 1b illustrates the equivalent results for diabetic patients with neuropathy. The peak HRV values are all reduced in frequency and lie in the range 0.06 - 0.08 Hz. These results can be interpreted as the basis of our analysis of RSA (see earlier Chapter). As previously stated, the results of the parameter sensitivity tests model showed that the oscillation frequency is a function of the time delay of the baroreceptor feedback loop, the 0.1 Hz oscillation corresponding to a loop delay of 3.3 seconds. Applying the same criteria to the results of Figure 1b, defines loop delays in the range 4.3 - 5.5 seconds (0.06 - 0.08 Hz). This implies an increase in the loop delay of 1.0 - 2.2 seconds. The most likely cause of the increased delay would seem to be the decrease in

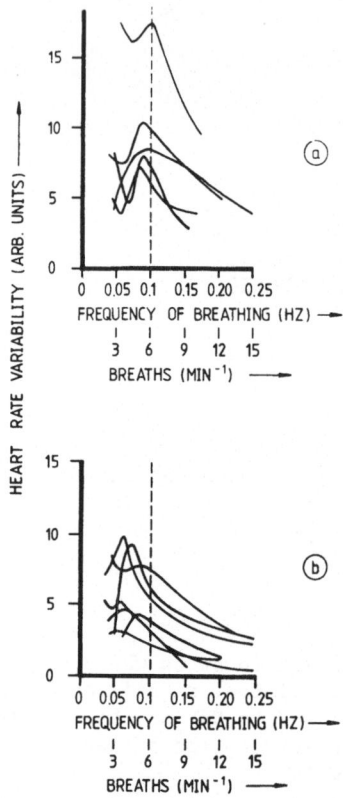

Fig. 1. Stimulus/response characteristics for respiratory sinus arrhythmia redrawn from Watkins and MacKay, 1980. (a) normal subjects (b) patients with peripheral and autonomic neuropathy.

neural conduction velocity or an increased delay at the neuro-muscular junction (Kitney, Byrne, Edmonds, Watkins and Roberts, 1982). On the basis of these results it is conceivable that the computer model/RSA analysis could form the basis of a clinical test for the degree of neuropathy by converting changes in HRV to a measure of changes in the loop delay.

HEART RATE VARIABILITY IN THE NEWBORN

As described in the previous Chapter, a considerable amount has been written about heart rate variability in adults. However, this is not the situation in the case of neonates and infants. We have applied to infants the type of nonlinear analysis techniques which have been described in relation to the work on adults. HRV and respiratory data were studied in 28 babies of average six weeks of age. Sections of data were selected from each baby during periods where breathing was relatively regular in rate and depth (possibly quiet sleep). These segments were chosen from chart records and as many sections as possible extracted from the 24-hour recording (x = 14 per infant).

The data were part of a prospective multicentered study involving 24-hour tape recordings of ECG and breathing movements on over 9000 infants, 29 of whom subsequently suffered SIDS (Southall et al., 1983). A sample of the recordings of thirteen infants who died, together with control recordings, provide the data. As this selection was made blind, it was not known which recordings were SIDS cases and which were controls.

The HRV records were subjected to Fast-Fourier Transform (FFT) spectral analysis. Figures 2a - 2e show the spectral layout used in the analysis. Figure 2 is the HRV time series of an episode of regular breathing (200 seconds duration, sampling rate 5 Hz). In order to study the "low" frequency and "high" frequency regions of the overall HRV power spectrum (0 - 2.5 Hz) (Figure 2b), spectra were subdivided by frequency into 0 - 0.2 Hz (Figure 2c), 0.02 - 0.2 Hz (Figure 2d), and 0.2 - 2.5 Hz (Figure 2e). The spectra of Figure 2c illustrate a section of data with a number of components spread throughout the range 0 - 0.2 Hz; in Figure 2b one can see a clear high frequency peak at 0.5 Hz (30 cycles per min.), possibly representing respiratory rate modulation. Other sections of regular breathing, from the same baby, showed a second type of HRV pattern (Figure 3). Referring to Figure 3c, there is a single dominant frequency component in the low frequency region. It is clear that such results were

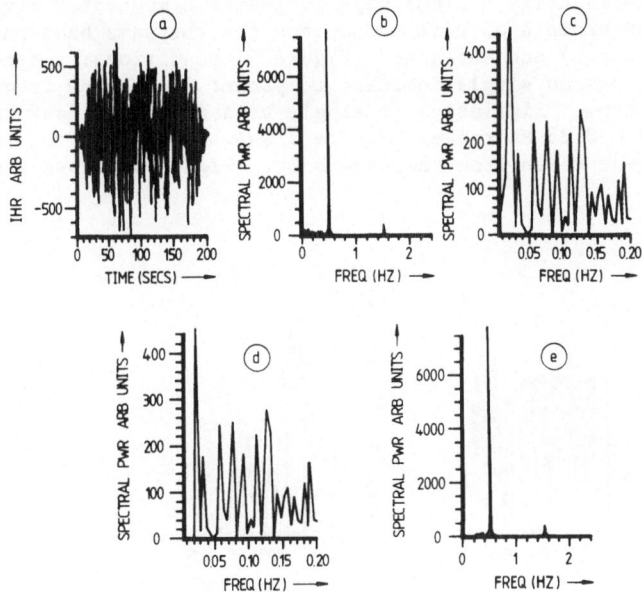

Fig. 2.   Example of the heart rate variability (HRV) data layout used in the analysis of baby data (a) 200-sec segment of HRV data; (b) power spectral density function (PSDF) of (a); (c) PSDF "b" with expanded frequency scale 0.02-0.2 Hz; (d) PSDF "b" with expanded frequency scale 0.02-0.2 Hz; and (e) PSDF "b" with expanded frequency scale 0.2-2.5 Hz.

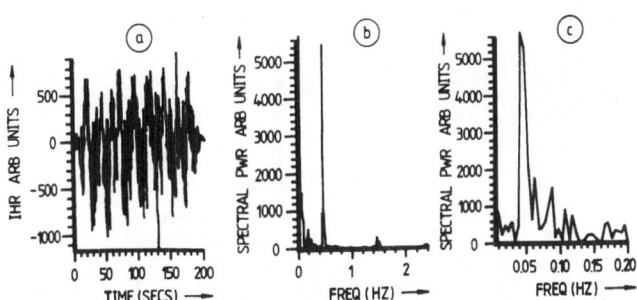

Fig. 3.   HRV data layout as Figure 2a - c but with a stable low frequency component at 0.05 Hz.

in a special category; comparing these results to earlier work on adults (Kitney, 1972; Hyndman, 1974; Kitney, 1980), could then represent examples of low frequency entrainment due to thermoregulation.

As stated previously, the spontaneous HRV spectrum in normal adults has three areas of activity (thermal around 0.05 Hz, blood pressure around 0.1 Hz, and respiration at the respiratory frequency). Because the respiratory frequency is higher in neonates, the HRV spectrum was divided for the purpose of analysis into low and high frequency regions; these regions were treated separately. For the two categories of data, i.e., entrained and non-entrained, the power of the largest component in the range 0 - 0.1 Hz was recorded and the mean calculated for all episodes from each 24-hour record. Similarly, the power in the largest corresponding component in the high frequency region (0.2 - 1.0 Hz, typically around 0.5 Hz) was recorded and the mean value for each 24-hour record determined. These two categories of data are termed 1 and 2. In many sections of the recording it was not possible to identify a clear high frequency component. Figures 4 and 5 illustrate an example of this phenomenon for the same baby under non-entrained (Figure 4) and entrained (Figure 5) conditions, respectively. In Figure 4b there was no single dominant component in the low frequency region of the spectrum. Similarly, no single high frequency peak was present in the 0.2 - 0.25 Hz range. Figure 5 shows an example of low frequency entrainment taken from the same baby. Figure 5b shows a dominant

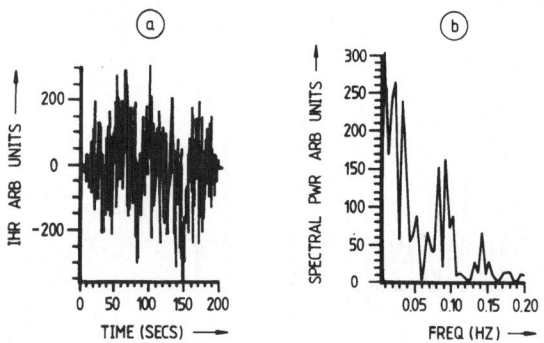

Fig. 4. Example of baby HRV data with no clearly dominant low or high frequency spectral peaks. (a) 200-sec segment of HRV data; (b) low frequency (LF) region of the HRV power spectrum (0-0.2 Hz).

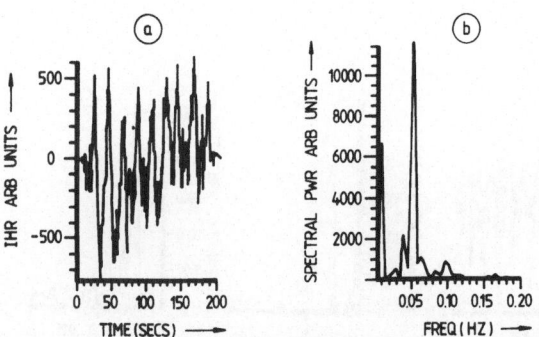

Fig. 5. Example of baby HRV data with a clearly dominant LF peak. (a) 200-sec segment of HRV data; (b) LF region of the HRV power spectrum (0.02 Hz) with a dominant frequency component (0.05 Hz).

single peak at 0.05 Hz, while there was no evidence of a single high
frequency component. Two new categories of data (3 and 4), non-entrained
and entrained, with no clear respiratory peaks can therefore be defined.

Because of the lack of a clear-cut high frequency component it was
important to establish the nature of any variability in the respiratory
signal both in terms of cyclic variation in amplitude and duration. The
amplitude and duration of each breath during every 200 seconds of HRV data
were therefore measured manually after being printed onto chart paper using
an ink-jet recorder. These data were then entered into the Cyber computer
system for further analysis. Time series of breath-by-breath duration and
amplitude variation were calculated. Figure 6 illustrates examples taken
from the same infant as Figures 4 and 5. Figure 6a is the time series of
amplitude variation and Figure 6b the corresponding Fourier power spectral
density function. Figures 7a and 7b illustrate the corresponding plots of
breath duration.

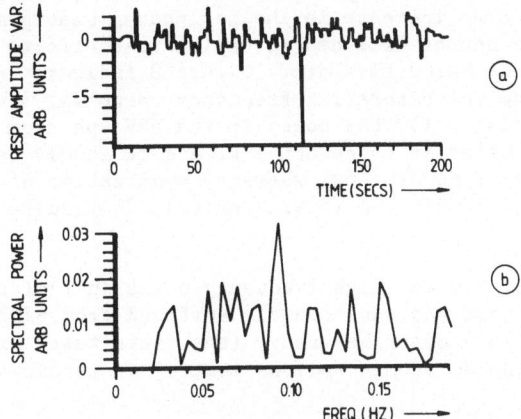

Fig. 6. Example of respiratory amplitude variability taken from the same
baby as Figures 16 and 17. (a) Time series of the amplitude
variation, (b) power spectrum of the time series.

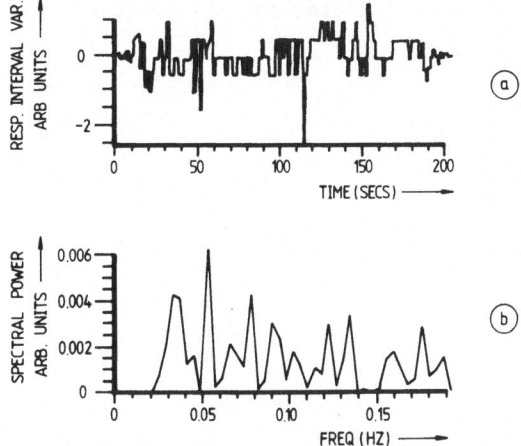

Fig. 7. Example of respiratory interval variation for the same segment of
data as Figure 6. (a) The time series of interval variation, (b)
the corresponding power spectrum.

349

Four separate categories were established for HRV data: (1) no low frequency entrainment, but a clear high-frequency component; (2) low frequency entrainment and a clear high frequency component; (3) no low frequency entrainment and no respiratory component; and (4) low frequency entrainment and no respiratory component.

ANALYSIS OF THE RESULTS

(a) Categories 1 and 2 Data

The frequency response of HRV to respiratory stimuli in normal adults shows a peak in the response at 0.1 Hz. As the respiratory frequency moves away from six breaths per minute, respiratory sinus arrhythmia decreases. The same is not true for patients with autonomic neuropathy where the results of similar studies have shown an increase in the response to low frequency stimuli (Kitney, 1981; Mackay, 1983). As discussed earlier, this can be attributed to a decrease in the natural frequency of the baroreflex arc arising from increased latency, due possibly to a reduction in nerve conduction velocity or an increase in the peripheral smooth muscle response time. This principle can be extended to explain the effects of other periodic stimuli on the baroreflex arc. Figure 8 indicates schematically the effect of shifting the baroreflex frequency response. Under normal conditions (characteristic 1), the power in the HRV spectrum for the same amplitude stimulus applied at frequencies f1 and f2 should be roughly comparable and ratios of powers low; whereas, application of the small stimuli under abnormal conditions (characteristic 2) results in a high ratio of power.

Identification of low and high frequency peaks in real time data from healthy infants and those who subsequently suffered from SIDS, suggested that the type of analysis described above (the ratio test) might be able to identify defects in the autonomic nervous control of cardiovascular and respiratory function.

Figure 9 illustrates the application of the ratio test to the entire sample of babies. For every 200 second period of regular breathing, the power of the largest component in the range (0 - 0.1 Hz) of the HRV spectrum was recorded together with the amplitude of the peak of high frequency region corresponding to the mean respiratory frequency as determined for analysis of breath-to-breath intervals. The ratio of powers for each episode was calculated and the average ratio for each baby

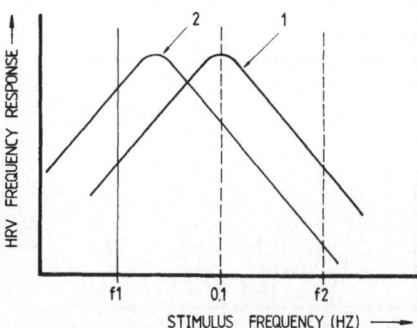

Fig. 8. Schematic representation of the RSA frequency response. Characteristic 1 shows the frequency response under normal conditions; characteristic 2 the frequency response with increased latency in the baroreflex arc.

determined. To avoid bias in low frequency amplitude selection, this part of the measurement was performed blind on all epochs in the raw data. Referring to the Figure where the ratios in individual infants are plotted against postnatal age, it can be seen that the results fall into three categories: (1) for average rate between 0 to 8, there are 9 controls and 2 deaths; (2) for the range 8 to 76 there are 11 deaths and 5 controls; and (3) above 76 there is one control. Hence in the first category, i.e., 0 to 8, there is a 4.5:1 bias towards controls, whilst in the second category there is a 2.2:1 bias towards SIDS. The control in the third category exhibits a high ratio (175) and shows respiratory amplitude and duration modulation, producing a diffuse respiratory pattern in the HRV spectrum. It is important to point out that there are no controls below 35 days of age.

(b) Categories 3 and 4 Data

A number of babies had no stable respiratory component and these were placed in categories 3 and 4, depending on whether or not LF entrainment could be observed. Again to locate the position of the respiratory component, particularly where no clear high frequency respiratory component can be seen (as in Figure 10), the breathing data were also analyzed. Figures 11a and 11b show the HRV waveform and its power spectrum; Figures 11c and 11d, the respiration amplitude variability signal and its power spectrum; and Figures 11e and 11f, the breath duration variability and its power spectrum. Comparing the three spectra, there is a dominant frequency component in Figure 11d which corresponds in frequency to the dominant component in the HRV signal (Figure 11b) (0.073 Hz). There is no large

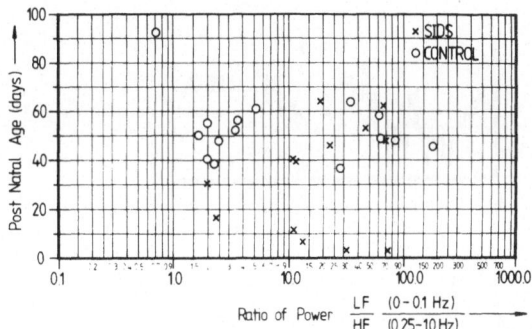

Fig. 9. Ratio diagram of the LF (0–0.1 Hz), HF (0.25–1.0 Hz) power in the HRV spectrum.

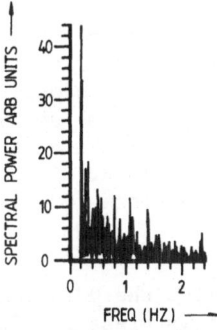

Fig. 10. Example of the HF power spectrum of a 200-sec section of spontaneous HRV data with no clear respiratory component.

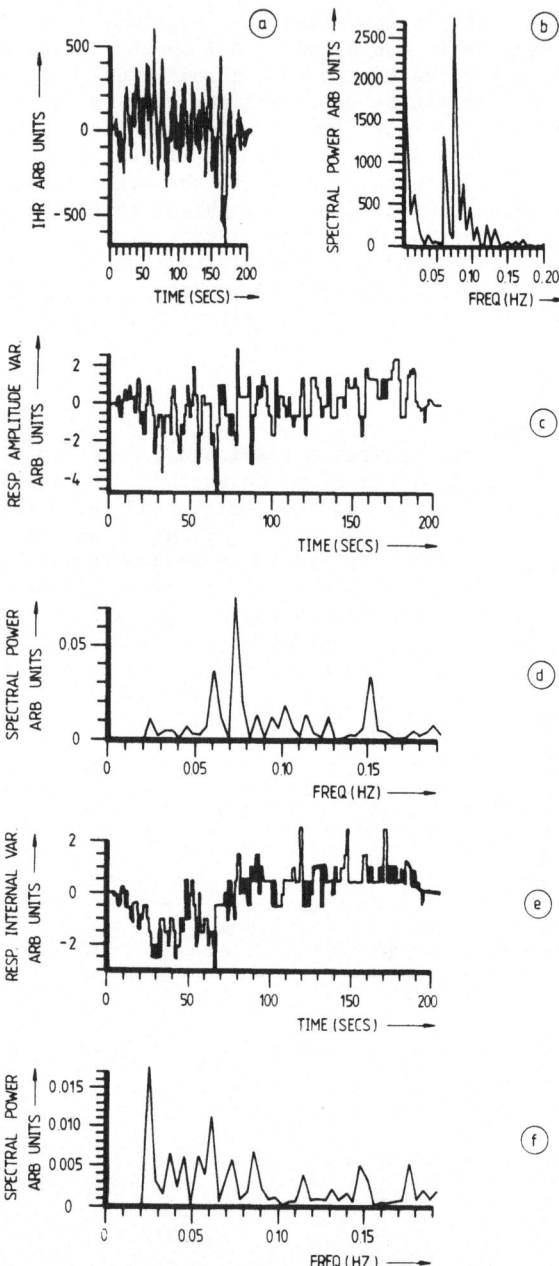

Fig. 11. Example of common frequency components in HRV, respiratory
amplitude and duration, variability.   (a) HRV data; (b) LF region
of the HRV power spectrum with a dominant component at 0.073 Hz;
(c) respiratory variability time series corresponding to (a); (d)
power spectrum of (c) with a dominant component at 0.073 Hz; (e)
corresponding respiratory interval variability time series; and
(f) power spectrum of waveform "e".

equivalent component in Figure 11f, the duration variability power spectrum, although a small component is present. If these results are compared
to a further category 4 episode in the same baby (Figure 12) some interesting differences are apparent. The layout of the Figure is identical to

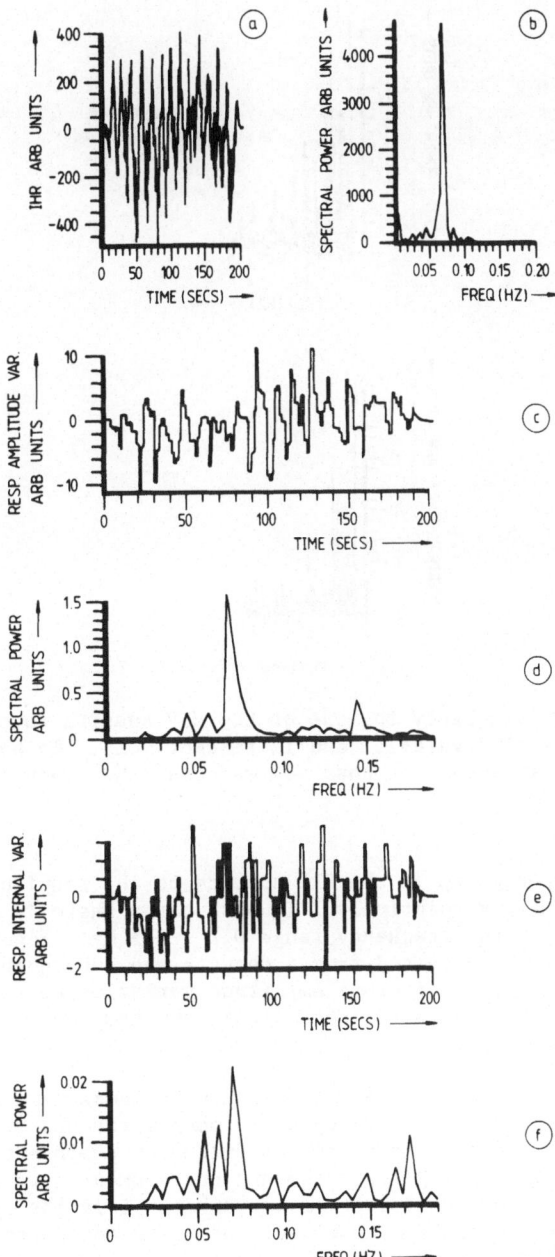

Fig. 12.   Second example of common frequency components in HRV, respiratory
amplitude and duration, variability (layout as Figure 11).   The
HRV, respiratory amplitude and respiratory interval power spectra
(Figures 12b, d and f, respectively) all have a large frequency
component at 0.073 Hz.

Figure 11.   First, comparing the HRV spectra (Figures 11a and 12b), it is
clear that in the latter case there is a single frequency component (at
0.073 Hz) which now completely dominates the spectrum.   The power spectrum
of respiratory amplitude variability shows a clear peak at 0.073 Hz
together with its second harmonic.   The power spectrum of respiratory
duration also has a large peak at 0.073 Hz.   Figures 13a and 13b illustrate

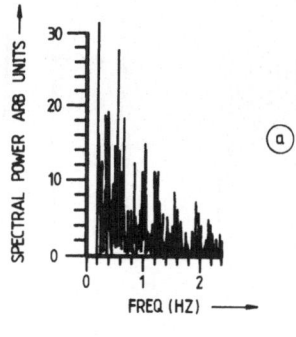

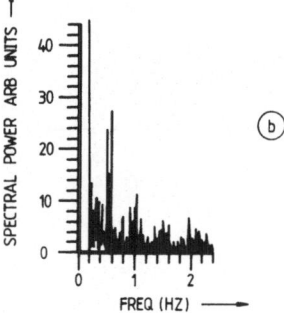

Fig. 13. The high frequency regions of the HRV spectra to the respiratory
episodes of Figures 11 and 12 respectively. In both cases there
is a large amount of power spread over the frequency range
0.2–2.5 Hz.

the high frequency regions of the HRV spectra to the respiratory episodes
of Figures 11 and 12, respectively. In both cases there is a large amount
of power spread over the frequency range 0.2 - 2.5 Hz. Figure 14 illustrates similar results obtained from a neonate who subsequently died from
SIDS. Again, the HRV, respiratory amplitude variation and respiratory
duration variability spectra all show clear components at the same frequency.

The results of category 3 and 4 data can be summarized as follows.
Under conditions of no low frequency entrainment, the HRV and respiratory
variability spectra comprise a number of frequency components spread
throughout the band. During low frequency entrainment, two basic conditions may occur. For low levels of entrainment only the respiratory
amplitude variability spectrum shows evidence of a component at the same
frequency as the HRV component. With high levels of entrainment, both the
respiratory amplitude variability and the respiratory duration variability
spectra have dominant frequency components corresponding to the dominant
frequency component in the low frequency region of the HRV spectrum.

DISCUSSION

The basic hypothesis of the study is that Sudden Infant Death Syndrome
(SIDS) is due to a lack of some form of cardio-respiratory control. Hence
the problem is one of studying the control of systems involved in order to
determine any differences in control function. As discussed earlier in the
Chapter, in adults these control systems have been studied in considerable
detail. In most of this work the control systems have been analyzed by
introducing a controlled, periodic stimulus of some form and observing its

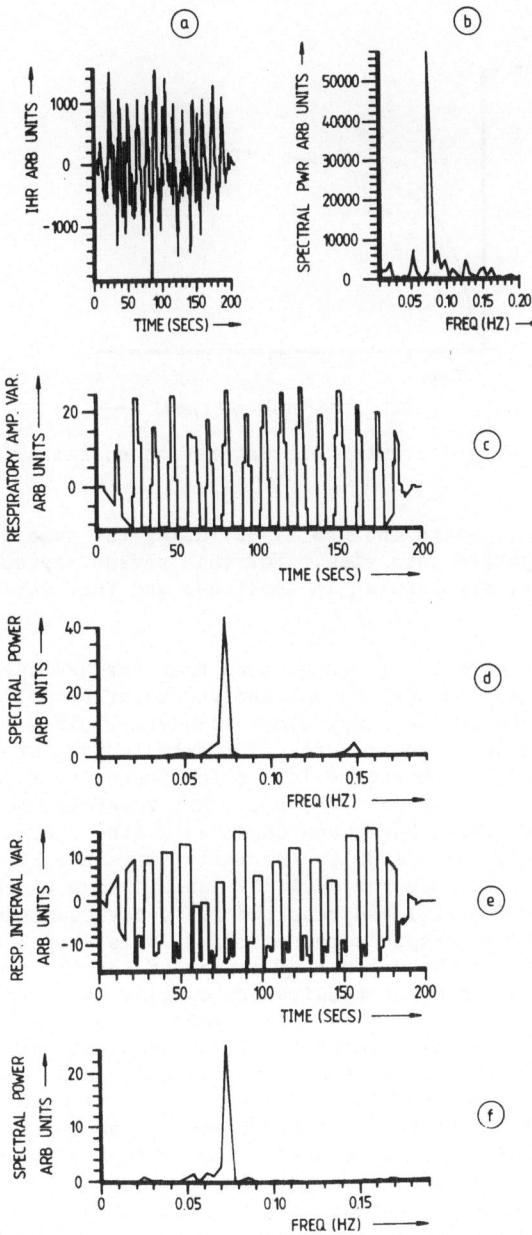

Fig. 14. The figure illustrates similar results to those of Figures 11 and 12; in this case, however, the baby subsequently died from SIDS.

effect on other physiological variables. To recapitulate, the results of these studies have shown that under spontaneous conditions, the blood pressure control system exhibits complicated interaction phenomena associated with the various rhythms present. For example, in either the blood pressure or heart rate records of healthy adults as the respiratory frequency approached the 0.1 Hz vasomotor component, the vasomotor component is pulled towards the respiratory component prior to full entrainment. It was therefore considered that for the best chance of success the analysis of spontaneous control activity in neonates required sections of data where the systems are in a relatively steady state. A previous analysis of quiet

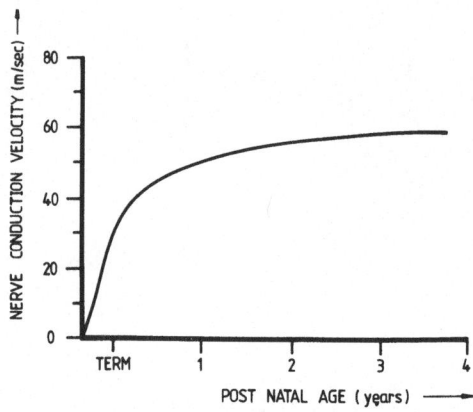

Fig. 15. Typical autonomic maturation characteristic.

sleep in full-term neonates (Holmes, 1982) using the same techniques as for the adult data supported this view. For this reason, episodes where breathing was relatively regular in amplitude and rate were chosen for analysis.

Referring to Figure 2, it can be seen that the HRV spectrum comprises low frequency activity in the thermal and vasomotor bands, and a clear higher frequency peak at the respiratory frequency. This is typical of category 1 data. Many of the records, for example that of Figure 3, showed a much simpler frequency structure in the low frequency region of the spectrum. Referring to Figure 3, both the HRV waveform and spectrum are identical to records which have been observed during thermal entrainment (for example, Kitney, 1974; 1980). Thermally entrained HRV records arise in adults from thermal vasomotor activity associated with the control of heat stress. Hathorn (1974) has reported frequency components in the range 0 - 0.1 Hz appearing in respiratory records. It is therefore possible that oscillatory activity in the 0 - 0.1 Hz region of the HRV spectrum under some circumstances might be of respiratory origin. Detailed analytical work on biological oscillations (e.g., Linkens, 1979a; 1979b) has shown that when one biological oscillator is entrained by another, the power of the self-frequency component of the entrained oscillator decreases relative to spontaneous level, as that in the entraining oscillator increases. This can be seen in relation to the thermal vasomotor component (Kitney et al., 1982). Hence the results in adults show that with RSA the power in the respiratory component of the HRV signal increases relative to the mean spontaneous level, while in thermal entrainment the opposite is true. Category 2 data, i.e., low frequency entrainment (thermal), with a clear respiratory component at the higher frequency were selected on this basis.

Another important aspect of the analysis of the HRV data is the question of frequency response. The research on adults (Hyndman et al., 1971; Kitney, 1979) has shown that the response of the baroreceptor reflex to periodic stimuli is very sensitive to stimulus frequency (Figure 1). The frequency response of HRV to respiratory stimuli was first described by Angelone and Coulter (1964) and subsequently by Hirsh and Bishop (1981) and Kitney et al. (1982a). These authors all describe a peak in the response at 0.1 Hz, and Kitney et al. (1982a) discussed the characteristic in terms of entrainment of the baroreflex. Hence in normal adults as the respiratory frequency moves away from six breaths per minute, RSA decreases.

The same is not true for patients with autonomic neuropathy (Kitney, 1981; Mackay, 1983; Kitney et al., 1982b; Weiling et al., 1982). The

356

results of studies on autonomic neuropathy have indicated that there is an increase in the response to low frequency respiratory stimuli. In terms of entrainment, this can be attributed to a decrease in the natural frequency of the baroreflex due to a decrease in neural conduction velocity or an increase in the peripheral smooth muscle response time (Kitney et al., 1982b; Van der Akker et al., 1983). This principle can be extended to explain the effect of other periodic stimuli on the baroreflex arc. Figure 15 indicates schematically the effect of shifting the baroreflex frequency response. Referring to Figure 8, under normal conditions (characteristic 1) the power in the HRV spectrum for the same amplitude stimulus applied at frequencies f1 and f2 should be roughly comparable, and the ratio of powers low. Under conditions of increased latency (characteristic 2) the ratio of LF to HF power would be high and there would be an increased likelihood of thermal entrainment.

Some infants did not produce stable high frequency components in the HRV spectra but did exhibit thermal entrainment; these data comprise categories 3 and 4 (non-entrained and entrained, respectively). Analysis of the respiratory amplitude and duration variability in some cases has shown that as the power in the LF component of the HRV spectrum during entrainment increases, first LF amplitude modulation of respiration occurs and later this is accompanied by frequency modulation of possibly a similar origin. Hathorn (1977) discussed oscillations of this type and noted that they occurred in both tidal volume and breathing frequency. His view was that these LF oscillations in V_t and f_b (tidal volume and instantaneous breathing frequency) could be due to different control systems. Hathorn also noted that oscillations in amplitude and frequency were out of phase producing overall negative correlation between rate and depth of breathing, thus keeping ventilation constant. The results of the present study show that as the stability of entrainment increases (i.e., the LF system has a greater and greater effect on heart rate variability), a series of events occur which may be explained by entrainment theory (Linkens, 1979a; 1979b; Kitney et al., 1982). Thus (1) LF entrainment may occur in the presence of stable respiratory activity (Figure 2, earlier Chapter). Here there is considerable separation between HF (respiratory) and LF peaks and the amplitude of the LF component is too small to influence the respiratory component. (2) As the amplitude of the LF component increases, the amplitude of the respiratory waveform is modulated by the LF HRV component (Figures 11c and 11d), but the duration of each breath is unaffected (Figures 11e and 11f). Finally, at high levels of LF entrainment, both the amplitude and frequency of breathing are modulated by the LF, possibly thermal vasomotor component.

One possibility is that as heat stress, as possibly evidenced by thermal entrainment, increased in the neonate, respiratory activity becomes directly affected, possibly by panting. This is first seen in modulation of the amplitude of breaths, but in order to regulate the levels of blood gases, the negative correlation mechanism described by Hathorn (1977) is activated. Hence a strong, possibly thermal component appears in both the respiratory amplitude variability spectrum (Figures 12c and 12d) and in the respiratory duration spectrum (Figures 12d and 12f). Figure 13 illustrates the "respiratory" region of the HRV spectra of Figures 11a and 12a. However, data from the newborn infants which we have analyzed (Giddens and Kitney, in press), indicate that the HRV is associated with breath amplitude variability (BAV) under stable or pseudostable states and not strongly influenced by the respiratory sinus arryhthmia seen in adults and in older infants. Nugent and Finley (1983) studied the correlation of periodic breathing with HRV. In their data the cross-spectra of respiration and heart rate records showed peaks at frequencies which coincided with the frequency of periodic breathing, a somewhat extreme manifestation of breath amplitude modulation. Also as described earlier, Kitney (1984) observed a common 0.073 Hz frequency in the spectra of HRV, respiratory amplitude and breath duration records of a six week old infant. In contrast, when we examined data from a young normal adult who was breathing rapidly (0.65 Hz) while modulating the tidal volume at 0.10 Hz, the major effect of tidal volume modulation was similar to that of a true AM response, i.e., the major HRV activity was in the ± 0.10 Hz neighborhood of the breathing rate itself while the oscillation magnitude at 0.10 Hz was significantly reduced.

It is difficult to identify unequivocally a baroreceptor self-oscillation frequency in the heart rate records of neonates since respiratory manipulation (e.g., breathhold) in efforts to isolate the effects of stimulation is not practical. However, in view of the fact that the average frequency activity in the LF region was 0.07 Hz and that the largest amplitude spectral peaks were in the 0.05 - 0.08 Hz range, the data from the neonates studied are consistent with the hypothesis that the latency time in the baroreceptor loop is longer than the 3.3 second adult value, and is appropriate for a 0.07 Hz self-oscillation.

The present study on neonates (Giddens and Kitney, in press) has shown a strong association in HRV and BAV behavior, the specific mechanisms of interaction of which have not been identified. One possibility is that the breathing amplitudes in neonates are easily exaggerated since the chest is rather complaint in comparison to adults, and thus thoracic stretch receptors may be sensitive to these amplitude changes. Another consideration is the possibility that venous return is modulated by the BAV. It is also conceivable that some higher level control mechanism, such as chemoregulation or thermoregulation, is acting simultaneously upon heart rate and respiratory control under stable conditions causing both to vary phasicly, yet somewhat independently. It is difficult to isolate specific effects in neonates due to the inability to control their breathing and spurious factors, such as crying, sucking and startling, which can all affect both respiration and heart rate. However, our future studies will address further the physiological implications of these findings, particularly with regard to mechanisms of interaction and to neurological maturation of the neonate.

REFERENCES

Van der Akker, T. J., Koelman, A. S. M., Hogenhuis, L. A. H., and Rompelman, O., 1983, Heart rate variability and blood pressure oscillations in diabetics with autonomic neuropathy, Automedica, 4:201-208.

Angelone, A., and Coulter, N. A., 1964, Respiratory sinus arrhythmia: a frequency dependent phenomenon, J. Appl. Physiol., 19:479-482.

Giddens, D. P., and Kitney, R. I., in press, Neonatal heart rate variability and its relation to respiration, J. Theoret. Biol.

Hathorn, M. K. S., 1974, Rate and depth breathing in newborn infants, in different sleep stages, J. Physiol., 243:101-113.

Hathorn, M. K. S., 1977, Analysis of the rhythm of infantile breathing, Br. Med. Bull., 31:8-12.

Hirsch, J. A., and Bishop, B., 1981, Respiratory sinus arrhythmia in humans: how breathing pattern modulates heart rate, Am. J. Physiol., 241:H620-629.

Holmes, A. K., 1982, A study of heart rate variability in neonates during sleep, MSc. Thesis, London University.

Hyndman, B. W., 1974, The role of rhythms in homeostasis, Kybernetik, 15:227-236.

Hyndman, B. W., 1980, Cardiovascular recovery to psychological stress: a means to diagnose man and task?, in: "The Study of Heart Rate

Variability", R. I. Kitney and O. Rompelman, eds., Clarendon Press, Oxford.

Kitney, R. I., 1972, The thermo-regulatory control system in man and its study by digital computer simulation, PhD Thesis, London University.

Kitney, R. I., 1974, The analysis and simulation of the human thermo-regulator control system, Medical & Biological Engineering, Jan. 57-65.

Kitney, R. I., 1979, A nonlinear model for studying oscillations in the blood pressure control system, J. Biomedical Engineering, 1:89-99.

Kitney, R. I., 1980, An analysis of the thermoregulatory influences on heart rate variability, in: "The Study of Heart Rate Variability", R. I. Kitney and O. Rompelman, eds., Clarendon Press, Oxford.

Kitney, R. I., 1981, Modelling respiratory sinus arrhythmia and its application to the study of neuropathy, in: "Computing in Medicine", P. J. Petel, ed., pp. 126-134.

Kitney, R. I., 1984, New findings in the analysis of heart rate variability in infants, Automedica, 4:289-310.

Kitney, R. I., Linkens, D. A., Selman, A. C., and McDonald, A. H., 1982, The interaction between heart rate and respiration: Part 2 - nonlinear analysis on computer modelling, Automedica, 4:141-153.

Kitney, R. I., Byrne, S., Edmonds, M. E., Watkins, P. J., and Roberts, V. C., 1982b, Heart rate variability in the assessment of autonomic diabetic neuropathy, Automedica, 4:155-167.

Linkens, D. A., 1979a, Theoretical analysis of beating and modulation phenomena in weakly intercoupled van der Pol oscillator systems for biological mdoelling, J. Theoret. Biol., 79:31-54.

Linkens, D. A., 1979b, Modulation analysis of forced nonlinear oscillations for biological modelling, J. Theoret. Biol., 77:235-251.

Lloyd-Mostyn, R. H., and Watkins, P. J., 1976, Total cardiac denervation in diabetic autonomic neuropathy, Diabetics, 25:748-751.

Mackay, J. D., 1983, Respiratory sinus arrhythmia in diabetic neuropathy, Diabetologia, 24:253.

Nugent, S. T., and Finlay, J. P., 1983, Spectral analysis of periodic and normal breathing in infants, IEEE Trans. Biomedical Engineering, BME-30, 10:672-675, October 1983.

Sayers, B. McA., 1973, Analysis of heart rate variability, Ergonomics, 16:17-32.

Sayers, B. McA., 1980, Signal analysis of heart rate variability, in: "The Study of Heart Rate Variability", R. I. Kitney and O. Rompelman, eds., Clarendon Press, Oxford.

Southall, D. P. et al., 1983, First report on the combined study of SIDS, Br. Med. J., 286:1092-1096.

Watkins, P. J., and Mackay, J. D., 1980, Cardiac denervation in diabetic neuropathy, Ann. Internal Med., 92 (Part 2):304-307.

Wheeler, T., and Watkins, P. J., 1973, Cardiac denervation in diabetics, Br. Med. J., 4:584-586.

Wieling, W., van Brederode, J. F. M., de Rijk, Borst, L. G., and Dunning, A. J., 1982, Reflex control of heart rate in normal subjects in relation to age: a data base for cardiac vagal neuropathy, Diabetologia, 22:163-166.

CONTRIBUTORS

J. Brener
University of Hull
Hull HU6 7RX
Yorkshire
England

B. T. Engel
National Institute of Health
National Institute on Aging
Gerontology Research Center
Baltimore City Hospitals
Baltimore
Maryland 21224
USA

L. J. Freeman
Department of Cardiology
Charing Cross Hospital
Fulham Palace Road
London W6 8RF
England

A. J. Gelsema
Department of Physiology
University of Amsterdam
m-01 Meibergdreef 15
1105 AZ Amsterdam
The Netherlands

P. Grossman
Institute for Stress Research,
  and Department of Physiological
  Psychology
Free University
De Boelelaan 1115
1081 HV Amsterdam
The Netherlands

K. Janssen
Tilburg University
Department of Psychology
225 Hogenschoollaan
Tilburg
The Netherlands

D. Johnston
University of Oxford
Department of Psychiatry
Warneford Hospital
Oxford OX3 7JX
England

J. M. Karemaker
Department of Physiology
m-01 Meibergdreef 15
1105 AZ Amsterdam
The Netherlands

R. I. Kitney
Engineering in Medicine Laboratory
Imperial College
London SW7
England

A. Langer
Syracuse University
Behavioral Physiology Laboratory
101 Stevens Place
Syracuse, N.Y. 13210
USA

P. Langhorst
Freie Universitaet Berlin
Institut Fuer Physiologie
im FB Natur- und
  Sozialwissenschaftliche
Grundlagenmedizin u. medizinische
  Oekologie
1000 Berlin
West Germany

S. A. Mortensen
Medical Department B
Rigshospitalet
Blegdamsvej 9
2100 Copenhagen
Denmark

S. W. Porges
University of Illinois
Department of Psychology
603 East Daniel Street
Champaign, Illinois 61820
USA

F. Raschke
Institute of Occupational Physiology
and Rehabilitation Research
Robert-Koch-Str. 7a
D-3550 Marburg
West Germany

O. Rompelman
Department of Electrical Engineering
Delf University of Technology
Postbus 5031
2600 GA Delft
The Netherlands

W. H. Sledge
P O Box 1842
CMHC
34 Park Street
New Haven, Connecticut 065183
USA

C. M. Stoney
Syracuse University
Behavioral Physiology Laboratory
101 Stevens Place
Syracuse, NY 13210
USA

S. Svebak
University of Bergen
Department of Somatic Psychology
Arstadveien 21
N-5000 Bergen
Norway

G. Turpin
Plymouth Polytechnic
Department of Psychology
Drake Circus
Plymouth, Devon PL 48L
England

D. Vaitl
University of Giessen
Department of Psychology
Otto-Behaghel-Str. 10
6300 Giessen
West Germany